COMMON PROBLEMS IN
VASCULAR SURGERY

COMMON PROBLEMS IN
VASCULAR SURGERY

DAVID C. BREWSTER, M.D.
Associate Clinical Professor of Surgery
Massachusetts General Hospital
Harvard Medical School Visiting Surgeon
Boston, Massachusetts

YEAR BOOK MEDICAL PUBLISHERS, INC.
CHICAGO • LONDON • BOCA RATON

2   3   4   5   6   7   8   9   0   KP   92   91   90

Library of Congress Cataloging-in-Publication Data

Common problems in vascular surgery.

Includes bibliographies and index.
1. Blood-vessels—Surgery.   2. Blood-vessels—
Surgery—Complications and sequelae.   1. Brewster,
David C.   [DNLM: 1. Vascular Surgery. WG 170 C734]
RD598.5.C63   1989   617'.413   88-10762
ISBN 0-8151-1222-X

Sponsoring Editors: Daniel J. Doody, Nancy E. Chorpenning
Assistant Director, Manuscript Services: Frances M. Perveiler
Production Manager, Text and Reference/Periodicals: Etta Worthington

COMMON PROBLEMS IN SURGERY SERIES

SERIES EDITOR

RICHARD F. KEMPCZINSKI, M.D.

Professor of Surgery
University of Cincinnati
Chief, Vascular Surgery
University Hospital
Cincinnati, Ohio

Additional volumes under development.

To Gloria

whose constant support, encouragement, and insight is a source of continued inspiration.

CONTRIBUTORS

WILLIAM M. ABBOTT, M.D.
Associate Professor of Surgery, Harvard Medical School; Chief of Vascular Surgery, Massachusetts General Hospital, Boston, Massachusetts

NELSON ANCALMO, M.D., F.A.C.S.
Chief of Surgery, Ochsner Clinic of Baton Rouge, Ochsner Foundation Hospital, New Orleans, Louisiana, Medical Center of Baton Rouge, Baton Rouge, Louisiana

RONALD J. BAIRD, M.D., M.S.(Tor.), F.R.C.S(C.), F.A.C.S.
Professor of Surgery, University of Toronto; Senior Surgeon, Toronto General Hospital, Toronto, Ontario, Canada

WILLIAM H. BAKER, M.D.
Professor of Surgery, Chief, Section of Peripheral Vascular Surgery, Stritch School of Medicine, Loyola University of Chicago; Chief, Peripheral Vascular Surgery, Director, Peripheral Vascular Laboratory, Foster G. McGaw Hospital, Maywood, Illinois

ROBERT W. BARNES, M.D.
Professor and Chairman, Department of Surgery, University of Arkansas for Medical Sciences; Attending Surgeon, University Hospital of Arkansas, Little Rock Veterans Administration Hospital, Arkansas Children's Hospital, Little Rock, Arkansas

HISHAM S. BASSIOUNY, M.D.
Cardiovascular Research Fellow, Instructor of Surgery, University of Chicago; Instructor of Surgery, University of Chicago Medical Center, Chicago, Illinois

JOHN J. BERGAN, M.D., F.A.C.S., Hon. F.R.C.S.(Eng.)
Magerstadt Professor of Surgery, Chief, Division of Vascular Surgery, Northwestern University Medical School; Attending Surgeon, Northwestern Memorial Hospital, Chicago, Illinois

VICTOR M. BERNHARD, M.D.
Professor of Surgery, Chief, Vascular Section, University of Arizona College of Medicine; Staff Surgeon, University Hospital, Tucson, Arizona

EUGENE F. BERNSTEIN, M.D., Ph.D.
Member, Division of Vascular Surgery, Scripps Clinical and Research Foundation, La Jolla, California; Adjunct Professor of Surgery, University of California, San Diego, California

BRUCE J. BRENER, M.D.
Chief of Vascular Surgery, Newark Beth Israel Medical Center, Newark, New Jersey

HARRY L. BUSH, Jr., M.D.
Associate Professor of Surgery, Cornell University Medical College; Full-Time Attending Surgeon, Division of Vascular Surgery, New York Hospital-Cornell Medical Center, New York City, New York

ALLAN D. CALLOW, M.D., Ph.D., Hon. D.Sc.
Consultant in Vascular Surgery, New England Medical Center, Emeritus Professor of Surgery, Tufts University School of Medicine, Boston, Massachusetts

RICHARD P. CAMBRIA, M.D.
Assistant Professor of Surgery, Harvard Medical School, Assistant Visiting Surgeon, Massachusetts General Hospital, Boston, Massachusetts

BENJAMIN B. CHANG, M.D.
Assistant Professor of Surgery, Department of Surgery, Vascular Service, Albany Medical College; Attending Surgeon, Albany Medical Center Hospital, Albany, New York

JOHN D. CORSON, M.B., Ch.B., F.R.C.S.(Eng.), F.A.C.S.
Associate Professor, Chief, Vascular Surgery, The University of Iowa Hospital and Clinics, Iowa City, Iowa

E. STANLEY CRAWFORD, M.D.
Professor of Surgery, Baylor College of Medicine, Senior Attending Surgeon, Methodist Hospital, Houston, Texas

BRUCE S. CUTLER, M.D.
Professor of Surgery, Chairman, Division of Vascular Surgery, University of Massachusetts Medical School, Director of the Vascular Laboratory, University of Massachusetts Medical Center, Worcester, Massachusetts

HERBERT DARDIK, M.D.
Clinical Associate Professor of Surgery, University of Medicine and Dentistry of New Jersey; Chief, General and Vascular Surgery, Englewood Hospital, Englewood, New Jersey

R. CLEMENT DARLING, Jr., M.D.
Associate Clinical Professor of Surgery, Harvard Medical School; Senior Vascular Surgeon, Chief of the Vascular Clinic, Massachusetts General Hospital, Boston, Massachusetts

R. CLEMENT DARLING III, M.D.
Clinical and Research Fellow, Harvard Medical School, New England Deaconess Hospital, Boston, Massachusetts

RICHARD H. DEAN, M.D.
Professor and Chairman, Department of Surgery, Bowman Gray School of Medicine of Wake Forest University; Chief of Staff, North Carolina Baptist Hospital, Winston-Salem, North Carolina

DOMINIC A. DELAURENTIS, M.D.
Professor of Surgery, University of Pennsylvania School of Medicine; Chief, Section of Vascular Surgery, Pennsylvania Hospital, Philadelphia, Pennsylvania

RALPH G. DEPALMA, M.D.
Professor and Chairman, Department of Surgery, George Washington University, George Washington University Medical Center, Washington, D.C.

JAMES A. DEWEESE, M.D.
Professor and Chairman, Division of Cardiothoracic Surgery, Chief of Vascular Section, and Associate Chairman, Department of Surgery. The University of Rochester, Cardiothoracic Surgeon-in-Chief, Strong Memorial Hospital, Rochester, New York

WILLIAM K. EHRENFELD, M.D.
Professor of Surgery, School of Medicine, University of California, San Francisco, California

ERIC D. ENDEAN, M.D.
Fellow, Section of Peripheral Vascular Surgery, Loyola University Medical Center, Foster G. McGaw Hospital, Maywood, Illinois

CALVIN B. ERNST, M.D.
Clinical Professor of Surgery, University of Michigan Medical School; Head, Division of Vascular Surgery, Henry Ford Hospital, Detroit, Michigan

WILLIAM E. EVANS, M.D.
Clinical Professor of Surgery, Ohio State University, Columbus, Ohio; Professor of Surgery, Meharry Medical College, Nashville, Tennessee

D. PRESTON FLANIGAN, M.D.
Professor of Surgery, University of Illinois College of Medicine at Chicago; Chief, Division of Peripheral Vascular Surgery, University of Illinois, West Side Veterans Administration Medical Center and Cook County Hospital, Chicago, Illinois

JOSE P. GARCIA, M.D.
Resident in Surgery, Brigham and Women's Hospital, Boston, Massachusetts

JONATHAN P. GERTLER, M.D.
Resident-Vascular Surgery, Clinical Fellow in Surgery, Massachusetts General Hospital, Harvard Medical School, Boston, Massachusetts

GARY W. GIBBONS, M.D.
Associate Clinical Professor of Surgery, Harvard Medical School, Clinical Director, Vascular Division, Co-Director, Vascular Laboratory, New England Deaconess Hospital, Boston, Massachusetts

JERRY GOLDSTONE, M.D.
Professor of Surgery, Chief of Vascular Surgery, University of California at San Francisco; Director, STAMP Program, Veterans Administration Medical Center, San Francisco, California

LAZAR J. GREENFIELD, M.D.
Professor and Chairman, Department of Surgery, University of Michigan; Chief of Surgery, University of Michigan Hospitals, Ann Arbor, Michigan

ROGER M. GREENHALGH, M.A., M.D., M.Chir., F.R.C.S.
Charing Cross and Westminster Medical School, Professor Department of Surgery, Charing Cross Hospital, London, England

JOHN W. HALLETT, Jr., M.D.
Associate Professor of Surgery, Mayo Medical School, Rochester Methodist Hospital and St. Mary's Hospital, Rochester, Minnesota

KIMBERLEY J. HANSEN, M.D.
Assistant Professor of Surgery, Department of Surgery, Bowman Gray School of Medicine of Wake Forest University, North Carolina Baptist Hospital, Winston-Salem, North Carolina

NORMAN R. HERTZER, M.D.
Head, Section of Cerebrovascular Surgery, Department of Vascular Surgery, The Cleveland Clinic Foundation, Cleveland, Ohio

ROBERT W. HOBSON, II, M.D.
Professor of Surgery, Chief, Section of Vascular Surgery, University of Medicine and Dentistry of New Jersey, New Jersey Medical School; Chief, Section of Vascular Surgery, University Hospital, Newark, New Jersey

L. H. HOLLIER, M.D.
Clinical Professor of Surgery, Louisiana State University and Tulane University Medical Schools; Chairman, Department of Surgery, Ochsner Clinic and Ochsner Foundation Hospital, New Orleans, Louisiana

ANTHONY M. IMPARATO, M.D., F.A.C.S.
Professor of Surgery, Director, Division of Vascular Surgery, New York University Medical Center; Attending Surgeon, New York University Hospital, Visiting Surgeon, Bellevue Hospital, New York City, New York

FREDRIC JARRETT, M.D.
Department of Surgery, University of Pittsburgh School of Medicine; Attending Surgeon, Montefiore Hospital and Shadyside Hospital, Pittsburgh, Pennsylvania

GEORGE JOHNSON, Jr., M.D.
Professor of Surgery, Roscoe B. G. Cowper Distinguished Professor of Surgery, University of North Carolina; Chief, Division of General Surgery, North Carolina Memorial Hospital, Chapel Hill, North Carolina

RICHARD F. KEMPCZINSKI, M.D.
Professor of Surgery, University of Cincinnati; Chief, Vascular Surgery, University Hospital, Cincinnati, Ohio

GLENN M. LAMURAGLIA, M.D.
Instructor in Surgery, Harvard Medical School, Assistant in Surgery, Massachusetts General Hospital, Boston, Massachusetts

ROBERT P. LEATHER, M.D.
Professor of Surgery, Chief of Vascular Surgery, Albany Medical College, Albany, New York

RONALD A. MALT, M.D.
Professor of Surgery, Harvard Medical School, Chief, Gastroenterological Surgery, Massachusetts General Hospital, Boston, Massachusetts

JOHN A. MANNICK, M.D.
Moseley Professor of Surgery, Harvard Medical School; Surgeon-in-Chief, Brigham and Women's Hospital, Boston, Massachusetts

JAMES O. MENZOIAN, M.D.
Associate Professor of Surgery, Boston University School of Medicine; Chief, Section of Vascular Surgery, University Hospital, Boston, Massachusetts

ASHBY C. MONCURE, M.D.
Associate Clinical Professor of Surgery, Harvard Medical School; Visiting Surgeon, Massachusetts General Hospital, Boston, Massachusetts

WESLEY S. MOORE, M.D.
Professor of Surgery, University of California at Los Angeles; Chief, Section of Vascular Surgery, UCLA Center for the Health Sciences, Los Angeles, California

JOHN L. OCHSNER, M.D.
Clinical Professor, Tulane University School of Medicine; Chairman Emeritus, Department of Surgery, Ochsner Foundation Hospital, New Orleans, Louisiana

THOMAS F. O'DONNELL, Jr., M.D.
Professor of Surgery, Tufts University School of Medicine; Chief, Vascular Surgery, Department of Surgery, New England Medical Center, Boston, Massachusetts

PATRICK J. O'HARA, M.D.
Staff Vascular Surgeon, Department of Vascular Surgery, The Cleveland Clinic Foundation, Cleveland, Ohio

LESLIE W. OTTINGER, M.D.
Associate Professor of Surgery, Harvard Medical School; Visiting Surgeon, Massachusetts General Hospital, Boston, Massachusetts

ALFRED V. PERSSON, M.D.
Associate Clinical Professor of Surgery, Clinical Instructor in Surgery, Boston University Medical School, Harvard University Medical School, Boston, Massachusetts, Staff Surgeon, Director, Noninvasive Vascular Laboratory, Lahey Clinic Medical Center, Burlington, Massachusetts, New England Deaconess Hospital, Boston, Massachusetts

MALCOLM O. PERRY, M.D.
The H. William Scott, Jr. Professor of Surgery, Chief, Division of Vascular Surgery, Vanderbilt University School of Medicine, Nashville, Tennessee

JOHN M. PORTER, M.D.
Professor of Surgery, Head, Division of Vascular Surgery, Oregon Health Sciences University, Portland, Oregon

NORMAN M. RICH, M.D., F.A.C.S.
Professor and Chairman, F. Edward Hébert School of Medicine, Uniformed Services University of the Health Sciences, Bethesda, Maryland

THOMAS S. RILES, M.D.
Associate Professor of Surgery, New York University; Associate Attending, Director of Vascular Laboratory, New York University Hospital, New York City, New York

ROBERT B. RUTHERFORD, M.D.

Professor of Surgery, University of Colorado Health Sciences Center, Chief, Vascular Surgery Section, University Hospital, Denver, Colorado

DONALD SILVER, M.D.

Professor and Chairman, Department of Surgery, University of Missouri-Columbia; Chief of Surgery, University of Missouri-Columbia Hospitals and Clinics, Columbia, Missouri

JAMES C. STANLEY, M.D.

Professor of Surgery, Head, Section of Vascular Surgery, University of Michigan Medical School, University of Michigan Medical Center, Ann Arbor, Michigan

BRENT L. STEFFEN, M.D.

Vascular Surgery Resident, University of Missouri Hospitals and Clinics, Columbia, Missouri

RONALD J. STONEY, M.D., F.A.C.S.

Professor of Surgery, Vascular Surgeon, University of California Medical Center, San Francisco, California

D. EUGENE STRANDNESS, Jr., M.D.

Professor of Surgery, University of Washington, School of Medicine; Head, Vascular Surgery Section, University Hospital, Seattle, Washington

DAVID S. SUMNER, M.D.

Professor of Surgery, Chief, Section of Peripheral Vascular Surgery, Southern Illinois University School of Medicine; Staff Surgeon, St. John's Hospital, Memorial Medical Center, Springfield, Illinois

JESSE E. THOMPSON, M.D.

Clinical Professor of Surgery, University of Texas Southwestern Medical School; Attending Surgeon and Former Chief of Surgery, Baylor University Medical Center, Dallas, Texas

JOHNATHAN B. TOWNE, M.D.

Professor of Surgery, Medical College of Wisconsin, Milwaukee County Medical Complex and Veterans Administration Medical Center, Milwaukee, Wisconsin

J. BENJAMIN TRIBBLE, M.D.

Chief Resident in Surgery, Bowman Gray School of Medicine of Wake Forest University, North Carolina Baptist Hospital, Winston-Salem, North Carolina

FRANK J. VEITH, M.D.

Professor of Surgery, Albert Einstein College of Medicine; Chief of Vascular Surgery, Montefiore Medical Center, Bronx, New York

WILLIS H. WAGNER, M.D.

Vascular Surgery Fellow and Clinical Instructor in Surgery, University of North Carolina, North Carolina Memorial Hospital, Chapel Hill, North Carolina

ANTHONY D. WHITTEMORE, M.D.

Associate Professor of Surgery, Harvard Medical School; Attending Vascular Surgeon, Brigham and Women's Hospital, Boston, Massachusetts

JAMES S.T. YAO, M.D.
Professor of Surgery, Northwestern University Medical School, Chicago, Illinois

CHRISTOPHER K. ZARINS, M.D.
Professor of Surgery, The University of Chicago Medical Center, Chicago, Illinois

SERIES INTRODUCTION

With the proliferation of medical and surgical monographs on every conceivable subject, it is difficult to embark on yet another publishing venture in the belief that such a contribution can be fresh and original. However, I believe this series, **COMMON PROBLEMS IN SURGERY,** achieves this unique goal. It departs from the traditional formula of assigning topics within a given area to recognized experts who then exhaustively review the medical literature and assemble a comprehensive, and, hopefully, definitive exposition of their subject. Rather, this series which is intended for busy, practicing surgeons and surgeons-in-training is designed to convey a maximum amount of *practical* information as succinctly as possible. The subject material of each volume is limited to those problems which are encountered in any active surgical practice and all discussions are built around illustrative clinical cases. More importantly, the mamagement of each case is approached entirely from the perspective of each consultant's personal experience. Accordingly, emphasis is on the transmission of useful, clinical information and literature citations are kept to a minimum.

Vascular surgery continues to comprise a significant component of many general surgeon's practices and is a discipline in which both diagnosis and therapy are rapidly evolving. Dr. Brewster has assembled a ''star studded'' list of contributors who are all nationally recognized experts in this field. He has compiled a comprehensive series of challenging clinical cases illustrating problems in the areas of cerebrovascular arterial occlusive disease, arterial aneurysms, infra-inguinal arterial occlusive disease, arterial trauma, venous disease and a variety of miscellaneous subjects which cover the gamut of situations likely to be encountered by the practicing surgeon. The discussion of each case clearly reflects the author's personal experience and offers a wealth of practical suggestions and guidelines in the management of these complex problems. This monograph clearly measures up to the exacting benchmark established by the other volumes in this series.

RICHARD F. KEMPCZINSKI, M.D.
Professor of Surgery
University of Cincinnati
Chief, Vascular Surgery
University Hospital
Cincinnati, Ohio

PREFACE

It is evident that the field of vascular surgery is one of the most rapidly expanding areas of surgical practice today. It has become a distinct and recognized specialty, with separate board qualifications, approved training fellowships, and a steadily increasing number of surgeons devoting the major portion of their practice to its unique problems. There has been tremendous growth both in methods of evaluating vascular diseases and in techniques for surgical correction of such problems.

As a consequence of such rapid evolution, it is not surprising that a variety of different approaches to management of specific problems exists. Such management alternatives may seem confusing and indeed bewildering to practitioners, particularly those less experienced in the care of vascular patients. Practical, succinct, and up-to-date advice on management decisions pertinent to a specific problem may be difficult to obtain from standard textbooks or the vast surgical literature that has developed in this field.

This book was assembled in the hope of meeting some of these needs. It is designed primarily to inform the clinical surgeon, surgical resident, or nursing staff caring for vascular patients. Primary care physicians, internists, or cardiologists, all of whom often first encounter patients with a vascular problem, may also benefit. This book is not meant to be a comprehensive textbook in the usual sense, or a review of various topics emphasizing a variety of opinions or alternatives. Rather, we sought to obtain the personal approaches of individual practicing surgeons, each an acknowledged and respected authority in their subject area. The emphasis is on practical, informal, and up-to-date advice based on each surgeon's own personal experience, and on opinion distilled from their own successes or failures with the wide array of alternative methods available. Inevitably, each chapter reflects the biases of the author. Similarly, some opinions will be controversial—I certainly did not agree with all. However, I believe such characteristics are a strength, not a weakness, of the book. Much of the value of the book is in learning what others would do when faced with a common problem.

The book is divided into six general areas, representing the broad spectrum of problems encountered by the practicing vascular surgeon. Within each section, separate chapters deal with specific clinical problems frequently seen in day-to-day practice by the surgeon. Each chapter is introduced by a brief clinical scenario, describing a patient and problem, and serving as a starting point for the discussion of patient management. Each author has supplied a bibliography at the conclusion of their chapter, meant to serve as a list of suggested references for further reading on the subject if desired. The emphasis, as the name of the volume implies, is on common problems, not rare situations likely to be seen "once in a lifetime" at a large center. Each contributor was encouraged to be brief and practical. As in any multiauthored book, some variation in length and style exists, but I believe each author has met the requirement of informing the reader how he or she would deal with the specific problem at hand.

   The value of the book is obviously attributable to the insight and experience of the contributors, each of whom took time from already overburdened schedules of clinical and academic activities. I am deeply indebted to each of them. I would like to acknowledge the invaluable secretarial, administrative, and proofreading assistance of Larissa Taylor, Rona Cavallaro, and Maureen Bidgood. Thanks also go to Susan Hunsberger, project editor at Editing, Design and Production, Inc., for helpful editing and production work. Finally, I express my gratitude to Dan Doody and Nancy Chorpenning of Year Book Medical Publishers, Inc., for their advice, encouragement, and thoughtful prodding.

DAVID C. BREWSTER, M.D.

CONTENTS

PART 2   ANEURYSMAL DISEASE 77

PART 3   OCCLUSIVE DISEASE 141

PART ONE

Cerebrovascular

1 Asymptomatic Carotid Bruit

A 59-year-old male is referred for evaluation and management of bilateral cervical bruits, noted by his internist during a recent routine physical examination. He has mild adult onset diabetes mellitus and a history of moderate left calf claudication. He denies any cardiac symptoms. Other than occasional light-headedness, he denies any neurologic symptoms.

Consultant: Wesley S. Moore, M.D.

ASYMPTOMATIC CAROTID DISEASE—WHY BE CONCERNED?

There are approximately 500,000 new strokes in the United States each year. Of those, 150,000 will die as a direct consequence of the cerebral ischemic event. Approximately 50% of all strokes are related to carotid bifurcation disease. If all patients had warning symptoms prior to the onset of stroke, there would be no need for concern about asymptomatic carotid artery lesions. Unfortunately, somewhere between 50 and 90% of all patients who suffer a stroke do so as a primary event. That is, they had no warning symptoms. As a consequence, there are approximately 150,000 patients each year who suffer a stroke from a lesion that had been previously asymptomatic.

RISK FACTORS

In order to identify those patients who are at risk of harboring a covert lesion that places the individual at risk for stroke, a number of risk factors in the patient's history can be identified. These include a history of cigarette smoking, hypertension, diabetes mellitus, and hypercholesterolemia. In addition, patients who have overt evidence of arterial disease in another system are also at risk for harboring lesions in their carotid arteries. Therefore, patients with a history of intermittent claudication or coronary artery disease should also be suspect for carotid artery disease.

Our patient has been identified as having two major risk factors, diabetes mel-

3

litus and calf claudication. We are not told whether or not he smokes cigarettes or has a history of hypertension. However, with his history of calf claudication, there is a high likelihood that cigarette smoking is a part of his history. The presence of multiple risk factors increases the likelihood of carotid artery disease in an exponential fashion.

PHYSICAL EXAMINATION

The most common physical finding that marks a patient at risk for covert carotid artery disease is the presence of a bruit heard over the carotid bifurcation. The presence of a bruit means that there is some lesion producing blood flow turbulence. However, the presence of a bruit or turbulence is not tantamount to a lesion that places the patient at stroke risk. In fact, a cervical carotid bruit turns out to be a better marker for subsequent myocardial infarction and death than it does for stroke. The lesions that place patients at high risk for stroke have been identified as high-grade stenoses involving the origin of the internal carotid artery (>75% occlusive) and large ulcerated or excavated lesions within the atherosclerotic plaque that have the potential for embolization. Previous studies correlating angiographic findings in patients with carotid artery bruit have demonstrated that only 20%, or one patient in five, with a carotid artery bruit will turn out to have a lesion of hemodynamic significance when a carotid angiogram is performed. Nonetheless, the presence of a carotid bruit, even though a nonspecific marker, must be evaluated to rule in or rule out a significant carotid artery lesion.

Other physical findings of importance include an elevated blood pressure, the detection of a difference in blood pressure between the two arms, abnormality or absence of a peripheral pulse, and bruit over a peripheral artery suggesting the presence of intraluminal atheromatous disease. In addition, a careful neurologic assessment should be carried out. While patients may be asymptomatic with respect to prior cerebrovascular symptoms, there may have been a subtle neurologic event about which the patient is unaware. A careful physical examination stressing a detailed neurologic assessment may uncover a defect that will identify the patient as, in fact, being symptomatic rather than asymptomatic.

Our patient is identified as having important physical findings by the presence of bilateral cervical bruit. While the rest of the physical examination is not reported, we may assume that it is negative with the exception of the pulse findings in the left leg. These are not detailed for us, and therefore no comment can be made other than to point out the fact that he is experiencing symptoms of left calf claudication and probably has abnormalities of the pulses on the left side.

NONINVASIVE ASSESSMENT OF THE CAROTID ARTERIES

We have now identified a patient who is at significant risk for harboring lesions in his carotid arteries that make him prone to stroke. Nevertheless, from prior experience, we recognize that proceeding with angiography at this point will only yield a 20% rate of patients with hemodynamically significant stenoses. Therefore, four out of every five patients undergoing an arteriogram based on available data to date will have needless study and, hence, needless exposure to the risk of angiography.

The use of screening in the noninvasive vascular laboratory will help to further identify the one patient in five with carotid artery bruit who has a lesion of hemodynamic significance. It will also help to reassure the four patients in five that, at present, a lesion of hemodynamic significance is not present. Finally, the noninvasive laboratory provides us with a risk-free vehicle for follow-up assessment of this latter group of patients.

Therefore, my next investigation in this patient would be to obtain a carotid artery duplex scan. A duplex scan will give me a great deal of information about the carotid bifurcations in this patient, the presence of pathology, and the nature of the pathologic lesion. B-mode will identify the carotid bifurcation and differentiate the internal from the external carotid artery. It will also identify the presence of atheromatous plaque in a critical location and, most important, will identify the nature of the plaque as to whether or not it is a smooth, hard lesion or a soft, irregular lesion. Once the bifurcation is identified, the common carotid artery, internal carotid artery, and external carotid artery can be insonated with the Doppler beam and spectral analysis can be obtained. From the spectral data, we can determine whether or not a lesion of hemodynamic significance is present in the extracranial internal carotid artery.

The lesions that concern me will be a stenosis involving the internal carotid artery in excess of 75% occlusive. In addition, a lesser stenosis made up of soft material and with an irregular surface may signal the presence of an ulcerative lesion that has embolic potential.

COMPUTERIZED TOMOGRAPHY OF THE BRAIN

If the patient is identified as having a critical arterial lesion, it may well be that cerebral infarction has already occurred and has either been forgotten by the patient or has taken place in a relatively silent area. A CT scan of the brain will be helpful in identifying evidence of cerebral infarction distal to a critical lesion. If there is evidence of cerebral infarction distal to a critical lesion, then this lesion is taken out of the asymptomatic category and is treated on its merit as a lesion having already produced brain damage. If the CT scan is negative, then this is important data for baseline purposes and future follow-up.

INDICATIONS FOR ANGIOGRAPHY

An angiogram is indicated when there is evidence of a hemodynamically significant lesion by noninvasive assessment and the patient has requested that we proceed with carotid endarterectomy if a lesion is proven by angiographic study. In essence, an angiogram is a preoperative test. Therefore, the indications for angiography are the same as the indications for operation.

While it might be feasible that patients will harbor an important ulcerative lesion of a low profile plaque that is missed by noninvasive assessment, at the present time we are not recommending routine angiography to discover these lesions.

INDICATIONS FOR OPERATION

My indications for carotid endarterectomy in asymptomatic patients are (1) the presence of a high-grade stenosis that is in excess of 75% occlusive and (2) the presence of a large ulcerative lesion, with or without stenosis, that fits our descriptive category of a grade B or C lesion. Suffice to say that the patient should be in otherwise reasonable health and be at satisfactory risk for general anesthesia and operation. Finally, the patient should have no comorbidity that would make his life expectancy less than five years.

The indications for carotid endarterectomy among experts in both neurology and surgery is at best controversial. Those who advocate a nonoperative approach argue that the risks of operation outweigh the benefits of stroke prevention. They point out that a significant percentage of patients will develop transient ischemic attacks in advance of stroke and therefore can be identified for elective operation at that time. They argue that the number of patients who present with stroke as their initial manifestation are few, and that the likelihood of major morbidity and mortality as a consequence of coronary artery disease exceeds that of stroke.

On the other hand, recent natural history studies have identified patient groups who are at high risk for stroke and who may well benefit from operation. Roederer, et al, following a group of 203 patients with duplex scanning, noted that 33% of patients with <50% stenosis progressed to lesions >50% stenosis within three years. They noted that 89% of patients who developed either TIA or stroke were preceded by a disease progression to >80% stenosis. Finally, if a lesion progressed to an 80% or greater stenosis, there was a 35% risk of symptoms or occlusion within six months and 46% risk at 12 months. D.J. Moore, et al, followed a group of 294 patients characterized by noninvasive assessment. There were 36 patients in this group that developed a stroke and only one was preceded by transient ischemic events. Those patients who initially had a 50% stenosis or greater had a 17% stroke rate within five years. They identified a subset of patients consisting of those over the age of 70, with a diagnosis of hypertension, and a stenosis in excess of 50%. This subgroup had a 49% stroke incidence in five years or a stroke rate of approximately 10% per year. Chambers and Norris, from the Toronto Asymptomatic Stenosis Study, noted a one-year cerebral ischemic event rate in patients with stenosis in excess of 75% to be 18%. The one-year stroke rate was 5%, and the one-year stroke rate without antecedent TIAs was 3%.

In an attempt to resolve the controversy, there are currently two randomized prospective studies in progress designed to compare medical and surgical management in patients with asymptomatic carotid stenosis. I support the need for these studies and, therefore, am willing to enter patients, who are willing to participate in this study, for randomization. However, for those patients not wishing to participate, I am willing to proceed with prophylactic carotid endarterectomy in lesions >75% occlusive.

The indications for operation on nonstenotic ulcerative lesions of the carotid bifurcation are based on a retrospective review of two patient groups. This review indicated that the risk of stroke in patients with category B ulcers was 4.5% per year and the risk of stroke with category C ulcers was 7% per year.

Our aggressive approach to prophylactic operation is based on a favorable experience with the operation. We have previously reported one series of operations on asymptomatic stenoses done without death or perioperative stroke. Late follow-up has demonstrated a stroke-free survival of up to 10 years. More recent experience has confirmed these data and, furthermore, has demonstrated that >95% of patients are still alive at the end of five-year follow-up. Therefore, patients do live long enough to enjoy the benefits of prophylactic operation.

PATIENT FOLLOW-UP

Following noninvasive assessment, if a patient is found is found to have a subcritical lesion, it is our recommendation that the patient be seen every six to 12 months for repeat duplex scanning. Lesions can and do change within a short time interval and a recent rapid progression can become an indication for operation.

For those patients having undergone prophylactic operation, we follow them at six-month intervals for the first two years utilizing duplex scanning and then yearly thereafter.

BIBLIOGRAPHY

1. Chambers BR, Norris JW: Outcome in patients with asymptomatic neck bruits. *N Engl J Med* 1986; 315:860–865.
2. Dixon S, Pais SO, Raviola C, et al: Natural history of nonstenotic asymptomatic ulcerative lesions of the carotid artery. *Arch Surg* 1982; 117:1493–1498.
3. Humphries AW, Young JR, Santilli PH, et al: Unoperated, asymptomatic significant internal carotid artery stenosis: A review of 182 instances. *Surgery* 1976; 80:695–698.
4. Kartchner MM, McRae LP: Noninvasive evaluation and management of the "asymptomatic" carotid bruit. *Surgery* 1977; 82:840–847.
5. Kartchner MM, McRae LP: Guidelines for non-invasive evaluation of asymptomatic carotid bruits. *Clin Neurosurg* 1981; 28:418–428.
6. Malone JM, Bean B, Laguna J, et al: Diagnosis of carotid artery stenosis: Comparison of oculoplethysmography and Doppler supraorbital examination. *Ann Surg* 1980; 191:347–353.
7. Mohr JP, Caplan LR, Melski JW, et al: The Harvard Cooperative Stroke Registry: A prospective registry. *Neurology* (NY) 1978; 28:754–762.

8 *Cerebrovascular*

8. Moore DJ, Miles RD, Gooley NA, et al: Noninvasive assessment of stroke risk in asymptomatic and nonhemispheric patients with suspected carotid disease: Five-year follow-up of 294 unoperated and 81 operated patients. *Ann Surg* 1985; 202:491–504.
9. Moore WS, Bean B, Burton R, et al: The use of ophthalmosonometry in the diagnosis of carotid artery stenosis. *Surgery* 1977; 82:107–115.
10. Moore WS, Boren CB, Malone JM, et al: Natural history of nonstenotic, asymptomatic ulcerative lesions of the carotid artery. *Arch Surg* 1978; 113:1352–1359.
11. Moore WS, Boren C, Malone JM, et al: Asymptomatic carotid stenosis: Immediate and long term results after prophylactic endarterectomy. *Am J Surg* 1979; 138:228–233.
12. Roederer GO, Langlois YE, Jager KA, et al: The natural history of carotid arterial disease in asymptomatic patients with cervical bruits. *Stroke* 1984; 15:605–613.
13. Sergeant PT, Drom F, Berzsenye G, et al: Carotid endarterectomy for cerebrovascular insufficiency: Long term follow-up of 141 patients followed-up to sixteen years. *Acta Chir Belg* 1979; 79:309–316.
14. Thompson JE, Patman RD, Talkington CM: Asymptomatic carotid bruit: Long term outcome of patients having endarterectomy compared with unoperated controls. *Ann Surg* 1978; 188:308–316.
15. West H, Burton R, Roon AG, et al: Comparative risk of operation and expectant management for carotid disease. *Stroke* 1979; 10:117–121.
16. Wolf PA, Kannel WB, Sorlie P, et al: Asymptomatic carotid bruit and risk of stroke. The Framingham Study. *JAMA* 1981; 245:1442–1445.
17. Ziegler DK, Zileli T, Dick A, et al: Correlation of bruits over the carotid artery with angiographically demonstrated lesions. *Neurology* (NY) 1971; 21:860–865.

2   Asymptomatic Carotid Bruit in Patient Requiring Coronary Bypass Surgery

You are asked to see a 62-year-old man who has been admitted for coronary artery bypass grafting the following day. He has severe angina and three-vessel coronary disease. On admission, a carotid bruit is detected and you are consulted.

Consultant: D. Eugene Strandness, Jr., M.D.

This clinical presentation is an extremely common one which all surgeons and cardiologists are forced to deal with. First, it must be recognized that it is impossible to define either the basis for the bruit or the degree of stenosis from the physical examination alone. While it is true that bruits of carotid bifurcation origin tend to be heard most prominently in the midneck region with radiation to the base of the skull, it is necessary to verify by some independent means the location and extent of involvement.

The traditional approach to studying the carotid bifurcation is angiography. With newer developments in angiographic methods, it is now possible to select the approach most reasonable for a particular patient. When first introduced, intravenous digital subtraction techniques were highly touted as the ideal method, since catheterization of the arterial system is not required. While it is possible to obtain films of diagnostic quality in most patients, at least 20% will be totally unsatisfactory. This is not acceptable and makes the method unsuitable for this application. Much better filming can be obtained by either intraarterial digital methods or conventional arteriography, but these are not warranted unless the patient is symptomatic, which this patient is not. Furthermore, its performance usually requires postponing of the planned cardiac operation for an additional day in most cases.

The only reasonable approach given the situation is to use a suitable noninvasive test. The simplest are the supraorbital Doppler and the OPG-GEE. Both of these tests become positive only when the lesions result in a decrease in pressure and flow. However, they are not sensitive to lesser degrees of disease and do not identify the sites of involvement.

My own preference is to perform ultrasonic duplex scanning. This method has a sensitivity of greater than 95% and a specificity of 90%. It not only provides precise localization of the disease but also permits its categorization into rather broad categories which appear to have clinical relevance. In my laboratory we define the following categories: (1) normal; (2) 1% to 15%—wall roughening; (3) 16% to 49%; (4) 50% to 79%; (5) 80% to 99% stenosis; and (6) total occlusion. These categories are presented in terms of diameter reduction, not cross-sectional area.

When such screening is done in patients with coronary artery disease, the chance of finding carotid artery lesions will be quite high. For example, in a study we did of patients with coronary artery disease who had bruits, 54% were found to have a stenosis of greater than 50% diameter reduction noted on the side of the bruit. If the screening is done in patients without a bruit, the yield for greater than 50% stenoses is considerably less, being in the 5% to 10% range.

Our initial studies on examining this problem consisted of two groups of patients. One group included patients with detected bruits who had duplex studies requested. There were 24 patients in this group—13 had a greater than 50% stenosis. There were an additional 78 patients studied who did not have a bruit (the unrequested group). In this cohort, only five of 78 (6%) had the moderately high-grade lesions found.

Endarterectomy was performed in five of the requested group (two synchronously and three prior to the cardiac procedure). All of these patients had a history of ischemic cerebrovascular events. All did well. The remaining 97 patients underwent coronary bypass without carotid endarterectomy. There were two perioperative events—one stroke and a TIA, both occurring in the unrequested group of patients. Neither of these patients had high-grade carotid lesions.

Based on this initial small study, we proposed the following hypothesis: No patient should have carotid endarterectomy in conjunction with aortocoronary bypass grafting unless the patient had a focal ischemic cerebrovascular event appropriate to the finding of a carotid bifurcation lesion. Furthermore, duplex scanning should be done prior to the procedure only if the patient was found to have a bruit or had a history of ischemic cerebrovascular events.

During a 31-month period, a total of 1,433 patients underwent coronary artery bypass in the University Hospital at the University of Washington. There were 94 patients with a carotid bruit identified who underwent duplex scanning. The results of this study can be summarized as follows:

1. Nine patients had a carotid bruit, a history of TIAs and a ≥50% diameter reducing stenosis. All underwent endarterectomy prior to or simultaneous with the operation. There was one neurological death in this group;

2. There were 16 asymptomatic patients with a greater than 50% stenosis. These patients underwent cardiopulmonary bypass without developing a neurological event;

3. There were 66 patients with asymptomatic bruits who had a less than 50% stenosis. All underwent coronary bypass without a neurological event;

4. The remaining 1,339 patients who were free of bruits and did not undergo duplex scanning had a neurological event rate of 0.7% subsequent to the aortocoronary bypass procedure. We concluded that there was no need for consideration of carotid endarterectomy either prior to or with coronary bypass grafting unless the patient was symptomatic. Is this the proper approach?

While it is always dangerous to compare results with other published series, Hertzer, et al, reported a mortality of 5.7% and a stroke incidence of 9.7% in patients undergoing simultaneous repair. There were 331 patients in this study with 52% being asymptomatic. It must be noted that their patients tended to be unstable with poor left ventricular function and a left main coronary stenosis. Rice, et al, reported a stroke rate of 3.9% with no deaths in 54 patients undergoing simultaneous repair. In a similar study, Craver and associates reported a stroke rate of 7.5% in 68 patients. There were no deaths.

This stance with regard to the incidental finding of carotid artery disease does not mean that the problem ought to be ignored. While the issue of management remains a controversial one, certain facts are beginning to emerge. Before considering some of the current trials, it is important to briefly review what we know about the natural history of atherosclerotic lesions wherever they occur.

While the pathogenesis of these lesions remains obscure, the plaque appears to progress from the uniform, largely smooth muscle lesion—the fibrous plaque—to that which is found in patients with clinical problems. The "clinical plaque" is described as complicated because of the many features which distinguish it. These include loss of surface covering, necrosis, hemorrhage, calcification, cholesterol crystallization, and fibrosis. One of the key occurrences which often leads to clinical events when it occurs is thrombosis. It is now known that high-grade arterial stenoses, whether occurring in the coronaries, peripheral arteries and carotid arteries, can have this as the sudden event which may lead to catastrophic tissue ischemia.

Our own studies and those of others have shown that it is the high-grade stenosis (>80%) which appears to be the most dangerous lesion. In our initial study, 47% of asymptomatic patients with high-grade stenotic lesions sustained an event (TIA, stroke, or total occlusion) usually within six months of discovery of the lesion.

These observations have led to two major recommendations. If a patient has a stenosis discovered which is less than 80% in terms of diameter reduction, it is safe to follow the patient with repeat studies every six months. For this group of patients, the event rate will be on the order of 4% per year. On the other hand, if a high-grade stenosis is discovered (>80%), prophylactic endarterectomy is recommended and should be done relatively quickly after discovery of the lesion.

Thus, in an asymptomatic patient with a severe carotid stenosis, our current approach would be to proceed with the carotid operation four to six weeks after the coronary bypass procedure. We prefer this to doing the endarterectomy before the bypass since it is important to have optimized cardiac function for the neck procedure. While the mortality rate from carotid procedures is low, the main cause of death is myocardial infarction.

BIBLIOGRAPHY

1. Breslau PJ, Fell G, Ivey TD, et al: Carotid arterial disease in patients undergoing coronary artery bypass operations. *J Thorac Cardiovasc Surg* 1981; 82:765–767.
2. Craver JM, Murphy DA, Jones E, et al: Concomitant carotid and coronary artery reconstruction. *Ann Surg* 1982; 195:712–720.
3. Hertzer NR, Loop FD, Taylor PC, et al: Staged and combined surgical approach to simultaneous carotid and coronary vascular disease. *Surgery* 1978; 84:803–811.
4. Ivey TD, Strandness DE Jr, Williams DB, et al: Management of patients with carotid bruit undergoing cardiopulmonary bypass. *J Thorac Cardiovasc Surg* 1984; 87:183–189.
5. Rice PL, Pifarre R, Sullivan HJ, et al: Experience with simultaneous myocardial revascularization and carotid endarterectomy. *J Thorac Cardiovasc Surg* 1980; 79:922–925.
6. Roederer GO, Langlois YE, Jager KA, et al: The natural history of carotid arterial disease in asymptomatic patients with cervical bruits. *Stroke* 1984; 15:605–613.

3 Carotid Stenosis with Unstable Fluctuating Neurologic Deficit

A 55-year-old man is admitted with a 24-hour history of difficulty speaking and right-sided weakness. His symptoms improved within several hours of onset, but later redeveloped, prompting him to come to the hospital. He was placed on heparin and again symptoms largely resolved. On the morning after admission, aphasia and right hemiparesis were again noted and you are asked to see the patient.

Consultant: Roger M. Greenhalgh, M.A., M.D., M. Chir., FRCS

The first point in the management of such a patient is to begin with a thorough assessment which, as always, implies that a most careful history should be taken. Ideally, this patient should be seen by a neurologist for baseline assessment of history, physical signs, and specific diagnosis. It is best if a neurologist and a vascular surgical service can work in harmony and decide together how to proceed. I shall outline how our group would approach this problem.

TERMINOLOGY

The Marseilles classification was an attempt to standardize some terms and define them more thoroughly. It was decided that the only way to categorize stroke was on clinical presentation. The term "transient ischemic attack" (TIA) is in common usage and was endorsed. It implies a neurologic deficit which resolves, usually in minutes, but certainly within 24 hours. A key issue of the diagnosis of a transient ischemic attack is that the neurological deficit entirely disappears between attacks. If the neurologic deficit persists for more than 24 hours but disappears within a three-week period, the term "transient stroke" was recommended since terms such as PRIND or RIND stood for a variety of terms with a variety of definitions. If a stroke persists after three weeks, the term "established stroke" was recommended and this could either have a good recovery or bad recovery. The term "progressing stroke" also means different things to different people, but I have recommended that its use should be reserved for those patients who have evidence of progression of neurologic deficit for more than 24 hours. Progressing stroke can be one of two types. If the progression is of a gradual nature without any fluctuation of deficit, the term "stroke in evolution" has been used. On the other hand, occasionally, there is a fluctuation of deficit superimposed on a progressing stroke with progressing deficit over 24 hours, at least. The term "stuttering hemiplegia" has been recommended for this type of progressing stroke.

The 55-year-old man under question here had an improvement of symptoms within several hours of onset and careful questioning would be required to establish whether the improvement was complete or partial. A neurologist would not have examined him at that stage because he didn't come into the hospital until his symptoms redeveloped. The critical issue in this patient is to assess his clinical status at once and to note from hour to hour whether the status improves and returns to the base line, in which case he is suffering from transient ischemic attacks. The term crescendo transient ischemic attack is usually reserved for patients who have more frequent TIAs or more severe TIAs implying a crescendo of deficit of attacks or a crescendo of frequency of attacks. On the evidence of this patient this might be the situation here but at the time of admission it would be difficult to be certain.

INVESTIGATION

While a period of observation of such a patient and thorough moment-to-moment assessment is vital, investigation can safely proceed and we would recommend this in every patient. Our vascular laboratory would be the first port of call. We would perform continuous wave spectral analysis of the common, internal and external carotid arteries on both sides and from this, gain an idea of the degree of stenosis of the carotid vessels. Using a separate instrument we would proceed to a duplex scan to check the original frequency analysis findings and also to image the carotid vessels noninvasively in order to assess the degree of stenosis and also the quality of the artery wall.

At this point the patient would be sent for a CT scan in our X-ray department. In our facility this is very close and the patient is not inconvenienced and receives rapid assessment.

Working with a neurologist, later on the first day of admission, we would reassess the clinical status of the patient to see if his attack had resolved, in which case the immediate urgency would be diminished. We would look at the CT scan, and, of course, if there was any evidence of intracranial hemorrhage, the heparin would be stopped immediately. Heparin, in any case, is frequently unwise in a patient who is hypertensive. We would be inclined to give it only if we know that a patient has a tight stenosis and would probably not give it for its own sake on admission, but rather perform noninvasive tests and CT scan first. If the noninvasive tests showed no abnormality, we would be disinclined to proceed to an angiogram. Having compared the noninvasive tests with angiography in our own hospital, we can place some reliance on their findings, and if we assess noninvasively that carotid blood flow is normal and there is minimal if any disease at the carotid bifurcation, an angiogram would not be requested, and the patient would have control of risk factors and would be considered to be managed medically, either on anticoagulants or antiplatelet therapy. On the other hand, if a demonstrable lesion was found on noninvasive tests, as is usually the case, we would confirm this by angiography.

ANGIOGRAPHY

Carotid stab angiography had its obituary some years ago, and conventional arch angiography with selective catheterization of the carotid arteries has an unacceptable morbidity. I can understand the reluctance of neurologists to investigate a patient such as this 55-year-old man if the only facility for investigation is an arch angiogram with selective carotid views. The risk of dislodging atheroma from the arch of the aorta or from the great vessels, or from placement of a catheter in the carotid vessels from the arch, produces an unacceptable risk, and this has inclined many neurologists to avoid proper investigation of these patients. However, digital subtraction angiography (DSA) is of tremendous value in a patient such as this. Intravenous DSA can produce a good outline, better in some hospitals than others, but we feel that the quality of the image is below par. I prefer to pass a small 5 French gauge catheter through a femoral artery under local anesthetic and to release contrast from the arch of the aorta without selective carotid views. This is no more invasive than intravenous DSA in which a small catheter is passed from the arm to the right atrium. The views of an arch flush DSA with intraarterial injection of contrast are greatly superior. Views in more than one plane are essential. The amount of contrast used can be kept to a minimum. The arch, carotid great vessels, carotid vessels, vertebral vessels, and intracranial vessels can all be visualized quite satisfactorily.

CLINICAL EXPERIENCE

Findings in Patients Presenting with Crescendo TIA

It is significant that despite an interest in this field, we have only seen eight patients, five male and three female (age range 55 to 72 years, mean age 63.6 years). One of these patients was hypertensive. There are undoubtedly more such patients in the community, but the referring doctor is unaware that these patients might be investigated to great effect. Another possibility is that general physicians are seeing the patients and not referring them on either to a neurologist or vascular surgeon. We had CT scan information on six of the eight patients with crescendo TIA and only one of the six had no evidence of cerebral infarction at that stage. The CT findings do not influence our management. All eight crescendo TIA patients had very significant carotid disease on noninvasive assessment and arch angiography. Seven had a stenosis of greater than 90% in the ipsilateral carotid artery and one had a most irregular carotid artery with marked kinking. In other words, all of the series had an extracranial demonstrable and correctable lesion.

Findings in Patients Presenting with Progressing Stroke

We have seen 15 patients with progressing stroke, seven men and eight women (age range 46 to 80 years, with a mean age of 65.7 years). Seven of the patients were hypertensive. Of the 15, seven of the patients had previously suffered crescendo TIAs which had moved on to a progressing stroke. This implies that the patient first started with a transient ischemic attack and that the attacks became either more frequent, or more severe, but after a period of observation, even with the use of heparin between attacks, the patient did not recover completely his neurologic deficit. This is why the thorough assessment of this 55-year-old man described in this case history is vital. Three of our patients had a previous history of an established stroke which was not operated on and after a variable period of time, they developed a progression of stroke on the ipsilateral side. Five of the 15 had no previous neurologic symptoms; the progressing stroke came out of the blue.

We had CT information on 13 of the 15 and only two of these 13 had no infarct demonstrable at the initial stage. However, 11 had evidence of ipsilateral infarction and in one patient, observed for three days by a conservative physician, there was evidence of progression of infarct on the CT scan on each successive day. Seven of the 15 patients had an ipsilateral stenosis of greater than 90%, three greater than 70%, three greater than 50%, and one greater than 40%. In the fifteenth patient, the carotid artery was aneurysmal and there was evidence of embolization from within the aneurysm. In other words, there was a demonstrable and correctable extracranial lesion on all of the patients.

The Natural History Studies

Performing a carotid endarterectomy in a patient with acute neurologic deficit has been controversial for more than 22 years. Early reports suggested a high incidence of complications when surgery was performed in the first few days after the development of an acute deficit. These complications were believed to be associated with the restoration of flow to an area of ischemic brain producing hemorrhage in an area of infarction. The Joint Study of Extracranial Arterial Occlusion in 1969 reviewed data on 255 acute stroke patients with altered consciousness. Of these, 187 were admitted in coma, semicoma or stupor and were treated medically. At the time of discharge, 53% improved, 22% were the same, 5% were worse, and 20% had died during the period of hospitalization. Fifty patients were operated on within the first two weeks of acute stroke and of these 34% were improved, 18% were unchanged, 6% were worse, and 42% died. In other words, the surgically treated group had a mortality twice as great as the medically treated group. The surgically treated group appear to be comparable with the nonsurgical group, although a random allocation study was not performed. Concerning operation for total internal carotid artery occlusion, the Joint Study made no definite conclusions regarding indications for operation, the greater the chance of reestablishing patency and the higher the risk of converting "anemic infarct" into the much more lethal "hemorrhagic infarct." This experience has provided the backbone of prevailing thought for two decades.

There are no control studies of the efficacy of operation for CTIAs or progressing stroke, but nonoperative series have been reported. Millikan reviewed the natural history of 204 consecutive patients with progressing stroke. This series served as a control for a clinical study evaluating the effects of carbon dioxide inhalation in patients with progressing stroke caused by carotid artery disease. At the end of 14 days, only 12% were normal, 69% hemiparetic, 5% monoparetic, and 14% of the patients had died. Mentzer, et al, identified 55 patients with fluctuating neurologic deficits from the records of 485 consecutive patients with cerebral ischemia. The fluctuation deficits were either CTIAs or progressing stroke, similar to the patient under review in this case. Of the 55 patients, 31 were managed nonoperatively and 24 had emergency operation. The operative and nonoperative groups had similar age and sex distribution and incidence of associated medical problems. Of the five nonoperative CTIA patients, one recovered completely, three were moderately to severely impaired at the time of discharge, and one died of complications of cerebral infarction. Seven operated CTIA patients recovered completely and were free of symptoms at the time of discharge. For progressing stroke, the operative and nonoperative groups were comparable for degree of neurologic deficit at the time of diagnosis. Of the 26 nonoperated progressing stroke patients, only two had a complete neurologic recovery, three had a mild residual deficit, 17 a moderate to severe deficit, and four patients died. In the operative group of 17 patients described as having progressive stroke, only 12 were admitted to hospital with the primary condition, while four developed signs after arteriography and one after an elective carotid endarterectomy. However, after surgery, four of the 17 had complete neurologic recovery and eight were left with a mild deficit, four with a moderate to severe deficit, and one patient died. In other words, 12 out of 17 of the operative group (70.6%) against five of the 26 of the nonoperative (19.2%) were in the mild to normal category with respect to the degree of neurologic deficit at the time of hospital discharge.

The Charing Cross Experience

We operated on the eight CTIA patients and the 15 progressing stroke patients, but we did not operate on patients in whom a total occlusion of the ipsilateral carotid artery was demonstrated. The carotid procedure used has been described elsewhere. The salient features are that the patient is operated on under a general anesthetic and PO_2 and PCO_2 levels are maintained at the normal levels. A skin crease incision is used to approach the carotid artery and very careful dissection is performed and, in particular, a gentle sling is placed around the common carotid artery and external carotid artery, but not around the internal carotid artery, which is left totally undisturbed in its bed. The carotid bifurcation is never handled. The patient is given an intravenous bolus of heparin of approximately 5000 units and after a three-minute period, a needle is placed in the external carotid artery for the purpose of measuring back pressure. A clamp is placed distal to the position of the needle such that the arterial trace from the needle is not interfered with. The common carotid artery is then clamped at the proximal end of the incision and far away from the carotid bifurcation. At this point, without clamping the internal carotid artery, an arteriotomy is made at the carotid bifurcation and advanced into the origin of the internal carotid artery. The internal carotid artery is allowed to bleed backward to remove any material which is loose. A Javid intraluminal shunt was inserted for all of the crescendo TIA patients, as back pressures were 50 or less and back pressure wave forms were flat in all patients. However, eight of the 15 patients with progressing stroke had a back pressure of 50 or greater and, of more significance to us, the back flow tracing was pulsatile. This implied to us that in those eight patients undergoing progressive stroke, the progression was more likely to be coming from recurrent embolization, and we considered that it was not necessary to use a shunt in these patients. We are aware that this decision is controversial and many surgeons would prefer to use a shunt in these circumstances. Our data would not incline us to recommend the use of shunt in these eight patients.

OUTCOME OF SURGERY

The outcome of surgery for crescendo TIAs is listed in Table 3–1 in which it can be seen that five of the eight patients recovered and were completely normal after the operation. One patient who had had a previous stroke and developed a fluctuating deficit had this fluctuating instability stabilized by the operation, and we feel that six out of eight (75%) of this small series justified surgery. The seventh patient emerged with a minor deficit and management of this patient was no different from

TABLE 3–1.
Crescendo TIA: Outcome of Surgery

	8 patients	
5 Normal	⎫	6 (75%)
1 Stabilized (previous stroke)	⎬	justified surgery
1 Moderate deficit (stable)	⎪	
1 Fatal stroke	⎭	
(occluded ICA at operation)		

the other six. It is difficult to explain why the outcome here was different as most of the patients had a positive CT scan at the time of the fluctuating deficit. In any event, this patient's deficit was stabilized and he was able to leave the hospital after a week, was able to walk and had only a minor deficit in his upper limb. The suspicion is that he could have been much worse than this if the operation had not been performed. We are not justified in making this conclusion so we have not placed him in the successful group. The eighth patient suffered a fatal stroke. She was not hypertensive and presented with CTIAs without any previous stroke or symptoms. The CT scan demonstrated infarction and angiography showed a 99% stenosis. Six hours after this, surgery was performed, and at operation, the internal carotid artery was found to be occluded with a recent clot in the lumen beyond the atherosclerotic stenosis. There was no alternative but to remove the clot in the lumen beyond the atherosclerotic stenosis and to allow it to be flushed out, which occurred quite easily. The patient was already heparinized and a Javid intraluminal shunt was inserted to restore flow to the brain after it was imagined that all clot had been flushed backward. A standard endarterectomy was performed and good flows into the internal carotid artery were monitored with electromagnetic flow probe and checked with the intraoperative Doppler probe. The patient did not recover and the error that occurred here was thought to be related to the development of thrombosis after the angiogram and with the elapse of the six hours before the operation was performed. Since this experience, I have been unwilling to operate on patients with a fluctuating deficit with a known internal carotid occlusion. In addition, we perform noninvasive assessment of the carotid vessels immediately before surgery to be certain that a silent internal carotid artery occlusion has not occurred within hours before the operation.

The progressing stroke patients' outcome of surgery is reviewed in Table 3–2. It should be remembered that these patients had a deficit at the time of operation and the object of surgery was to prevent the deficit from getting worse and to stabilize the patient with a known surgically correctable lesion. Six of the 15 patients not only had their deficit stabilized, but the deficit improved so that as far as the patients were concerned, they were completely normal within days of the procedure and any remaining deficit was either completely absent or minimal. Eight patients had their deficit stabilized and no further progression of the stroke took place from the moment of surgery. Improvement occurred after the operation but after some weeks, the neurologists were able to detect a significant neurologic deficit. However, it is considered that these 14 patients would undoubtedly have been

TABLE 3–2.
Progressing Stroke: Outcome of Surgery

6 normal or almost normal	
8 improved	93% justified surgery
1 progression	
(arrested then stroke	
after one week)	

worse had the operation not been performed, implying the justification of surgery in 93% of the series. In the remaining patient, the progression of stroke was halted for a week after surgery and then a stroke in the ipsilateral territory occurred. Carotid imaging was performed for this patient but no abnormality was detected a week after the operation. This patient was a 63-year-old woman, was not hypertensive and had developed a gradual stroke in evolution, without previous TIA or stroke. At operation the stump pressure was 45 mm Hg and a shunt was used. It is very difficult to explain why this patient suddenly had an established stroke one week after surgery and this patient is considered to be the only one of the 15 patients who had an undesirable outcome.

CONCLUSION

Indications and timing of carotid surgery are under threat. To justify carotid surgery under any circumstances, one needs evidence to demonstrate that the intervention is better than the likely natural history of the condition. Many carotid operations are being performed at the present time for asymptomatic indications, but we have not recommended surgery for asymptomatic bruit after rigorous comparison with a control series. Carotid surgery for TIA and established stroke is also being scrutinized. It takes courage to operate on a patient with a fluctuating deficit, be it for crescendo TIAs or progressive stroke. The reason for this is the prevailing attitude over the last 20 years and the fear of converting an anemic into a hemorrhagic infarction. Our experience has demonstrated that the majority of patients do have an infarct at the time that I have operated on them and that the majority of patients have done well as a result of emergency carotid surgery. This series is small and would only have been half as large if half the patients had been randomly allocated to conservative approach. The problem is that no single vascular surgeon sees enough of these patients to do the definitive clinical trial. From the data which I have presented, I am of the opinion that the skilled carotid surgeon is likely to produce a better result in patients with fluctuating deficits than can be achieved by conservative measures alone. It stands to reason, however, that the surgeon performing these controversial procedures should have a good track record of carotid surgical results for other indications, by which I would hope to see a combined perioperative stroke and mortality rate in the region of 3% for transient ischemia attacks and established stroke. If a surgeon can achieve results in this order, in my view his patients with a fluctuating deficit will fare better with a surgical approach than being managed conservatively.

BIBLIOGRAPHY

1. Blaisdell WF, Clauss RH, Galbraith JG, et al: Joint study of extracranial arterial occlusions. *JAMA* 1969; 209:1889–1895.

2. Courbier R (ed): *Basis for a Classification of Cerebral Arterial Disease.* Amsterdam, Excerpta Medica, 1985.
3. Ellis MR, Greenhalgh RM: Management of asymptomatic carotid bruit. *J Vasc Surg* 1987; 5:869–873.
4. Goldstone J, Moore WS: A new look at emergency carotid artery operations for the treatment of cerebrovascular insufficiency. *Stroke* 1978; 9:599–602.
5. Greenhalgh RM: Carotid endarterectomy, in Greenhalgh RM (ed): *Vascular Surgical Techniques.* London, Butterworth, 1984, pp 41–48.
6. Greenhalgh RM, McCollum CN, Bourke BM, et al: Emergency carotid endarterectomy, in Bergan JJ & Yao JST (eds): *Vascular Surgical Emergencies.* New York, Grune & Stratton, 1987, pp 139–152.
7. Mentzer RM, Finkelmeier BA, Crosby IK, et al: Emergency carotid endarterectomy for fluctuating neurological deficits. *Surgery* 1981; 89:60–66.
8. Meyer FB, Piepgras DG, Sandok BA, et al: Emergency carotid endarterectomy for patients with acute carotid occlusion and profound neurological deficits. *Annals Surg* 1986; 203:82–89.
9. Millikan CH: Clinical management of cerebral ischaemia, in MacDonnell FL, Brennan RW (eds): *Cerebral Vascular Disease—Eighth Conference.* New York, Grune & Stratton, 1973, pp 209–235.
10. Wylie EJ, Hein MF, Adams JE: Intracranial hemorrhage strokes. *J Neurosurg* 1964; 21:212–215.

4 Carotid Stenosis With a Completed Stroke

You are consulted by the medical service to see a 66-year-old woman who has been admitted 48 hours previously with a stroke. Within the past six months, she has had several transient ischemic attacks. Two days prior to admission she developed moderate weakness of the left upper extremity. A right cervical bruit has been auscultated.

Consultant: Allan D. Callow, M.D., Ph.D., Hon. D. Sc.

The evidence presented suggests that this patient has suffered a thromboembolic ischemic episode to the territory of the right middle cerebral artery as a consequence of occlusive disease in the right internal carotid artery. The history of several transient ischemic attacks within six months and a neurologic deficit limited to moderate weakness of the left upper extremity 48 hours prior to admission are important in selecting optimal management.

The incidence of stroke following a transient ischemic attack is approximately 10% in the first six months. More than half the number of patients, as illustrated by this case, who have suffered a stroke and have coexisting carotid disease, will give a history of prior transient ischemic attacks of carotid origin. These patients are at risk for further stroke unless, in the course of the disease, the involved carotid has undergone occlusion. Among patients with a completed stroke in the carotid territory, approximately 45% will have a second carotid territory stroke, and stroke is the eventual cause of death in approximately 50% of patients suffering a carotid territory stroke. Thus, there is a strong argument in favor of evaluation of this patient with a view toward prompt carotid endarterectomy. It is presumed that this patient is in a stable state with a small stroke.

DIAGNOSIS AND EVALUATION

A careful history and thorough physical examination including a complete neurologic evaluation are essential. The nature of the previously suffered transient ischemic attacks, the course of progression of the admission deficit, as well as the presence or absence of other symptoms such as headache, loss of consciousness, nausea and vomiting, and rapidity of onset, often give information concerning the mechanism of stroke. Ischemic stroke as a consequence of cerebral embolism or thrombotic occlusion is the cause in approximately 80% of individuals presenting with these signs and symptoms, whereas subarachnoid hemorrhage and intracerebral hemorrhage account for only approximately 10%, respectively. Transient ischemic attacks in the same territory are not only a common precursor of thrombotic stroke, but when identical in repetition virtually identify the mechanism. Thus, if the patient's several ischemic attacks always involve the left side, one can be fairly certain that the TIAs and the stroke are the consequences of thrombotic occlusion in the right carotid territory. An episode of partial or total amaurosis of the right eye would further secure the location.

In addition to left motor weakness, there may be neglect of the left visual space manifested by difficulty in drawing or copying figures presented to the patient with left visual field defect and poor left conjugate gaze—elements in the physical examination not likely to be identified unless specific examination is made.

In this stable patient, a CT scan of the brain to rule out intracranial hemorrhage is essential. Noninvasive evaluation, preferably duplex scanning, should be performed to assess the status of the carotids. If disease is identified and if intracerebral hemorrhage can be excluded, arteriography should be done without delay. Intravenous digital subtraction arteriograms are disappointing because of lack of high resolution. We prefer the standard three- or four-vessel arch approach with visualization of both the extra and intracranial vessels. Properly performed intraarterial digital subtraction arteriography may be sufficient if the major intracranial vessels can also be visualized. Careful cardiac evaluation is mandatory for it is the leading cause of morbidity and mortality in the carotid endarterectomy patient.

MANAGEMENT

Because of the presence of the carotid bruit and of occlusive disease presumably to be confirmed by noninvasive testing, a cardiac source of embolus is not likely. Because the possibility of reembolization and stroke are high and because the patient with a minimal or limited deficit may suffer a massive deficit with such reembolization, I favor urgent endarterectomy in certain circumstances. If there is severe preocclusive stenosis, with or without evidence of intraluminal thrombus, I would recommend immediate operation upon establishment of the diagnosis. These are the patients at highest risk. Prompt but not emergent operation is recommended for the patient with a lesser degree of stenosis whose major risk factor is an unstable plaque due to intraplaque hemorrhage or intraluminal thrombus. These patients are placed on intravenous heparin and are operated on as soon as conveniently possible during the same admission. For the patient with a small stable stroke and with no infarct seen on CT scan, or if present and of small size, we no longer defer operation for

CONDITIONAL SURVIVAL
(DEATHS DUE TO STROKE ONLY)

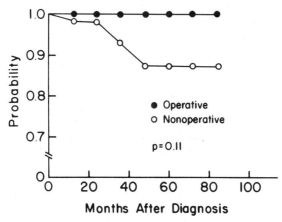

Months After Diagnosis

FIG 4–1.
Probability of not dying from stroke (conditional survival). (Data from McCullough JL, Mentzer RM, Harman PK, et al: Carotid endartectomy after a completed stroke: Reduction in long-term neurologic deterioration. *J Vasc Surg* 1985; 2:7–14.)

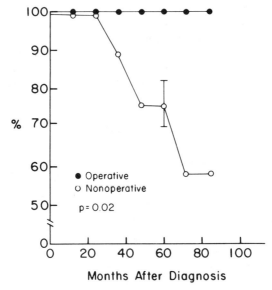

Months After Diagnosis

FIG 4–2.
Cumulative probability of remaining free from recurrent deficits. (Data from McCullough JL, Mentzer RM, Harman PK, et al: Carotid endartectomy after a completed stroke: Reduction in long-term neurologic deterioration. *J Vasc Surg* 1985; 2:7–14.)

the traditional six to eight weeks after onset of the neurologic deficit. The opportunity to remove the plaque and the risk of reembolization may be lost due to thrombosis of the internal carotid artery and fibrous organization of the clot. Restoration of flow then is usually impossible.

Hypotension, hypertension, and cardiac arrhythmias and cerebral hypoperfusion must be avoided. Blood pressure must be carefully monitored and care taken to prevent and promptly treat arrhythmias. The use of a routine shunt is strongly recommended, for in patients with a history or evidence of stroke or a cerebral infarct by CT scan, we noted a 25% incidence of intolerance to cross-clamping by EEG monitoring. Perioperative stroke in this group of patients, however, was no higher when cerebral hypoperfusion was detected by EEG and a shunt was inserted, than in patients without evidence of cerebral infarction. Perioperative stroke is 4.1% in patients with a history of stroke compared to 0.8% in patients with a normal neurologic status at operation or with a history of TIA only.

The primary element in this recommendation for carotid endarterectomy is the high risk of recurrent cerebral infarction in the patient who suffers an acute stroke and enjoys maximum recovery. In one series of 118 stroke patients with mild to severe permanent neurologic deficit, half were managed without operation and half with carotid endarterectomy. The long-term follow-up averaged approximately 42 months. Although the overall survival rate of both groups was comparable with nine deaths in the medically managed and eight in the surgically managed group, the incidence of new neurologic deficits was significantly different. Of the 59 unoperated patients, 12 developed new neurologic deficits and three died at 12, 36, and 48 months as a result of recurrent stroke. In the 59 surgically managed patients, only two developed neurologic deficits and there were no stroke related deaths. The cumulative probability of freedom from recurrent deficits among surviving patients at six years revealed that all of the operated group remained free of new neurologic events as compared to only 58% of the unoperated patients. The late annual stroke rate in this series was 1% per year, less than the 3% to 4% per year customarily reported. This retrospective study strongly suggests, therefore, that patients with a complete stroke and with a fixed mild to moderate neurologic deficit on the basis of a carotid lesion derive substantial protection from recurrent neurologic events by carotid endarterectomy. Finally, increasing anecdotal evidence suggests that conversion of an ischemic to a hemorrhagic infarct as a consequence of carotid endarterectomy is less likely if operation is done within the first 48 to 72 hours of onset of the deficit than when done a week later (Figs 4–1 and 4–2).

BIBLIOGRAPHY

1. Matsumoto N, Whisnant J, Kurland L, et al: Natural history of stroke in Rochester, Minnesota, 1955–1969. *Stroke* 1973; 4:20–29.
2. McCullough JL, Mentzer RM, Harman PK, et al: Carotid endarterectomy after a completed stroke: Reduction in long-term neurologic deterioration. *J Vasc Surg* 1985; 2:7–14.

3. Moore WS: Indications for operative repair of lesions of the extracranial arterial tree, in Rutherford RB (ed): *Vascular Surgery,* Philadelphia WB Saunders, 1984, pp 1245–1247.
4. Whittemore AD, Mannick JA: Fixed stroke secondary to carotid artery atherosclerosis, in Ernst CB, Stanley JC (eds): *Current Therapy in Vascular Surgery,* Toronto, BC Decker, 1987, pp 9–10.

5 Acute Postoperative Neurologic Deficit Following Carotid Endarterectomy

You perform a left carotid endarterectomy in a 71-year-old man with an irregular 80% left internal carotid stenosis and transient ischemic attacks. The procedure is uneventful, and the patient appears to awaken appropriately. One hour after arrival in the recovery room, you are called regarding onset of apparent right-sided weakness.

Consultants: William H. Baker, M.D. and Eric D. Endean, M.D.

The case presented is a tragic example of a patient having a stroke following carotid endarterectomy. While carotid endarterectomy has been shown to be effective for the prevention of stroke in high-risk patients, stroke is a known complication of the procedure. Fortunately, its occurrence is rare. The incidence of postoperative stroke should be in the 1% to 3% range, but some reports indicate a much higher complication rate. Acute postendarterectomy neurologic deficits range in severity from mild and temporary to major strokes resulting in significant morbidity and mortality. There are no large series in the literature describing the treatment of this complication due both to its infrequency and the surgeon's reluctance to report "bad" results. Nonetheless, guidelines for the diagnosis and management of these patients can be stated.

ETIOLOGY

The etiology of postendarterectomy central nervous system deficits can be classified under four general categories: thrombotic, embolic, hemorrhagic, and metabolic. The thromboembolic group is of particular interest to the vascular surgeon for two reasons. First, a postendarterectomy thromboembolic stroke may implicate a technical misadventure occurring either during operation or as a result of operation. In order to *prevent* these strokes, the surgeon needs to carefully review each detail of his operative technique. Second, the surgeon may have a short-lived opportunity to effectively *treat* a patient with a thrombosed internal carotid artery. Thrombectomy of the occluded carotid artery may reverse or prevent further neurologic deficit. This is a decision that may have to be made with minimal and sometimes insufficient data if the patient is to be benefited. Embolic strokes or TIAs cannot be treated per se, but if the source of embolus is identified and treated (reoperation, anticoagulants), then future neurologic events may be avoided. Hemorrhagic infarcts may be the result of uncontrolled hypertension and/or the result of inappropriate timing of operation. Operative evaluation of the hematoma may be required and anticoagulation is contraindicated. A metabolic etiology implies that neuronal tissue has been deprived of oxygen and nutrients, leading to ischemia and/or infarction. This is a central nervous system manifestation of a systemic disorder and treatment is directed toward correction of the systemic problem. While somewhat arbitrary, this classification forms a useful differential diagnosis to work from in order to establish a diagnosis and formulate a rational treatment plan for these patients.

THROMBOTIC STROKE

Thrombotic strokes encompass a wide range of postoperative deficits from transient ischemic attacks to major strokes. Thrombosis, a potentially treatable obstructive lesion, can occur at anytime intraoperatively or in the postoperative period. Wound closure takes so little time that most thromboses become manifest postoperatively, usually within the first few hours of operation although thrombosis has been reported to occur days later. Total and abrupt occlusion may result in a "major" stroke manifested by profound contralateral hemiparesis, sensory changes, altered sensorium, and coma. The patient under discussion may fit into this category as he has awakened appropriately but now develops a right-sided weakness. Lesser degrees of neurologic dysfunction seen are dependent on the extent of collateral blood flow. For example, patients with a patent Circle of Willis and well-developed collaterals as a result of a preexisting severe stenosis may thrombose an internal carotid artery and remain asymptomatic. On the other hand, patients with an inadequate Circle of Willis and poorly developed collateral circulation may develop more profound neurologic symptoms. It is this latter group of patients in which an aggressive approach is promulgated to reverse the neurologic condition of the patient. Because the accuracy of noninvasive testing in the immediate postoperative period has not been well established, and because angiography requires at least an hour in most settings, these diagnostic studies are avoided. The patient is immediately returned to the operating room for reexploration of the carotid artery. Although data is lacking, we prefer to use local anesthesia. If thrombosis is found, the arteriotomy is opened, the internal carotid artery is back bled, the endarterectomy site is thrombectomized, and a shunt is placed immediately to reestablish blood flow to the ischemic hemisphere. If a patent carotid artery is palpated, intraoperative angiography is performed (Fig 5–1). Technical reasons for the thrombosis are carefully sought out including, but not limited to, an unrecognized intimal flap, retained plaque, kinking of the vessel, thrombus propagating from the external carotid artery orifice, clamp injury, or narrowing from the closure of the arteriotomy. If one of these reasons is found, it is corrected. A patch is routinely used in the closure to assure wide patency. It is again emphasized that *immediate* reoperation is needed to optimize the chances of neurologic recovery. Good results have been reported if cerebral flow is reestablished within one hour after the onset of symptoms. For this reason the diagnostic test of choice is reexploration. To waste time with noninvasive testing and angiography would defeat the reason for thrombectomy.

We assume that patients who have a stroke immediately upon awakening (no

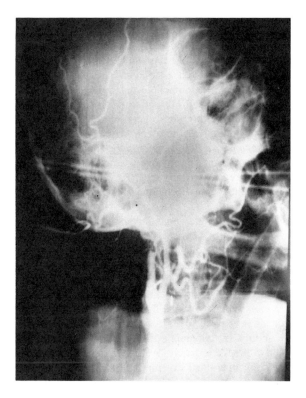

FIG 5–1.
An operative arteriogram that shows a complete occlusion at the distal end of the endarterectomy site. At exploration a pulse was readily palpable in the proximal internal carotid artery. A distal flap of intima was seen at reoperation. (Reproduced with permission from Baker WH, Management of stroke during and after carotid surgery, in Bergan JJ, Yao JST (eds): *Cerebrovascular Insufficiency*, Grune & Stratton, Inc., New York, 1983, pp 481–495.

lucid period) do not have a thrombosed carotid but have had a metabolic or embolic event during the operation. These patients are not usually reexplored especially if an excellent quality postendarterectomy angiogram or ultrasound examination has revealed a good technical result.

A delay in making the diagnosis of carotid occlusion does sometimes occur, especially if the thrombosis forms days after the endarterectomy was done, or if the symptoms are minimal. Emergent reoperation and thrombectomy under these conditions is hazardous because of the high risk of converting an ischemic, benign infarct into a hemorrhagic infarct. These patients are usually diagnosed using the usual criteria of noninvasive testing, angiography, and CT scanning.

EMBOLIC STROKE

Postoperative strokes may be the result of platelet aggregates, thrombus, or plaque material which have embolized. Signs and symptoms vary in this group of patients depending on the size of the embolus, the number of emboli, and the area of brain affected. Most patients present with a "minor" stroke, that is, a stroke which is manifested by focal findings. The embolic event can occur intraoperatively or postoperatively. Intraoperatively, rough dissection of the carotid artery and especially the carotid bulb may dislodge thrombus or loose plaque. Use of a shunt does not protect against cerebral emboli as these can arise from plaque disruption during shunt placement, or retained air bubbles within the shunt. Postoperatively, the endarterectomized artery is a highly thrombogenic surface and can be a nidus for the formation of platelet aggregates or thrombus. Prevention of embolic stroke emphasizes the necessity for meticulous technique and careful dissection of the carotid artery.

Patients suspected of having an embolus undergo a diagnostic workup to identify the embolic source. Carotid duplex scanning can be done quickly at the bedside. This examination may be of limited usefulness because of pain and swelling at the operative site. Identification of intraluminal thrombus or total occlusion would prompt immediate anticoagulation and reexploration. Normal noninvasive studies are followed by angiography, attempting to identify a surgically correctable problem such as a clamp injury, intimal flap, or retained plaque. If such a lesion is identified, consideration is given for surgical correction. Patients who have temporary deficits and minimal arteriographic findings are usually treated with anticoagulation. Patients with severe deficits are also treated medically. Those patients who have transient ischemic attacks or minimal neurologic deficits, no change on their CT scans, and a dangerous-looking lesion on their arteriogram are reexplored. Anticoagulation in any patient is not maintained unless a CT scan of the head is obtained to exclude intracerebral hemorrhage. If preoperative arteriograms have been incomplete, the postoperative arteriogram should seek to identify common carotid or distal internal carotid and cerebral artery lesions. Cardiac sources of emboli should be ruled out by the usual methods.

INTRACEREBRAL HEMORRHAGE

Intracerebral hemorrhage results in a sudden, sometimes devastating stroke. This problem is frequently related to either inappropriate timing of endarterectomy or uncontrolled hypertension. Patients with recent stroke or stroke in evolution who undergo carotid endarterectomy may convert an ischemic infarct into a hemorrhagic infarct. A clue to diagnosis occurs if the patient develops an exacerbation or sudden worsening of previous deficits, often accompanied by hypertension. A second group of patients at risk for intracerebral hemorrhage are those with severe uncontrolled hypertension, usually having a systolic blood pressure in excess of 200 mm Hg. These patients often have had severe carotid stenosis corrected by endarterectomy. The resultant combination of hypertension together with increased cerebral blood flow may predispose to cerebral hemorrhage. The patient may initially complain of a headache followed by neurologic deterioration. CT scan confirms the diagnosis. Anticoagulation is an absolute contraindication. Consideration is given for craniotomy and evacuation of hematoma.

METABOLIC ETIOLOGY

Hypoperfusion and hypoxia of the brain, due to any cause, can be a cause of postoperative stroke. Many patients with a metabolic cause of stroke or TIA will have generalized symptoms such as increased drowsiness, slurred speech, decreased vision, and obtundation. However, patients with preexisting but compensated neurologic damage may manifest local symptoms. This may occur, for example, in a patient with transient ischemic attacks who has CT scan evidence of an infarct but no permanent neurologic deficit. Any metabolic derangement may be tolerated by most of his brain, but not by the previously damaged area. Therefore, when he becomes hypoxic, he may manifest a focal deficit.

Patients undergoing endarterectomy without a shunt rely on collateral circulation to provide adequate flow to that hemisphere of the brain during the period the clamps are applied. While most patients tolerate temporary carotid clamping without ill effect, there are those patients with insufficient collateral circulation who will develop postoperative stroke. Patients who may be at particular risk are those with inadequate collateral circulation as, for example, is more likely in a patient with an occluded or severely stenosed contralateral carotid artery. These patients are identified on the basis of preoperative angiography. Care should be exercised to assure adequate cerebral flow through the use of a shunt, or the adequacy of collateral circulation should be verified by EEG monitoring or stump pressure measurements. Patients with intraoperative hypoperfusion ordinarily awake with their deficit. Unlike the patient presented here, they do not have a lucid postoperative period without dysfunction.

Other causes of hypoperfusion include arrhythmias, inadequate fluid administration, overly aggressive treatment of hypertension, hypotension associated with induction of anesthesia, and myocardial infarction resulting in compromised cardiac output. These conditions should be identified and aggressively managed. Preoperative placement of a radial arterial catheter is useful for continuous blood pressure monitoring and early detection of hypotension. Our practice is to maintain the systolic blood pressure at a level greater than the lowest recorded preoperative blood pressure, less 10% by means of fluid administration and pharmacologic support when needed.

Hypertension has been previously mentioned in association with intracerebral hemorrhage. However, hypertension by itself can contribute to edema formation in ischemic brain leading to neurologic deficit or seizure activity. Again, monitoring blood pressure and maintaining a systolic blood pressure less than the highest recorded preoperative blood pressure plus 10% is done through pharmacologic manipulation. Our drug of choice is Nitroprusside because of its immediate onset of action and the ability to titrate its effect.

Hypoxia is usually manifested by global symptoms, but in an area with tenuous blood supply focal symptoms may result. The causes of hypoxia are many, and include premature extubation after general anesthesia, narcotic overdose, and pulmonary edema. Immediate support with supplemental oxygen or even mechanical ventilation is instituted and the primary cause of the hypoxia is addressed secondarily.

RESULTS

Results obtained following the treatment principles presented are difficult to access due to the limited number of patients having the problem and the multiple etiologies associated with postoperative stroke. Although the algorithm (Fig 5–2) detailing our approach to this problem is supported by many vascular surgeons, it cannot be backed with solid data, and other surgeons prefer to avoid early reoperation entirely in this group of patients. Reports of good to complete neurologic recovery have been demonstrated in those patients with a thrombosed endarterectomy site if cerebral flow is reestablished within one hour. Flow established after two hours of occlusion appears to be of little benefit and may be detrimental. Because emboli can be platelet aggregates, thrombus, or plaque of varying sizes, a resultant neurologic event can be permanent or transient. These patients, by and large, have a better prognosis and good functional recovery is anticipated. Identification of the source of embolus and its treatment would be indicated to prevent recurrent and possibly more devastating emboli. Intracerebral hemorrhage tends to be a devastating stroke resulting in profound neurologic deficit. Some success has been reported with evacuation of a hematoma, but this is inconsistent and the overall prognosis continues to be poor. Metabolic causes of postoperative stroke should always be sought, as their correction usually leads to neurologic recovery.

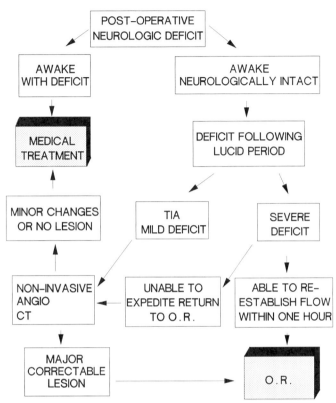

FIG 5–2.
Algorithm of care.

TREATMENT PLAN FOR THE PATIENT

We would recommend that this patient who develops a neurologic deficit one hour after his carotid endarterectomy be returned to the operating room immediately. It is to be emphasized that he has not awakened with his deficit but has developed the deficit after a lucid period of one hour. The object of returning to the operating room is to find an occluding thrombus in the internal carotid artery. Hopefully by performing an immediate thrombectomy, cerebral blood flow will be restored prior to permanent neurologic damage. Because timing is so important in the management of this problem, otherwise helpful diagnostic studies such as ultrasonography and angiography are not performed. In the operating room if a thrombus is not found, operative angiography would be performed. Any potential source of an embolus would be corrected. An intraluminal shunt would be used under all circumstances. Although this is our preferred method of treatment, it should be emphasized that data establishing reexploration as a preferred treatment modality is lacking. In our experience recovery is not the rule, but it is our feeling that this approach offers the best hope of neurologic recovery.

BIBLIOGRAPHY

1. Collins GJ, Rich NM, Anderson CA, et al: Stroke associated with carotid endarterectomy. *Am J Surg* 1978; 135:221–225.
2. Hafner DH, Smith RB, King OW, et al: Massive intracerebral hemorrhage following carotid endarterectomy. *Arch Surg* 1987; 122:305–307.
3. Imparato AM, Ramirez A, Riles T, et al: Cerebral protection in carotid surgery. *Arch Surg* 1982; 117:1073–1078.
4. Jernigan WR, Hamman JL: The causes and prevention of stroke associated with carotid artery surgery. *Am Surg* 1982; 48:79–84.
5. Kwaan JHM, Connolly JE, Sharefkin JB: Successful management of early stroke after carotid endarterectomy. *Ann Surg* 1979; 190:676–678.
6. Najafi H, Hushang J, Dye WS, et al: Emergency carotid thromboendarterectomy. *Arch Surg* 1971; 103:610–614.
7. Owens ML, Wilson SE: Prevention of neurologic complications of carotid endarterectomy. *Arch Surg* 1982; 117:551–555.
8. Perdue GD: Management of postendarterectomy neurologic deficits. *Arch Surg* 1982; 117:1079–1081.
9. Rosenthal D, Zeichner WD, Lamis PA, et al: Neurologic deficit after carotid endarterectomy: Pathogenesis and management. *Surgery* 1983; 94:776–780.
10. Steed DL, Pettzman AB, Grundy BL, et al: Causes of stroke in carotid endarterectomy. *Surgery* 1982; 92:634–641.
11. Towne JB, Bernhard VM: The relationship of postoperative hypertension to complications following carotid endarterectomy. *Surgery* 1980; 88:575–580.
12. Treiman RL, Cossman DV, Cohen JL, et al: Management of postoperative stroke after carotid endarterectomy. *Am J Surg* 1981; 142:236–238.

6 Bilateral Carotid Stenoses with Nonlateralizing Symptoms

You admit a 69-year-old male with complaints of dizziness, intermittent confusion and impairment of memory. Bilateral carotid bruits have been evaluated by noninvasive studies which suggest significant bilateral disease. Arteriography confirms bilateral severe internal carotid stenoses.

Consultant: Jesse E. Thompson, M.D.

This case represents the problem of management of a patient with transient diffuse or generalized cerebral ischemia. Symptoms of this syndrome include dizziness, vertigo, blackout spells, fainting, confusion and mental impairment, and are nonspecific and nonlateralizing. They result from a reduction in cerebral blood flow below the level required for normal brain function. The critical level of cerebral blood flow is 15–20 ml/100g/min, or approximately 30% of normal flow (50 ml/100g/min). Below this level cerebral circulation becomes insufficient to support cerebral metabolic activity and changes occur in the EEG. Practically, such reduction in flow occurs with severe extracranial obstructions, especially when multiple, as in the case presentation, where severe bilateral carotid stenoses were demonstrated. Under these circumstances, retinal artery pressures will also be low.

Since dizziness is also a symptom of vertebrobasilar disease, one must consider lesions in this area of the vasculature as well as in the carotid system. The symptoms described may accompany disease states other than cerebrovascular insufficiency. True vertigo, implying an illusion of motion, is a vestibular symptom which can arise from a number of nonvascular lesions such as brain tumor, Meniere's syndrome, hypertension, etc. The symptoms of transient diffuse cerebral ischemia may also be caused by cardiac arrhythmias. Loss of memory may be due to senile dementia or Alzheimer's disease, as well as to chronic cerebral ischemia.

WORKUP

As a result of the foregoing discussion, the workup of this patient must include, besides a complete history and physical, a neurologic examination and a cardiac evaluation including an ECG. The arteriogram must include biplane views of the carotid system in the neck as well as views of the aortic arch, great vessels, vertebral arteries and also biplane views of the intracranial vessels. A CT scan of the brain would be helpful to rule out infarct or other brain lesions. If not already done, an OPG-GEE should be performed to measure retinal pressures and determine the functional severity of the carotid stenoses, lateralizing the more severe one if possible. The risk factors of hypertension, diabetes and smoking, in addition to cardiac problems, should be noted.

Following the workup described above, if no other conditions are found to account for the patient's symptoms, one may assume that the patient has transient generalized cerebral ischemia, in this case due to severe bilateral carotid stenoses with reduction in cerebral blood flow. Obstructive lesions may also be present in one or both vertebral arteries, contributing further to the total cerebral blood flow reduction.

TREATMENT

The problem is now one of treatment. There is no adequate medical treatment for such a case since relief of symptoms depends on restoration of adequate cerebral blood flow, which can only be accomplished by carotid endarterectomy. The risks of no treatment are further cerebral deterioration and possible stroke. The statistical chance of subsequent stroke in patients with transient cerebral ischemia due to extracranial lesions is approximately 40%, if patients are followed three to five years or longer. The hazard of total occlusion with severe stenoses is great. There is a strong correlation between acute total carotid occlusion and acute profound stroke. Patients with bilateral total carotid occlusions nearly all exhibit neurologic deficits of varying degrees. It is extremely rare to see a patient with bilateral total carotid occlusions with a normal neurologic status. Therefore, the therapeutic recommendation in this case, provided the other risk factors of diabetes, hypertension and cardiac disease are absent or minimal, is bilateral carotid endarterectomy performed in stages.

I prefer to perform this operation under general anesthesia although some surgeons prefer local or regional block supplemented by tranquilizers. For cerebral protection I routinely use a temporary inlying shunt, especially under the present circumstances of severe bilateral stenoses. Some surgeons would use the shunt selectively if the stump pressure at operation is found to be less than 50 mm Hg, if EEG changes occurred during carotid clamping, or if under local anesthesia the patient exhibits any sign of neurologic deficit or dysfunction. Careful arteriotomy closure without a patch graft following endarterectomy is quite satisfactory unless the artery is very small.

Another question is which side should be operated on primarily. Several factors are involved in this decision. If one lesion appears worse than the other on the arteriogram and confirmed by OPG, then the most severe lesion may be operated on first. If the two lesions are of equal severity, then an examination of the intracranial cross-filling is done. If the cross-filling is from left to right, the right artery should be operated on first. If the cross-filling is from right to left, then the left artery should be operated on first. If cross-filling is equal, the artery to the dominant hemisphere is usually operated on primarily. These considerations are based on safety factors related to the patient's own collateral circulation.

I believe this patient should have bilateral carotid endarterectomies even though symptoms may be relieved after the first side has been operated on. The patient has severe lesions on both sides and is thus at increased risk if left untreated. A number of studies have shown that in patients with an unoperated second-side lesion, even if asymptomatic, the incidence of subsequent transient ischemic episodes is 15% to 17% and the incidence of subsequent strokes is 4% to 5%. Risk may be greater than this for the patient under discussion who has severe stenoses. Long-term studies have also shown that patients having bilateral carotid endarterectomies have a lower rate of subsequent stroke than patients having unilateral endarterectomy, when followed five years postoperatively.

The second operation in this case should be done one to two weeks following the first operation. For mild lesions I would wait three to four weeks to allow for longer recovery before performing the second side, but with a severe lesion one runs the risk of a total occlusion on the unoperated side. Thus at one to two weeks the second side should be done provided the patient's general condition is otherwise satisfactory. He should be on aspirin (325 mg daily) and Dipyridamole (50 mg TID) in the interval between operations.

Simultaneous bilateral carotid endarterectomy is never done under elective circumstances. It is rarely indicated under emergency circumstances unless, for some reason, bilateral acute total occlusions are present, or an acute total occlusion occurs on the unoperated side during the performance of carotid endarterectomy, when the second side must then be done as an emergency immediately following the first operation. Except for these unusual circumstances, bilateral carotid operation in a single stage is not recommended because of the complications that may ensue, including respiratory difficulties, postoperative hypertension, cerebral ischemia, and aggravation of neurologic deficits.

Under the circumstances of this case results of carotid endarterectomy should be quite satisfactory. Mortality should be no more than 1% to 2% and neurologic deficits related to operation should be in the same range. Dizziness and intermittent confusion should be totally relieved and memory loss has about a 30% chance of improvement. Symptomatic recurrent carotid stenosis should be no more than about 1% and chances of the patient being asymptomatic at five years should be in the vicinity of 95%.

This patient may have been demonstrated to have occlusive disease in the vertebral vessels. Even so, experience has shown that restoration of carotid blood flow under these circumstances will relieve vertebrobasilar symptoms in 90% of cases without further surgery to the vertebral vessels themselves. In a few cases, with persistent or recurrent vertebrobasilar symptoms, appropriate vertebral reconstruction may be required at a later date.

BIBLIOGRAPHY

1. Lord RSA: *Surgery of Occlusive Cerebrovascular Disease,* St. Louis CV Mosby Co, 1986.
2. Millikan CH: Treatment of occlusive cerebrovascular disease, in FH McDowell and LR Caplan, (eds): *Cerebrovascular Survey Report,* Bethesda, MD, 1985, pp 149–187.
3. Podore PC, DeWeese JA, May AG, et al: The asymptomatic contralateral carotid artery stenosis: A five-year follow-up study following carotid endarterectomy. *Surgery* 1980; 88:748–752.
4. Riles TS, Imparato IM, Mintzner R, et al: Comparison of results of bilateral and unilateral carotid endarterectomy five years after surgery. *Surgery* 1982; 91:258–265.
5. Rosenthal D, Cossman D, Lebig CB, et al: Results of carotid endarterectomy for vertebrobasilar insufficiency: An evaluation over ten years. *Arch Surg* 1978; 113:1361–1364.
6. Sundt TM, Sharbrough FW, Piepgras DG, et al: Correlation of cerebral blood flow and electroencephalographic changes during carotid endarterectomy. *Mayo Clin Proc* 1981; 56:533–543.
7. Thompson JE, Patman RD, Talkington CM: Carotid surgery for cerebrovascular insufficiency. *Curr Prob Surg* 1978; 15:1–68.
8. Thompson JE: Carotid endarterectomy, 1982—the state of the art. *Brit J Surg* 1983; 70:371–376.

7   Recurrent Carotid Stenosis

A 63-year-old man is seen for routine follow-up examination one year after right carotid endarterectomy for amaurosis fugax of the right eye. He has had no further symptoms. Auscultation reveals a soft right cervical bruit. Carotid noninvasive studies suggest severe recurrent stenosis involving the right internal carotid artery.

Consultant: Norman R. Hertzer, M.D.

Much of the current controversy about carotid endarterectomy concerns its perceived overuse by too many surgeons, its presumed risk outside major centers, and its long-term benefit in comparison to antiplatelet therapy alone. Until recently, recurrent carotid stenosis was not considered to be a practical liability of surgical treatment simply because reoperations have, at least from a historical perspective, rarely been necessary for its correction. Since the introduction and wide deployment of noninvasive cerebrovascular testing, however, a number of studies have suggested that early recurrence is far more common than had been suspected and that these findings may be a relative contraindication to carotid endarterectomy in patients who originally present with asymptomatic stenosis. Irrespective of whether the magnitude of this problem really is as serious as some have implied, recurrent disease clearly contradicts the purpose of carotid endarterectomy in those who do experience it.

INCIDENCE

Information concerning the incidence of recurrent carotid disease often is confusing because related data may be defined, collected and calculated in several different ways. As indicated in Table 7–1, a low recurrence rate (<4%) traditionally has been reported for retrospective clinical series in which late atherosclerotic lesions generally were discovered only if they became symptomatic and consequently warranted reoperations. In comparison, the incidence of early hyperplastic stenosis has been estimated to be substantially higher (8% to 21%) in small prospective studies employing serial objective imaging. Nevertheless, most patients have remained

TABLE 7–1.

Representative Data Concerning Recurrent Carotid Stenosis Detected by Clinical Assessment or Prospective Noninvasive Testing

SERIES CLINICAL ASSESSMENT	ORIGINAL OPERATIONS	MAXIMUM FOLLOW-UP (YRS)	RECURRENT CAROTID STENOSIS		
			INCIDENCE %	ASYMPTOMATIC %	REOPERATION %
Cossman, et al[6]	361	2	3.6	—	3.6
Piepgras, et al[11]	1,992	12	1.7	NA	1.7
Stoney and String[12]	1,654	13	1.5	0.1	1.5
Das, et al[7]					
Noninvasive Testing	2,742	14	2.1	NA	2.1
Baker, et al[1]	133	4	9.7	8.3	2.6
Cantelmo, et al[2]	199	8	12.1	7.5	2.0
Colgan, et al[5]	80	4	12.5	11.2	NA
Kremen, et al[9]	173	12	9.8	8.1	2.3
O'Donnell, et al[10]	276	15	12.3	9.8	1.4
Thomas, et al[13]	257	5	14.8	13.2	2.3
Turnipseed, et al[14]	80	3	8.8	8.8	NA
Zbornikova, et al[15]	113	9	23.9	21.2	NA
Zierler, et al[16]	89	4	14.6	5.6	NA

NA: Data not available

asymptomatic and the reoperation figures in these surveys are no higher than in the larger retrospective investigations that preceded them.

Whatever their incidence, the *implications* of such incidental findings for the most part are unknown. Although surprisingly high recurrence rates have been documented by Doppler ultrasound (duplex) scanning, its results do not always correlate with those of angiography (Fig 7–1). Furthermore, Zierler, et al, reported that nine (41%) of 22 hyperplastic lesions actually regressed in severity during follow-up examinations. Both of these observations are consistent with the possibility that normal steps in arterial remodeling may sometimes be mistaken for recurrent stenosis merely because the noninvasive technology to witness them has not previously been available.

ETIOLOGY

While myointimal hyperplasia may be only the precursor to atherosclerosis under different circumstances, each has distinct clinical features and appears to act independently in the etiology of recurrent carotid stenosis.

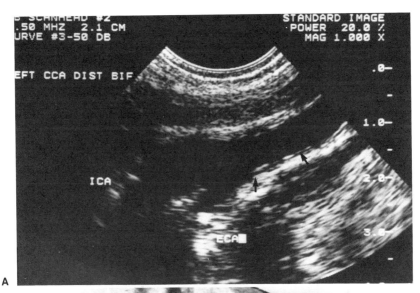

A

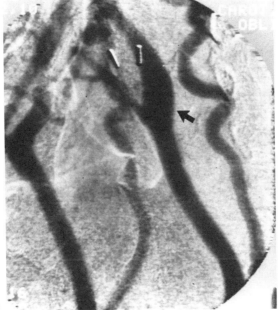

B

FIG 7–1.
Noninvasive imaging performed two years after left carotid endarterectomy and vein patch angioplasty: **A,** Recurrent stenosis (arrows) compromising the lumen by approximately 50% was interpreted on the basis of a Doppler ultrasound (duplex) scan; **B,** Subsequent intravenous digital subtraction angiography instead demonstrated a normal result (arrow).

Myointimal Hyperplasia

Stoney and String were among the first to conclude that myointimal hyperplasia is the predominant cause for recurrent stenosis within the first few years after carotid endarterectomy. In an example of healing run amok, myofibroblasts occupying the medial layer of the arterial wall produce a dense collagenous scar that is pearly white on gross inspection and microscopically acellular (Fig 7–2A). Probably because their surface is smooth and discourages microembolization, hyperplastic lesions usually are asymptomatic and are discovered on the basis of new bruits or follow-up noninvasive studies. All reports concur that women are particularly susceptible to myointimal hyperplasia, and like atherosclerosis, it seems to be more common among smokers and hyperlipidemic patients as well.

Atherosclerosis

Atherosclerotic recurrence usually occurs in patients with appropriate risk factors several years after carotid endarterectomy. While they may even have withdrawn from routine examination because of the apparent durability of their original operations, such patients may eventually return with new neurologic symptoms caused by atheromatous emboli originating from typical ulcerated lesions (Fig 7–2B). In comparison to some of the uncertainties related to the treatment of asymptomatic hyperplasia, the indications for reoperation in this group are comparable to those applied to primary carotid disease.

PREVENTION

The control of such risk factors as smoking and hyperlipidemia is a worthwhile objective after carotid endarterectomy or any other vascular procedure, but adequate patient compliance often is unreliable. Although long-term antiplatelet therapy has been widely used in an empiric effort to prevent new hyperplastic lesions, its merit still is speculative. From a technical standpoint, intraoperative angiography or Doppler ultrasound scanning has been employed at some centers to identify correctable defects that could cause subsequent recurrence. While this approach presently is not feasible at every hospital, there are two additional options that may reduce the incidence of recurrent carotid stenosis in any setting. One of these (medial layer excision) offers at least theoretical advantages, and the other (vein patch angioplasty) appears to have practical importance as well.

Medial Layer Excision

In large arteries, the midmedial plane frequently is the most convenient and expeditious level for endarterectomy. Since the myointimal cell responsible for hyper-

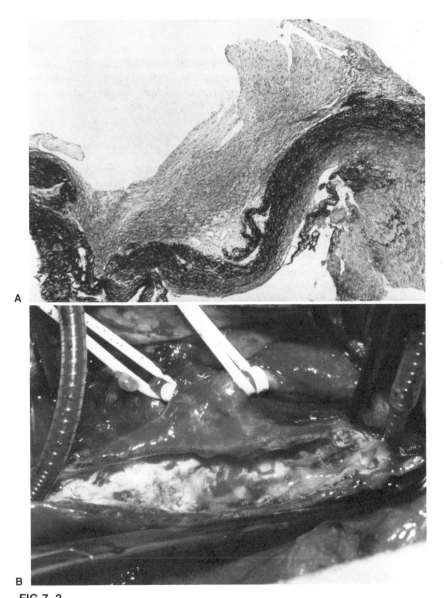

FIG 7–2.
A, The collagenous microscopic appearance of myointimal hyperplasia occurring eight months after endarterectomy; **B,** An ulcerated atheromatous lesion discovered in the eighth postoperative year.

plastic recurrence is found within the medial layer of the carotid bifurcation, it also seems reasonable to excise this layer completely during the primary procedure. If the original atheromatous plaque is dense and generally "mature," an alabaster subadventitial plane usually can be maintained throughout the endarterectomy. In patients who instead have eccentric or segmentally ulcerated disease, residual fibers of the medial layer must be peeled circumferentially from the proximal and distal limits of the arteriotomy once the plaque itself has been removed.

Vein Patch Angioplasty

Vein patching enlarges the diameter of the internal carotid artery and may enhance rapid reendothelialization. Because of these features, some experienced surgeons have encouraged its routine use in order to reduce the risk for both early and late recurrent stenosis. In our recent study of 917 carotid endarterectomies in 801 patients at the Cleveland Clinic (see #8), saphenous patch angioplasty was associated with an exceedingly low incidence of perioperative stroke (0.7%) or thrombosis (0.5%). Furthermore, the results of 332 operations in this series were reassessed by objective imaging (intravenous angiography or Doppler ultrasonography) during a maximum follow-up interval of three years (mean, 20 months). Recurrent defects representing ≥30% stenosis were identified in only 4.8% of the arteries that were patched (Table 7–2), compared to 14% of those that were not (P = 0.0137, Fisher exact test). The cumulative three-year recurrence rates were 9% and 31% (P = 0.0066), respectively, and actuarial calculations suggested that vein patching was especially advantageous among patients with asymptomatic carotid stenosis as their surgical indication (Fig 7–3).

Postoperative disruption occurred in three (0.7%) of the 434 patches in this study, each of which was harvested at or near the ankle. This serious complication

TABLE 7–2.
Recurrent Stenosis During an Interval of Three Years Following 896 Carotid Endarterectomies. (Operative Deaths and Early Occlusions Have Been Omitted.)[8]

RECURRENT CAROTID STENOSIS	NO PATCH (N = 466)		PATCH (N = 430)	
	No.	%	No.	%
Reoperations	7	1.5	3	0.7
Objective	146	31	186	43
Follow-up Imaging				
Documented Lesions	21	14	9	4.8
30–49%	5	3.4	4	2.2
50–69%	6	4.1	1	0.5
70–89%	6	4.1	1	0.5
≥90%	2	1.4	1	0.5
Occlusion	2	1.4	2	1.1

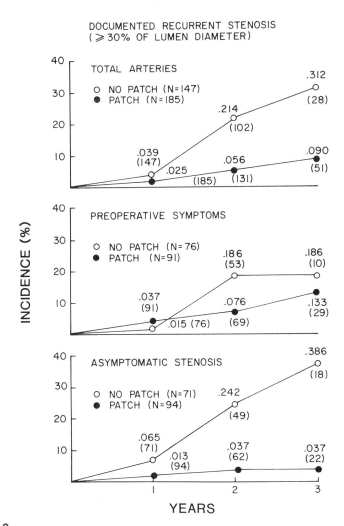

FIG 7–3.
The cumulative incidence of recurrent stenosis determined by intravenous angiography within three years after carotid endarterectomy performed with or without vein patch angioplasty at the Cleveland Clinic. (From Hertzer NR, Beven EG, O'Hara PJ, et al: A prospective study of vein patch angioplasty during carotid endarterectomy. Three-year results for 801 patients and 917 operations. *Ann Surg* 1987; 206:628–635. Used by permission.)

seems to be rare provided the vein is saturated with saline throughout the operation and is applied as a true patch rather than as an oversized "blister." Nevertheless, the use of a saphenous segment removed from the groin may be the only absolute precaution against early rupture because of its superior tensile strength.

TREATMENT

Since myointimal hyperplasia is most likely to be discovered within three years after the original operation, all patients receiving carotid endarterectomy at the Cleveland Clinic are encouraged to have annual objective studies during this interval and every 18 to 24 months thereafter. Because early hyperplastic lesions ordinarily remain asymptomatic and may stabilize or even regress with time, those of only intermediate severity (<70% stenosis) currently are managed with antiplatelet therapy and serial imaging every four to six months to detect further progression. Conceding that others might disagree, however, high-grade (≥70% stenosis) asymptomatic recurrences generally have been corrected by elective reconstruction at this center simply because their tendency for spontaneous occlusion is unpredictable. Individual surgical risk factors obviously may influence this decision, and preoperative angiography is virtually always obtained to confirm the results of noninvasive testing. Whatever its etiology, symptomatic disease represents a compelling indication for reoperation, especially if focal neurologic events have occurred despite the use of antiplatelet agents.

Surgical Considerations

Notwithstanding their relative difficulty in comparison to primary procedures, carotid reoperations still are associated with an early stroke rate of 5% at experienced centers. Approximately twice as many patients, however, sustain at least temporary dysfunction of the hypoglossal or vagus (recurrent laryngeal) nerves because of local traction injuries that may well be unavoidable. Preoperative inspection of the vocal cords should be considered for candidates who have had previous bilateral endarterectomies, since unsuspected paralysis of the contralateral cord could represent a contraindication to an elective reoperation for asymptomatic recurrent stenosis on the side opposite the paralysis.

Safe mobilization of the internal carotid artery beyond the current lesion is the most demanding aspect of the preliminary dissection, but if problems are anticipated, certain precautions may be taken to simplify the operation. First, nasotracheal intubation for general anesthesia facilitates the exposure of structures above the level of the mandible. Second, the omohyoid muscle may be divided in order to identify the common carotid artery below the perivascular scar, and the posterior belly of the digastric muscle may be sectioned to isolate the internal carotid artery above it. Once suitable control of these two vessels has been established, the remainder of the bifurcation can be cautiously sculptured from surrounding fibrosis and the adjacent cranial nerves.

With few exceptions, the rest of the remedial procedure generally is performed in much the same way as standard carotid reconstruction (Fig 7–4), particularly if the recurrent lesion is atherosclerotic in origin. Routine shunting is an appropriate measure because an extended period of clamp occlusion may be necessary. A patch should always be used to close the arteriotomy, and the fact that this approach virtually eliminates the possibility of further recurrence can be interpreted as additional evidence that it probably should be employed more frequently during con-

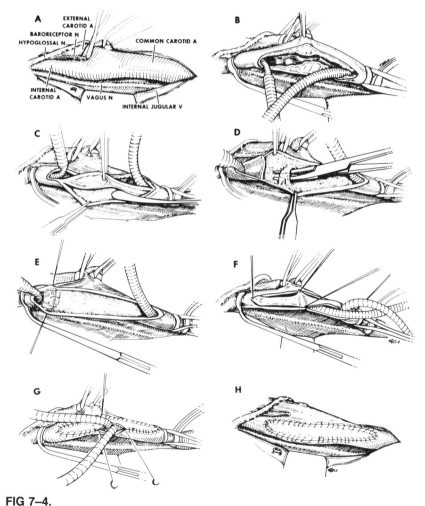

FIG 7–4.
The technique for carotid endarterectomy and vein patch angioplasty currently employed for either primary or recurrent disease at the Cleveland Clinic.

ventional endarterectomy. Unlike recurrent atherosclerosis, myointimal hyperplasia occasionally cannot be excised without irreparable damage to the remaining arterial wall. Under these circumstances, the best solution may be either a simple patch angioplasty or an interposition vein graft to exclude the area of previous endarterectomy altogether.

BIBLIOGRAPHY

 1. Baker WH, Hayes AC, Mahler D, et al: Durability of carotid endarterectomy. *Surgery* 1983; 94:112–115.
 2. Cantelmo NL, Cutler BS, Wheeler HB, et al: Noninvasive detection of carotid stenosis following endarterectomy. *Arch Surg* 1981; 116:1005–1008.
 3. Civil ID, O'Hara PJ, Hertzer NR, et al: Late patency of the carotid artery after endarterectomy. Problems of definition, follow-up methodology and data analysis. *J Vasc Surg,* in press.
 4. Clagett GP, Rich NM, McDonald PT, et al: Etiologic factors for recurrent carotid artery stenosis. *Surgery* 1982; 93:313–318.
 5. Colgan MP, Kingston V, Shanik G: Stenosis following carotid endarterectomy: Its implication in management of asymptomatic carotid stenosis. *Arch Surg* 1984; 119:1033–1035.
 6. Cossman D, Callow AD, Stein A, et al: Early restenosis after carotid endarterectomy. *Arch Surg* 1978; 113:275–278.
 7. Das MB, Hertzer NR, Ratliff NB, et al: Recurrent carotid stenosis. A five-year series of 65 reoperations. *Ann Surg* 1985; 202:28–35.
 8. Hertzer NR, Beven EG, O'Hara PJ, et al: A prospective study of vein patch angioplasty during carotid endarterectomy. Three-year results for 801 patients and 917 operations. *Ann Surg* 1987; 206:628–635.
 9. Kremen JE, Gee W, Kaupp HA, et al: Restenosis or occlusion after carotid endarterectomy. A survey with ocular pneumoplethysmography. *Arch Surg* 1979; 114:608–610.
10. O'Donnell TF Jr, Callow AD, Scott G, et al: Ultrasound characteristics of recurrent carotid disease: Hypothesis explaining the low incidence of symptomatic recurrence. *J Vasc Surg* 1985; 2:26–41.
11. Piepgras DG, Sundt TM Jr, Marsh WR, et al: Recurrent carotid stenosis. Results and complications of 57 operations. *Ann Surg* 1986; 203:205–213.
12. Stoney RJ, String SJ: Recurrent carotid stenosis. *Surgery* 1976; 80:705–710.
13. Thomas M, Otis SM, Rush M, et al: Recurrent carotid artery stenosis following endarterectomy. *Ann Surg* 1984; 200:74–79.
14. Turnipseed WD, Berkoff HA, Crummy A: Postoperative occlusion after carotid endarterectomy. *Arch Surg* 1980; 115:573–574.
15. Zbornikova V, Elfstrom J, Lassvik C, et al: Restenosis and occlusion after carotid surgery assessed by duplex scanning and digital subtraction angiography. *Stroke* 1986; 17:1137–1142.
16. Zierler RE, Bandyk DF, Thiele BL, et al: Carotid artery stenosis following endarterectomy. *Arch Surg* 1982; 117:1408–1415.

8   Vertebral Artery Disease

A 73-year-old lady is admitted with several episodes of blurred vision and near syncope. Cerebral arteriography reveals a moderate 40% to 50% stenosis of the left internal carotid artery, and a widely patent right carotid bifurcation. There is a tight stenosis at the origin of the dominant right vertebral artery. The left vertebral is small and appears diffusely diseased.

Consultants: Anthony M. Imparato, M.D. and Thomas S. Riles, M.D.

This case history illustrates a symptom complex frequently encountered in patients of advanced years which often is ascribed to causes other than surgically correctible extracranial occlusive vascular disease. Indeed, our experience indicates that cerebral angiographic studies are infrequently performed in such individuals who may have nonlocalizing symptoms. Despite the seemingly nonthreatening character of symptoms, "the dizzies," as they are referred to, may be associated with extensive though correctible extracranial arterial occlusive disease. It is the number of vessels involved and the extent of involvement which will ultimately determine outcome, be it catastrophic stroke or sudden death, rather than the nature of the premonitory symptoms.

Our approach to the problem presented is to perform carotid endarterectomy first if there are flow restricting carotid lesions producing 70% or greater stenosis. If nonlocalizing or clearcut vertebrobasilar territory symptoms persist after a period of one or two months, we proceed to correction of vertebral arterial lesions unilaterally by subclavian vertebral angioplasty for the usual ostial lesions, in preference to reimplantation or bypass procedures. The reasoning for this approach will be presented in some detail in view of the controversies regarding the need to perform vertebral operations.

INTRODUCTION

The marked discrepancy between the number of operative procedures performed on the extracranial carotid arteries compared to those performed on the vertebrals is explained by several factors. First is the collateral circulation through the Circle of Willis in protecting the brain from multivessel occlusions. Only one of the four extracranial arteries may suffice to maintain cerebral blood flow because of this arrangement. An incomplete circle combined with multiple extracranial arterial occlusions is required, therefore, for flow to the brain stem to be significantly decreased. Secondly, differences exist in progression of the pathologic process which afflicts each artery. The carotid bifurcation develops lesions which, though initially fibrous, become friable, ulcerate, give rise to emboli, and subsequently thrombose; in contrast, lesions of the vertebral system tend to be fibrotic producing stenoses, rarely ulcerating and embolizing. Another factor is the difficulty of clearly demonstrating radiographically, during routine cerebral angiography, the site of most frequent involvement of the vertebrals, namely their origins. In addition, symptoms of brain stem ischemia can often be relieved by correcting carotid bifurcation stenoses. Lastly, what constitute significant symptoms of vertebral arterial insufficiency and their prognostic significance is debated.

Potent arguments are raised against serious consideration of the vertebrals as a source of cerebral ischemia based on facts of the physiology of cerebral blood flow which may be misleading. It is estimated that only 11% of total cerebral blood flow is by way of the vertebral arteries. One vertebral, however, may provide sufficient blood flow to maintain the integrity of the entire brain illustrated by the finding of triple vessel occlusions; totally occluded internal carotids and occlusion of one vertebral. A single vertebral artery therefore, whose average flow normally may be 45 cc per minute may compensate for the 750 to 830 cc per minute total cerebral blood flow measured under physiologic conditions.

The high incidence of surgically accessible extracranial vertebral lesions was demonstrated during the Joint Study of Extracranial Arterial Occlusions. The experience in that study, since confirmed by others, indicated that correction of carotid lesions frequently improved vertebrobasilar and nonlocalizing cerebral symptoms. Yet there remains a cohort of patients in whom this does not occur and another cohort of symptomatic patients in whom only vertebral lesions are present.

PATHOLOGY

Four-vessel cerebral angiographic studies performed in symptomatic patients show that the most commonly encountered occlusive lesions are due to atherosclerosis, that they occur at stereotyped locations characteristic for each artery involved, and that stenoses predominate over occlusions. The carotid bifurcations are most frequently involved. The origins of the vertebrals are second in incidence.

Since the most commonly encountered vertebral lesions are due to atherosclerosis at the origins, it is noteworthy that plaques rarely extend beyond the proximal 3 mm of the vertebral origins and are actually lesions of the subclavian artery which may be quite pronounced and impinge on the vertebral origins, while the remainder of the vertebrals distally may be smooth and totally uninvolved.

SELECTION OF PATIENTS FOR OPERATION

The syndromes encountered in patients with extracranial occlusive arterial lesions are complex. Symptoms may be focal and recognizable in terms of areas of the brain involved or they may be nonfocal and nonlocalizing, raising serious questions regarding which part of the brain is involved. Arterial lesions rarely occur singly, but rather tend to be multiple, involving the anterior and posterior circulations, though fortunately most often in the accessible extracranial portions. The frequency of operative intervention, however, does not match the incidence of vertebral involvement. Indeed, only 5% of operations on the extracranial cerebral arteries are performed on vertebrals in our vascular service. The decision to operate on a vertebral artery rests on the symptoms with which the patient presents, the radiographic findings of significant vertebral arterial involvement, and whether or not symptoms fail to be relieved by correction of flow impeding carotid lesions, if present.

Clinical Symptoms

Symptoms of carotid arterial insufficiency are usually focal, resulting in contralateral motor and sensory disturbances, ipsilateral visual disturbances, and speech disorders if the dominant cerebral hemisphere is affected. Symptoms of vertebrobasilar insufficiency are less easily recognized. Characteristically, they are bilateral, although on occasion unilateral. They may be intermittent. Embolization is rarely recognized in contradistinction to the frequency with which the diagnosis of embolization is made in the anterior circulation. If vertebral occlusive lesions are associated with carotid disease there may be combinations of cerebral and brain stem symptoms.

The variability of the Circle of Willis renders accurate diagnosis of the pattern of arterial lesions impossible without complete angiographic survey. Angiographic study is done for obvious cerebral hemispheric symptoms and for symptoms of basilar artery insufficiency such as bilateral motor or sensory disturbances occurring during the same attack, ataxia of gait or clumsiness of both extremities, diplopia, dysarthria, or bilateral homonymus hemianopsia. For less specific symptoms such as vertigo, tinnitus, dizziness, drop attacks, syncope and transient global amnesia, cerebral angiographic studies have been done when other possible causes have been excluded since even mild and seemingly nonspecific symptoms can be associated with extensive, correctible extracranial lesions, often involving multiple vessels. This is illustrated by the present case description.

Arteriographic Findings

Diagnosis of vertebrobasilar insufficiency syndromes depends on an accurate assessment of the entire cerebral circulation starting at the aortic arch, including the origins of the vertebrals to their intracranial terminations. Other causes of brain stem symptoms must be excluded. While oculoplethysmography and duplex scanning of the neck are invaluable in assessing lesions of the carotid bifurcations, they are of limited value in assessing the condition of the vertebrobasilar circulation so that ultimately radiographic visualization is needed.

Conventional arch angiographic survey via percutaneously introduced catheters supplemented with selective injection of arch vessels has been the most reliable technique for producing satisfactory studies. When the vertebral origins are not clearly visualized, retrograde brachial arterial injections are used with careful positioning of the patients to project the vertebral origins unobscured by opacified subclavian arteries. A single vertebral of acceptable dimension free of obstructing lesions is considered sufficient to maintain brain stem circulation. If so visualized, the contralateral vertebral is often not studied unless embolization is suspected. Digital subtraction angiography following intravenous injection of a bolus has been unsatisfactory for delineation of the vertebrobasilar circulation.

The angiographic criteria for unilateral vertebral surgical intervention are diagramatically shown and can be summarized by stating that *bilateral* flow-impeding lesions must be present (Fig 8–1).

Whether symptoms are of cerebral hemispheric or brain stem origin, "significant" lesions of the carotids are corrected first. If symptoms persist, be they cerebral hemispheric or brain stem, after a suitable period of observation of usually one to three months, correction of vertebral lesions is undertaken.

If, on the other hand, symptoms are not focal and/or are clearly vertebrobasilar in origin, one of paired vertebral arteries with tight stenoses is operated on if these are the only lesions present. Dizziness of great severity, syncope, bilateral visual disturbances, diplopia, drop attacks, periodic four-extremity motor or sensory symptoms constitute the most common symptoms which have precipitated isolated vertebral artery reconstruction.

Patients with extensive fixed neurologic deficits cannot be expected to be relieved by either carotid or vertebral operations. Patients with catastrophic brain stem strokes with coma and quadriplegia are not considered surgical candidates.

SURGICAL OPTIONS

The surgical procedures utilized to correct extracranial arterial lesions are determined by the sites of arterial inoement, the surgical accessibility of the artery, and the nature of the pathologic process. We consider all of these factors before deciding which specific surgical approach to use. Most often, vertebral arterial reconstructive procedures can be performed through supraclavicular incisions. The mediastinum need not be entered. Various options of surgical therapy include thromboendarterectomy of the subclavian vertebral junction, subclavian vertebral angioplasty, transplantation of the vertebral origin into the side of the common carotid artery, either subclavian or carotid to vertebral bypass with autologous sa-

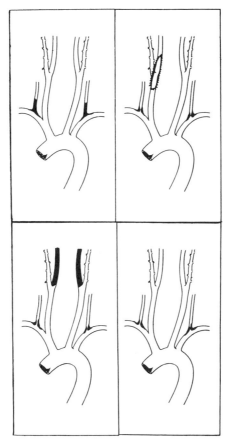

FIG 8–1.
Examples of the most commonly encountered lesions which serve as indications for unilateral vertebral arterial reconstructions. (From Imparato AM, Riles TS, Kim GE: Cervical-vertebral
angioplasty for brain stem ischemia. *Surgery* 1981; 90:842–852. Used by permission.)

phenous vein, and various procedures on the second portion of the vertebral within
the bony canal.

Direct ostial endarterectomy performed through subclavian arteriotomies is
possible through supraclavicular incisions with exposure of the subclavian artery
and its branches. The localized nature of the atherosclerotic process at the subclavian vertebral junction makes possible its disobliteration. Following endarterectomy, the subclavian artery may be friable and difficult to control, and the procedure does not correct the rather marked kinking and tortuosity often found in the
first portion, a major factor in causing intermittent symptoms in some.

Subclavian vertebral angioplasty can be performed by exposure of the subclavian artery and its branches through a supraclavicular incision. The anterior scalene muscle is divided. The branches of subclavian artery, the vertebral, the internal mammary, the thyrocervical trunk, and the costocervical trunk are exposed and controlled. The vertebral artery is dissected from its origin to its entrance into the foramina transversaria. The thyrocervical trunk origin is resected, extending the resultant subclavian arteriotomy upward toward the vertebral across its origin to beyond the most distal kink before its entrance into the bony canal. The kink may be corrected by plication sutures to shorten the vertebral and at the same time cover the plaque at the subclavian vertebral junction with normal vertebral artery intima. The subclavian vertebral openings are then closed with a patch of autologous saphenous vein (Fig 8–2).

Vertebral transposition to a new origin may be preferred. Suture of the vertebral arteriotomy to a new site on the subclavian artery does result in correction of the kinking as well as correction of the stenosis. It has limited application, however, since the wall of the subclavian artery may be thick and calcified. On occasion, the proximal vertebral may be transected with reanastomosis to the thyrocervical trunk just beyond its origin. The thyrocervical trunk origin may have an atherosclerotic plaque as prominent as the one in the vertebral origin, however, and the procedure is often technically difficult.

Vertebral transposition to the common carotid artery is most common and with a surgical approach similar to that described for subclavian vertebral angioplasty. The anterior scalene muscle, however, does not have to be divided. A segment of common carotid artery, approximately 1½ inches in length, must be exposed in order to perform a lateral arteriotomy and affect a suture between the transected end of the vertebral and the common carotid artery.

This procedure suffers from the disadvantage of requiring clamping of the common carotid artery, introducing the risk of cerebral embolization. The wall of the common carotid may be quite thick and anastomosis of the small vertebral to the thick-walled carotid may introduce technical difficulties and perhaps predispose to ostial intimal hyperplasia or even acute thrombosis. To overcome this problem, a roof patch angioplasty of the common carotid artery with a segment of autologous saphenous vein has been done. This anastomosis of the transected vertebral is performed to an incision made in vein roof patch.

Vertebral bypass grafts. Alternatively, vertebral artery lesions may be treated by a variety of bypass grafts from the subclavian or carotid artery to proximal or distal aspects of the vertebral. The proximal bypasses which have been performed in our vascular service have been for total occlusions of the first portion of the vertebral artery and have terminated at the intraosseous portion of the artery which requires unroofing one or more segments of the roof of the foramina transversaria. Such procedures do not appear to enjoy favor at this writing. Most often, distal vertebral bypass is preferred. The vertebral artery is surgically accessible at the C2 level. The vertebral artery between the transverse processes C1, C2 is exposed. End-to-end-to-side anastomosis between a segment of reversed autologous vein

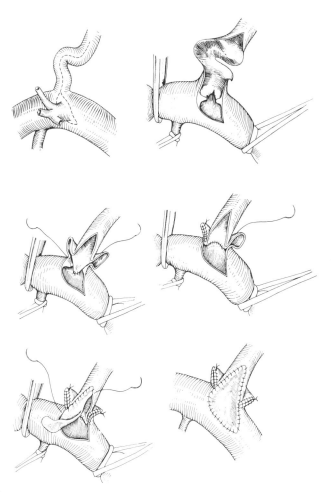

FIG 8–2.
The technique of subclavian vertebral angioplasty. (Proceeds from left to right, top to bottom.) (From Imparato AM, Riles TS: Surgery of vertebral and subclavian artery occlusions, in Bergan JJ, Yao JST (eds): *Cerebrovascular Insufficiency*, New York, Grune & Stratton, Inc., 1983. Used by permission.)

whose inflow is provided from end-to-side anastomosis to either the common carotid or the subclavian arteries, is done.

Since the exposure of the vertebral artery between the bony segments is somewhat limited, and since end-to-end anastomosis to a collapsed vertebral artery may be difficult, exposure has been improved by unroofing the bony canal at C2, performing the difficult dissection of the periarterial veins. This permits end-to-side anastomosis between the end of the saphenous vein and the side of the vertebral artery.

RESULTS OF SURGICAL TREATMENT

Results of surgical interventions on the vertebrobasilar circulation are difficult to fully evaluate since there is no control series of patients whose symptoms and arterial lesions have been radiographically documented and natural history determined. In addition, firm conclusions often cannot be drawn since each series describes a variety of conditions, without differentiating between intrinsic and extrinsic lesions, and a variety of operative procedures. Three series attempt to evaluate survival and late strokes. Both Roon and Reul indicate that survival for the operative group approached normal and late strokes were unusual.

Our own series tends to support their conclusions. Remarkably, 88% of our patients were alive at five years; 69% at ten years and 69% at 15 years. Stroke occurred at the rate of one yearly between the second and the ninth years, with an additional stroke at the second and another at the fifth year. Sixty-nine percent of the patients were alive and essentially symptomfree, except for occasional mild dizziness at the fifteenth year. Twenty-one patients who experienced syncopal episodes were relieved of these episodes by cerebral revascularization alone. An additional seven required additional procedures including cardiac pacemakers and aortic valve replacement for severe aortic stenosis.

CONCLUSIONS

It is not known whether vertebral artery lesions occurring in isolated fashion carry the same prognosis as that associated with carotid arterial lesions. Nevertheless, patients with intrinsic lesions of the vertebral arteries have complex patterns of extracranial arterial involvement with combined carotid and vertebrobasilar insufficiency symptoms. Correction of carotid lesions frequently relieves the vertebrobasilar symptoms. When neurologic symptoms, be they cerebral hemispheric or vertebrobasilar, are not relieved by carotid endarterectomy procedures and bilateral occlusive vertebral involvement is present, correction of the occlusive process in a single vertebral artery is sufficient to relieve symptoms and appears to have a beneficial effect on late stroke rate and survival.

There is a group of patients in whom vertebral revascularization is the only procedure possible because of occlusion of both the carotids. Or, symptoms of probable vertebrobasilar insufficiency may be noted in patients without carotid artery disease. Again, if bilateral vertebral disease is present, unilateral vertebral revascularization may relieve symptoms.

BIBLIOGRAPHY

1. Berguer R: Distal vertebral bypass: Technique, the occipital connection: Potential uses. *J Vasc Surg* 1985; 2:621–626.
2. Edwards WH, Mulherin JL Jr: The surgical reconstruction of the proximal subclavian and vertebral artery. *J Vasc Surg* 1985; 2:634–639.
3. Hass WK, Fields WB, North RR, et al: Joint study arterial occlusion II: Arteriography, techniques, sites and complications. *JAMA* 1968; 203:961–968.
4. Imparato AM, Riles TS: Surgery of vertebral and subclavian artery occlusions, in Bergan JJ, Yao STY (eds): *Cerebrovascular Insufficiency*, New York, Grune & Stratton, 1963, pp 521–542.
5. Imparato AM: Vertebral arterial reconstruction: A nineteen-year experience. *J Vasc Surg* 1985; 2:626–634.
6. Imparato AM: The carotid bifurcation plaque: A model for the study of atherosclerosis. *J Vasc Surg* 1986; 3:249–255.
7. Moufarrij NA, Little JR, Furlan AJ, et al: Basilar and distal vertebral artery stenosis: Long-term follow-up. *Stroke* 1986; 17:938–942.
8. Reul GJ, Coolery DA, Olson SK, et al: Long-term results of direct vertebral artery operations. *Surgery* 1984; 96:854–862.
9. Roon AJ, Ehrenfeld WK, Cooke PB, et al: Vertebral artery reconstruction. *Am J Surg* 1979; 138:29–36.
10. Whisnant JP, Cartlidge NEF, Elvebach LR: Carotid and vertebral transient ischemic attacks: Effects of anticoagulants, hypertension and cardiac disorders on survival and stroke—a population study. *Ann Neurol* 1978; 3:107–115.

9   Symptomatic Patient with Tandem Lesions

A 75-year-old man is admitted with recurrent episodes of weakness and numbness of the left hand. These symptoms have continued despite his taking aspirin and dipyridamole. Cerebral angiography shows significant occlusive lesions involving both the right carotid bifurcation and right internal carotid siphon intracranially.

Consultant: D. Preston Flanigan, M.D.

This patient presents with a classic syndrome of transient ischemic attacks. Apparently he has been placed on antiplatelet agents prior to this presentation (presumably for the same or similar symptoms), but these agents have been unsuccessful. We shall assume that additional studies to rule out causes other than cerebrovascular disease as a cause of the symptoms have been performed. We are presented, then, with a patient with documented cerebrovascular transient ischemic attacks and tandem carotid lesions involving the appropriate carotid artery for the symptom complex.

SURGICAL CONSIDERATIONS

For a long time, many believed that the presence of tandem lesions was a contraindication to carotid endarterectomy, especially if the siphon stenosis was more severe than the bifurcation lesion (Fig 9–1). The logic was that there would be greater morbidity associated with operation and that a carotid siphon stenosis would still exist which might be responsible for ongoing symptoms.

A careful review of the literature revealed that there was no objective data to support these beliefs. It has been our belief for years that the presence of siphon disease does not affect the results of carotid endarterectomy, and in a recent review we confirmed this impression. In Schuler's review of patients with and without tandem lesions undergoing carotid endarterectomy there was no difference in the stroke or death rates. Forty-four of 91 (48%) carotid arterial systems subjected to endarterectomy had carotid siphon stenosis of greater than 20%, suggesting that the

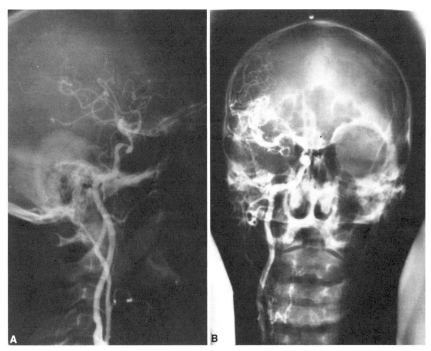

FIG 9–1.
A, Right lateral arteriogram of symptomatic patient with tandem lesions. Note the relatively minor degree of proximal internal carotid stenosis as compared to the severe siphon stenosis (arrow). **B,** Anteroposterior arteriogram of the same patient. Endarterectomy of the carotid bifurcation and proximal internal carotid artery have produced complete relief of preoperative symptoms for 19 months.

presence of tandem lesions intracranially is not at all infrequent in patients undergoing conventional carotid endarterectomy. In the patients with tandem lesions the intraoperative stroke rate was 4.5% which was not statistically significantly different from the zero stroke rate in the group without tandem lesions. Likewise, the 9.1% operative death rate in the tandem lesion group was not significantly different from the 2.1% rate seen in the patients with bifurcation lesions only (Table 9–1). While patients with tandem lesions tended, in general, to fare more poorly than those patients with carotid bifurcation disease alone with respect to operative stroke rate, operative mortality, and late mortality, none of the above-mentioned differences was statistically significant. In this study, the only discernible difference between the two groups was a higher incidence of bilateral extracranial carotid disease severe enough to require operation in the group of patients with tandem lesions. This difference may be indicative of a generally more extensive or widespread distribution of atherosclerotic occlusive disease in patients with tandem lesions.

TABLE 9–1.
Results of Carotid Endarterectomy

	BIFURCATION LESION ONLY		TANDEM LESIONS	
	n	%	*n*	%
Operative stroke	0/47	0	5/44	11.4
Intraoperative stroke	0/47	0	2/44	4.5
Stroke within 30 days of operation	0/47	0	3/44	6.8
Immediate relief of symptoms	41/41*	100	29/29†	100
Late stroke referable to operated side	4/46	8.7	2/39	5.1
Late development of symptoms referable to operated side	3/46	6.5	2/39	5.1
Late development of symptoms referable to unoperated side	1/42‡	2.4	2/28§	7.1
Late stroke referable to unoperated side	2/42‡	4.8	0/28§	0
Operative deaths	1/47	2.1	4/44	9.1
Late deaths	0/46	0	3/40	7.5

*Excludes five carotid birfurcation lesions that were asymptomatic prior to surgery and one nonstroke-related operative death.
†Excludes eight carotid bifurcation lesions that were asymptomatic prior to surgery, five operative strokes, and two nonstroke-related operative deaths.
‡Excludes two patients who underwent staged bilateral carotid endarterectomies one to three weeks apart and one operative death.
§Excludes six patients who underwent staged bilateral carotid endarterectomies one to three weeks apart and four operative deaths.

To further assess these groups, patients with tandem lesions having siphon stenoses greater than 50% stenotic were compared to similar patients having siphon lesions less than 50% stenotic and patients with bifurcation lesions only. By such a comparison, we evaluated the possibility that differences in stroke rate, mortality, or relief of symptoms are related to the absolute amount of carotid siphon stenosis. The patients with the more severe siphon lesion had an operative stroke rate of 7.1% which was not significantly different than the 5.2% rate seen in the other patients. The patients with greater than 50% siphon stenosis had no operative mortality while the other patients had a not significantly different operative mortality rate of 6.5% (Table 9–2).

When patients were subgrouped to compare those patients whose siphon stenosis was greater than their bifurcation stenosis to those patients whose bifurcation stenosis was greater than their siphon stenosis, similar results were obtained. Eighteen of 91 carotid systems (19.8%) had carotid siphon stenosis more severe than proximal internal carotid stenosis. Results in this group of patients were compared to the results of operation in the combined groups of 73 patients with bifurcation lesions only and those with siphon lesions less severe than bifurcation stenosis. The operative stroke rate for those patients whose siphon stenosis was more severe was

TABLE 9–2.

Results of Carotid Endarterectomy in Patients with Carotid Siphon Stenosis

	SIPHON STENOSIS < 50%		SIPHON STENOSIS > 50%	
	n	%	*n*	%
Operative stroke	4/77	5.2	1/14	7.1
Intraoperative stroke	2/77	2.6	0/14	0
Stroke within 30 days of operation	2/77	2.6	1/14	7.1
Immediate relief of symptoms	58/58*	100	12/12†	100
Late stroke referable to operated side	5/72	6.9	1/13	7.7
Late development of symptoms referable to operated side	4/72	5.6	1/13	7.7
Late development of symptoms referable to unoperated side	2/58‡	3.4	1/12§	7.1
Late stroke referable to unoperated side	2/58	3.4	0/12	0
Operative deaths	5/77	6.5	0/14	0
Late deaths	3/72	4.1	0/14	0

*Excludes 12 carotid bifurcation lesions that were asymptomatic prior to surgery, four operative strokes, two nonstroke-related operative deaths, and one death six weeks after operation resulting from unknown causes.
†Excludes one carotid bifurcation lesion that was asymptomatic prior to surgery and one operative stroke.
‡Excludes seven patients who underwent staged bilateral carotid endarterectomies and five operative deaths.
§Excludes one patient who underwent staged bilateral carotid endarterectomy.

11.1% and was not significantly different from the 4.1% stroke rate seen in the patients with the more severe bifurcation lesion. Similarly, the operative death rate was not significantly different, 5.6% vs 5.5%, respectively (Table 9–3).

Of further importance was the postoperative course of the patients regarding relief of symptoms. All patients in both groups were relieved of their symptoms following carotid endarterectomy (Table 9–1). This information supported the tenet that carotid bifurcation disease is by far the most common source of symptoms in patients with cerebrovascular disease. Also, the uniform relief of symptoms in patients with tandem lesions undergoing carotid endarterectomy, in whom the siphon lesion was more stenotic than the bifurcation lesion, further supported embolization rather than stenosis as the main pathology responsible for symptoms in patients with cerebrovascular disease (Table 9–3). These findings also are supported by the data reported by Roederer, et al. The above information also supports the use of duplex scanning in lieu of arteriography in patients with carotid territory symptoms if one follows the approach of performing carotid endarterectomy in patients with tandem lesions since, in this situation, the detection of tandem lesions would not alter the therapeutic course.

Technical considerations during surgery are not different in patients with tan-

TABLE 9–3.
Results of Carotid Endarterectomy

	SIPHON STENOSIS > BIFURCATION STENOSIS		BIFURCATION STENOSIS > SIPHON STENOSIS	
	n	%	*n*	%
Operative stroke	2/18	11/1	3/73	4.1
Intraoperative stroke	1/18	5.6	1/73	1.4
Stroke within 30 days of operation	1/18	5.6	2/73	2.7
Immediate relief of symptoms	12/12*	100	58/58†	100
Late stroke referable to operated side	1/17	5.9	5/68	7.4
Late development of symptoms referable to operated side	1/17	5.9	4/68	5.9
Late development of symptoms referable to unoperated side	2/17	11.8	1/53‡	1.9
Late stroke referable to unoperated side	0/17	0	2/53‡	3.8
Operative deaths	1/18	5.6	4/73	5.5
Late deaths	1/17	5.9	2/69	2.9

*Excludes four carotid bifurcation lesions that were asymptomatic prior to surgery plus two operative strokes.
†Excludes nine carotid bifurcation lesions that were asymptomatic prior to surgery, three operative strokes, two nonstroke-related operative deaths, and one death six weeks after operation resulting from unknown causes.
‡Excludes eight patients who underwent staged bilateral carotid endarterectomies one to three weeks apart and four operative deaths.

dem lesions. The author does not routinely employ a shunt except in patients with residual neurologic deficits. The presence of tandem lesions does not appear to indicate the need for a shunt since the siphon lesion does not add to the effect of common carotid artery clamping alone. Extracranial to intracranial bypass has been suggested in patients with symptomatic intracranial cerebrovascular disease. A recent large multicenter study has indicated that this procedure is not efficacious. In patients with tandem lesions the procedure is seldom, if ever, indicated because of the nearly uniform success of carotid endarterectomy in relieving symptoms.

POSTOPERATIVE CARE

Once carotid endarterectomy is performed on a patient with tandem lesions, there is no evidence that subsequent care should be other than that rendered to carotid endarterectomy patients. Fields has indicated that the incidence of postoperative TIA may be less if patients are placed on aspirin postoperatively. It is the author's approach to utilize one baby aspirin daily on all postoperative vascular patients including those having carotid endarterectomy. Asymptomatic recurrent carotid disease can be expected in 10% of patients while symptomatic recurrence occurs in 1% to 2% of patients. Indications for surgery in patients with asymptomatic recurrent disease have not yet been defined.

LATE RESULTS

The overall late results in patients with tandem lesions is not different from that seen in patients with bifurcation disease alone. In our analysis there was no significant difference in late stroke referable to the operated side (8.7% vs 5.1%), late development of symptoms referable to the operated side (6.5% vs 5.1%), late stroke referable to the unoperated side (2.4% vs 7.1%), or late development of symptoms referable to the unoperated side (4.8% vs 0) between patients with bifurcation lesions only and patients with tandem lesions, respectively (Table 9–1). Similarly no difference in these parameters was seen when the patients were further subdivided based on the degree of their siphon stenosis (Table 9–2) or when subdivided according to whether the bifurcation lesion or the siphon lesion was more severe (Table 9–3).

CONCLUSIONS

Several conclusions may be drawn from the observations noted above. First, approximately half of all patients with symptoms of cerebrovascular disease have some degree of tandem disease, and approximately 20% have a greater degree of intracranial carotid siphon stenosis than proximal internal carotid stenosis. Second, although patients with tandem disease tend to have somewhat less favorable outcomes, those with tandem lesions do not have a statistically significant higher rate of operative stroke, operative mortality, or late mortality as compared to patients without tandem lesions. Finally, all patients with tandem lesions were uniformly relieved of symptoms by carotid endarterectomy alone. For all of these reasons, it would seem unwise to deprive a symptomatic patient with tandem lesions the proven benefits of carotid endarterectomy because of the theoretical possibility of continued symptoms originating from the carotid siphon. Hence, in the patient presented at the beginning of this section, I would certainly proceed with right carotid endarterectomy and anticipate a favorable result.

BIBLIOGRAPHY

1. Goodson SF, Flanigan DP, Bishara RA, et al: Can carotid duplex scanning supplant arteriography in patients with focal carotid territory symptoms? *J Vasc Surg* 1987; 5:551–558.

2. Roederer GO, Langlois YE, Chan ARW, et al: Is siphon disease important in predicting outcome of carotid endarterectomy? *Arch Surg* 1983; 118:1177–1181.
3. Schuller JJ, Flanigan DP, Lim LT, et al: The effect of carotid siphon stenosis on stroke rate, death, and relief of symptoms following elective carotid endarterectomy. *Surgery* 1982; 92:1058–1067.
4. The EC/IC Bypass Study Group: Failure of extracranial-intracranial arterial bypass to reduce the risk of ischemic stroke: Results of an international randomized trial. *N Engl J Med* 1985; 313:1191–1200.

10 Symptomatic Patient with "Negative" Carotid Arteriography

A fifty-five-year old executive is admitted for recurrent episodes of disturbed vision of the right eye typical of amaurosis fugax. Carotid arteriography, however, reveals minimal occlusive disease of both the extracranial and intracranial vessels.

Consultant: William E. Evans, M.D.

DISCUSSION

With the limited data available, it appears the patient probably has an embolic source producing the symptoms. The arteriogram, if more typical of lesions usually associated with amaurosis, with more significant stenosis and particularly with surface irregularity would make decision-making relatively simple. The finding, in this case and others in the past, of a normal or only minimally involved carotid raises additional considerations. Neurologic consultation is particularly important in this setting. In addition to tumors and seizure disorders, multiple sclerosis and atypical migraine have on occasion provided confusion.

Assuming that other neurologic syndromes have been eliminated, and emboli still appear to be the most likely explanation for the symptoms, the next consideration is the source of emboli.

The minimal nature of the carotid changes on the arteriogram raises the possibility of an alternate source. Central neurologic considerations require CT scan, EEG, and careful and thorough neurologic consultation. Obviously, review of the arteriogram is needed to rule out innominate artery lesions as the source, and lastly, potential cardiac sources should be sought. Electrocardiography, echo cardiography and cardiology consultation should be carried out. Assuming no suspicions exist concerning the innominate artery, proximal carotid, heart, or cerebral neurologic problems, by exclusion, amaurosis fugax appears to be embolic in origin—most probably from the carotid bifurcation.

The remaining problem is to clarify more precisely the nature and extent of the

65

"minimal" carotid lesion. Arch angiography may underestimate the real extent of bifurcation lesions, so selective studies, especially with multiple views are vital. The identification of definite arteriosclerotic plaque, particularly with wall irregularity, prompts a decision for carotid exploration. At surgery, occasionally the carotid is relatively normal, but, in the vast majority of instances, significant wall abnormality with subplaque hemorrhage, ulceration, and friable mural thrombus are found. In these cases, properly performed endarterectomy, relieved the symptoms and may have prevented the risk of subsequent major stroke.

The addition of duplex scanning is also of help in this group of patients with minimal stenosis. The identification of surface abnormalities and ulceration, particularly the finding of heterogeneous mixed plaque supports a surgical approach.

When left with the patient with clear-cut symptoms, who has either a "normal" carotid, or minimal lesion which is smooth by angiogram and homogeneous by duplex scan, the decision is less clear. A recent review of patients in this category provides some suggestions. Eighty-three patients with hemispheric TIA or amaurosis were followed from three to 132 months. Original reports at two years following the initial symptoms suggested a very benign course for this group, treated only with antiplatelet agents. With longer follow-up, patients faired less well. By three years, 4.8% suffered strokes, 8.4% at four, and 12.5% at six years. The data of Toole, et al, are similar.

In reviewing this data, no predictive value was noted between those with minimal versus "normal" carotids, nor were other risk factors of any help. The only finding that appeared to identify those at risk was the presence of multiple neurologic episodes prior to entry into the study.

In retrospect, all subsequent TIAs and strokes occurred in patients with multiple transient episodes. Patients with single episodes appear to have a very benign prognosis. By contrast, of the 31 patients with multiple episodes, 11 had further hemispheric neurologic episodes (35%), and six had strokes (20%).

Therefore, in patients with "normal" or minimally stenotic carotid lesions which are smooth and homogeneous, who have had a single episode, antiplatelet agents would appear to be the treatment of choice. Recurrence should prompt reevaluation and probably exploration.

In those with multiple events, exploration should be strongly recommended because of the rather poor long-term prognosis.

Obviously, additional data is required and as it becomes available, these guidelines may change, but at present they appear to be reasonable, based on the limited data available.

BIBLIOGRAPHY

1. Evans WE, Hayes JP: Life history of patients with transient ischemic attacks and essentially normal angiograms. *J Vasc Surg* 1987; 6:6;548–552.
2. Toole JF, Yuson CP: Transient ischemic attacks with normal arteriograms: Serious or benign prognosis? *Ann Neurol* 1977; 1:100–102.

11 Symptomatic Patient with Total Internal Carotid Artery Occlusion

A 61-year-old man had a right hemispheric stroke one year ago from which he fully recovered. Duplex scan at that time revealed a right internal carotid occlusion without any other cerebrovascular disease present. He has had three 30-minute episodes of left hemiparesis in the last month, each of which completely resolved.

Consultants: Jonathan P. Gertler, M.D. and David C. Brewster, M.D.

The incidence and significance of internal carotid artery (ICA) occlusion remains difficult to assess. ICA occlusion may be heralded by stroke or transient ischemic attack (TIA), or may be unrecognized and asymptomatic. The prognosis of the asymptomatic patient with an established, chronic ICA occlusion is enigmatic. Many factors contribute to the appearance of later symptoms, and it is difficult to predict which individuals will go on to develop neurologic problems.

The symptomatic patient with ICA occlusion, as described in the index case above, has a documented high risk of stroke. The progressive rate of stroke in this group of patients may be as high as 40% at three-year follow-up. Neurologic morbidity from diagnostic and surgical intervention is increased in the symptomatic patient. However, the otherwise poor outcome of these patients warrants an aggressive appraisal of available means for improving cerebral perfusion.

POTENTIAL MECHANISMS OF SYMPTOMS

Symptoms from an occluded ICA may be caused by several mechanisms. Embolic events, which predominate in stenotic ICA disease, also occur in the acute and/or chronic phase of ICA occlusion. The reconstituted ICA distal to the more proximal totally occluded segment often contains thrombus and atheroma which, due to turbulent flow and poor adherence to arterial sidewalls, can embolize distally into the

67

cerebral and retinal circulation. In addition, the threat of distal propagation of thrombotic and atheromatous occlusion is always present. However, such events are difficult to predict or study prospectively because a reliable means of imaging this arterial configuration does not exist. Propagation of occlusion clearly has been shown to determine the extent of, and outcome from, stroke as cerebral collaterals are progressively compromised.

Other potential sources of emboli are the external carotid artery (ECA) orifice or the stump of the proximal ICA which often persists despite total ICA occlusion above its origin. In the former situation, atheromatous debris from the ECA orifice travels through the enlarged periorbital and facial collaterals which often develop following ICA occlusion (Fig 11–1). Emboli lodge in either retinal or hemispheric arteries, resulting in classic TIAs or strokes. With an ICA stump or "cul-de-sac" (Fig 11–2A, 11–2B), atherothrombotic debris may be carried by turbulent flow retrograde into the ECA circulation, and henceforth into the cerebral and retinal vessels.

In the patient with diffuse cerebrovascular disease involving multiple vessels, collateral flow is also compromised. Internal carotid artery occlusion may represent

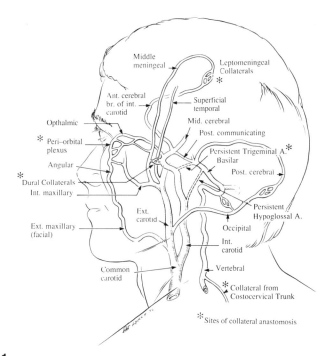

FIG 11–1.
Available ipsilateral collateral circulation in the setting of internal carotid occlusion. (From J Vasc Surg 1987; 6:158–67. Used by permission.)

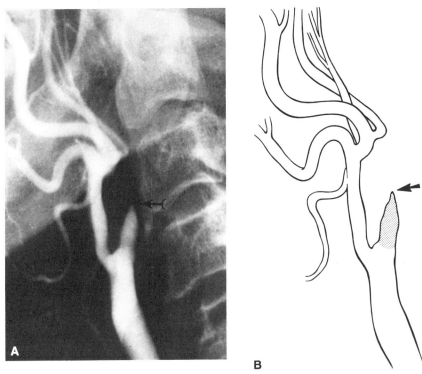

FIG 11–2.
A, Angiogram depicting ICA occlusion with remaining cul-de-sac. (From Neurovascular Laboratory, Massachusetts General Hospital. Used by permission.) **B,** Artist's depiction of ICA occlusion with remaining ICA cul-de-sac as source of thromboembolic debris.

a threshold hemodynamic event in these patients, resulting in immediate neurologic symptoms, or may predate the loss of other important cerebrovascular channels, ultimately resulting in inadequate cerebral blood flow and neurologic symptoms.

Recent reports, using cerebral blood flow studies as well as standard computerized tomographic scanning and angiography, have attempted to determine the subset of patients with chronic ICA occlusion at risk for stroke. It has been suggested that many so-called embolic events are in fact hemodynamic events, due to combinations of poor cardiac output and cerebrovascular occlusive disease. Other patients may have CT scans and angiograms consistent with emboli at the time of, or following, an occlusive event in the ICA. Though no prospective determination of patients at risk for stroke as yet exists, it is worthwhile to bear these different mechanisms in mind.

Carotid pseudo-occlusion must be mentioned for the sake of completeness.

Though in the patient described above it seems an unlikely situation, some individuals will have apparent ICA occlusion on noninvasive studies but a patent, though critically narrowed, ICA when studied angiographically. In this setting, systemic heparinization, early angiography, and urgent carotid endarterectomy markedly reduces the risk of stroke.

APPROACH TO THE PATIENT

The case presented suggests embolic events in the setting of adequate cerebral blood flow, as carotid noninvasive studies one year prior to the onset of the new neurologic symptoms revealed normal cerebral blood vessels except for the occluded ICA. This noninvasive evaluation, however, must be repeated. The patient's symptoms, following a known stroke ipsilateral to a known ICA occlusion, place him firmly in a group at high risk for progressive neurologic deterioration.

There is no question that angiography is necessary to assess these problems fully. Other studies should be obtained, however, to provide additional current neurologic information. These studies also will be useful for comparison with subsequent studies following any possible therapy for the patient's current symptoms. With this in mind, CT scan with and without contrast, repeat carotid noninvasive studies, and a full cardiac evaluation are indicated.

The CT scan may demonstrate the old infarct as well as discern any subtle infarcts in "inarticulate" areas of the brain. In addition, some symptoms previously thought to be TIAs may, in fact, have been small infarcts. Additional cerebral infarcts also place the patient at high risk for further stroke. This information is essential to determining the relative risk of surgery and provides further compelling indications for aggressive diagnostic and therapeutic intervention. Magnetic Resonance Imaging (MRI) and Positron Emission (PET) Scanning may be more sensitive for detecting both recent and old subtle infarcts and also can measure total cerebral blood flow. Their relative inaccessibility and expense renders them, as yet, not useful for evaluation or follow-up in the routine clinical setting.

Carotid noninvasives will provide a useful baseline for long-term assessment of cerebrovascular disease; however, their use does not provide adequate anatomic detail for surgical planning. Angiography is thus indispensable. The subtle findings of ECA stenosis, distal ICA thrombus, ICA cul-de-sac, cerebral cross-filling through the Circle of Willis, and carotid pseudo-occlusion will only be addressed by cerebral angiography. Common carotid occlusion with reconstitution of the extracranial ICA, may sometimes masquerade as ICA occlusion on noninvasive study and thus accurate anatomic information from angiography is critical. Similarly, the exact status of the vertebrals and contralateral carotid should be evaluated. Recognizing the limitation of noninvasive screening, however, does not preclude its use in the perioperative setting for both short-term and long-term follow-up.

Cardiac echo, Holter monitoring, and assessment of ventricular function exclude abnormalities that might have accounted for his original stroke. Cardiac emboli may lodge in and occlude the ICA, while arrhythmias and poor cardiac output may produce hemodynamic events which may be interpreted as classic anterior circulation TIAs or strokes.

Angiography, as mentioned above, remains the standard for diagnostic investigation. We favor an aortic arch and four-vessel assessment including selective carotid views. Intracranial views to delineate collaterals are also essential. In the patient with complete internal carotid artery occlusion, as well as the patient with a symptomatic stenosis, such extensive anatomic information has no substitute in its ability to guide the surgeon to the most appropriate therapeutic intervention.

SURGICAL AND MEDICAL THERAPY

Medical therapy is limited. The recently published "Extracranial-intracranial bypass trial" is the best prospective information on patients with ICA occlusion treated with aspirin. In this study a stroke rate of approximately 15% at one year was noted in patients treated with aspirin alone and was slightly higher in surgically treated patients. Anticoagulation with Coumadin has been utilized for patients with diffuse extracranial cerebrovascular disease as well as those with ICA occlusion. Anticoagulation in the setting of ICA occlusion and stroke may be helpful acutely, once CT scan has ruled out cerebral hemorrhage. When ICA occlusion occurs due to embolization from valvular, atrial, or ventricular thrombus rather than progression of a stenotic carotid lesion, the indication for anticoagulation is clearcut.

Surgical options are predicated on angiographic findings some of which are outlined in the algorithm (Fig 11–3). In situation A, no demonstrable extracranial vascular disease is identified except for an ICA occlusion. In a patient with hemispheric symptoms as described in the case, emboli from the thrombosed ICA must be considered the cause of the symptoms. Anticoagulation with Coumadin is logical in this setting to prevent propagation of clot and ongoing embolization.

In a patient with hemispheric or retinal symptoms ipsilateral to an ICA occlusion who has an ECA stenosis, ICA cul-de-sac, or both (Situations B & C), ECA endarterectomy with obliteration of the ICA orifice is an attractive possibility. Even if the contralateral carotid is diseased, if the symptoms are specifically referable to the side of the ICA occlusion and appropriate ECA anatomy is demonstrated angiographically, we would pursue this course. In a recent review of 218 published cases of ECA endarterectomy or bypass, we found a high percentage of patients with neurologic symptoms resolved (83%) or markedly reduced (8%). Even patients with vague neurologic complaints and these anatomic configurations, may still find their symptoms improved or resolved by this approach. However, a careful assessment of all extracranial vessels, as well as views of intracranial anatomy, are prudent before advising that ECA reconstruction would be of benefit in this group.

The technique of ECA reconstruction is depicted in Figure 11–4. The approach is similar to routine carotid bifurcation endarterectomy. We favor selective shunting using electroencephalographic intraoperative monitoring. A shunt can easily be

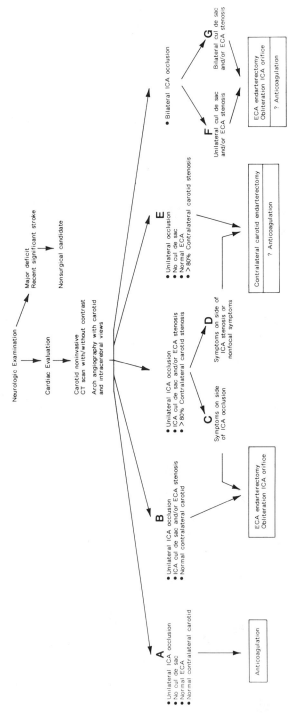

ALGORITHM - MANAGEMENT OF SYMPTOMATIC PATIENT WITH INTERNAL CAROTID OCCLUSION

Neurologic Examination

Cardiac Evaluation

Major deficit
Recent significant stroke

Nonsurgical candidate

Carotid noninvasive
CT scan with/without contrast

Arch angiography with carotid
and intracerebral views

A
• Unilateral ICA occlusion
• No cul de sac
• Normal ECA
• Normal contralateral carotid

Anticoagulation

B
• Unilateral ICA occlusion
• ICA cul de sac and/or ECA stenosis
• Normal contralateral carotid

ECA endarterectomy
Obliteration ICA orifice

C
Symptoms on side
of ICA occlusion

D
Symptoms on side of
ICA stenosis or
nonfocal symptoms

• Unilateral ICA occlusion
• ICA cul de sac and/or ECA stenosis
• >80% Contralateral carotid stenosis

E
• Unilateral occlusion
• No cul de sac
• Normal ECA
• >80% Contralateral carotid stenosis

Contralateral carotid endarterectomy

? Anticoagulation

• Bilateral ICA occlusion

F
Unilateral cul de sac
and/or ECA stenosis

G
Bilateral cul de sac
and/or ECA stenosis

ECA endarterectomy
Obliteration ICA orifice

? Anticoagulation

FIG 11–3.
Algorithm of patient management according to symptoms and anatomic finding of cerebral arteriography.

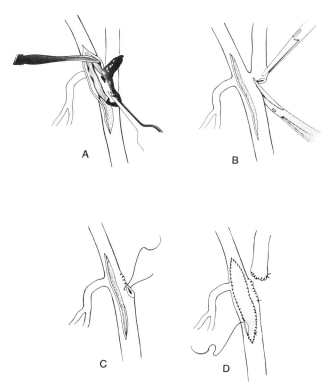

FIG 11–4.
Technique of external carotid endarterectomy with obliteration of ICA origin.

placed in the ECA, should EEG changes occur. An ECA shunt has been shown to increase internal carotid stump pressure in patients undergoing routine carotid endarterectomy. Accurate intraoperative neurologic monitoring or routine shunt insertion appear important in this high-risk group of patients, especially in those in whom hemodynamic rather than embolic sources of neurologic symptoms are suspected.

The essential maneuvers in this operation are exclusion of the ICA cul-de-sac and removal of ECA orificial disease. Many techniques have been applied, but we favor separation of the ICA from the bifurcation and careful closure of the orifice with fine everting interrupted sutures. Finally, to adequately widen the ECA orifice, especially in cases where ECA atherosclerosis appears to be responsible for symptoms, formal ECA endarterectomy, as well as use of a saphenous vein patch in closure of the arteriotomy, should ensure removal of atheromatous debris, as well as minimize the chance of recurrent stenosis in a critical remaining collateral vessel.

Certain patients will present with ICA occlusion and contralateral critical carotid stenosis (Situations D & E). Careful history and intracranial angiographic views are imperative to making the correct therapeutic choice. If the symptoms are ipsilateral to the ICA stenosis, or if vague neurologic complaints or vertebrobasilar insufficiency appear to be present, the symptoms may well be due to the hemodynamic sequelae of a critically narrowed remaining ICA or to emboli from this artery. In such situations, we would proceed with carotid endarterectomy of the remaining patent though diseased ICA to both alleviate symptoms and also to preserve the major source of cerebral blood flow. Anticoagulation might be a useful adjunct postoperatively in this group of patients.

In the setting of bilateral carotid occlusion with either unilateral or bilateral ECA stenosis and/or an ICA cul-de-sac (Situations F & G), we would proceed with ECA endarterectomy and obliteration of the cul-de-sac on the symptomatic side. If the patient were having nonfocal symptoms suggestive of inadequate cerebral perfusion, an attempt to correct the tighter ECA stenosis might be reasonable in an otherwise good risk patient. There are no prospective data to support this approach currently, and such intervention must be carefully considered and individualized.

Attempted disobliteration of the occluded ICA itself is controversial, but we would consider it in several settings. The rare patient will have a short segment of internal carotid artery occlusion with reconstitution of the distal ICA within reach of a cervical approach. If such a situation is documented by preoperative angiography, attempted endarterectomy or bypass to the distal extracranial ICA may be carried out. Criteria for endarterectomy should include angiographic evidence of a low plaque termination, such that a ''blind'' endarterectomy endpoint would not be present. Similarly, a patient with reconstitution of the ICA and ECA above a common carotid artery occlusion may be a candidate for bypass. As mentioned above, noninvasive studies are not always sensitive in picking up this anatomic configuration, and good quality preoperative arteriography with late filming of the cervical region are often necessary to visualize the patent carotid branches. Autologous tissue is preferred for the bypass, if available. Such bypasses may originate from the ipsilateral subclavian artery or contralateral common carotid, depending on the status of associated atherosclerotic disease in these vessels or preference of the surgeon. The ECA can sometimes be reattached end-to-side to the ICA graft to reconstruct the bifurcation if desired.

It is necessary to mention the extracranial-intracranial (EC-IC) bypass. While the recently published EC-IC prospective trial did not demonstrate a benefit to the procedure, the trial itself has generated much controversy. We would currently recommend neurosurgical consultation if cardiac sources of neurologic symptoms are excluded, the extracranial vessels are free of disease except for an occluded ICA, intracranial occlusive disease is noted on angiography, and the patient is symptomatic but otherwise a good operative risk. In general, however, it appears that extracranial procedures designed to augment cerebral inflow and exclude embolic sources are appropriate initial maneuvers in the setting of symptomatic ICA occlusion.

CONCLUSION

The treatment of a totally occluded internal carotid artery with continuing symptoms of cerebrovascular ischemia remains controversial, and little prospective data are available to clearly delineate the optimal method of management. Due to the heterogeneity of anatomic configurations causing neurologic symptoms in the setting of ICA occlusion, we emphasize again that thorough preoperative cerebrovascular and cardiovascular evaluation is necessary. If an anatomic configuration which correlates to physiologic derangements experienced by the patient is found, appropriate operative intervention should be carefully considered in these neurologically high-risk patients.

BIBLIOGRAPHY

1. Cote R, Barnett HJM, Taylor DW: Internal carotid occlusion: A prospective study. *Stroke* 1983; 14:898–906.
2. The EC/IC Bypass Study Group: Failure of EC-IC arterial bypass to reduce the risk of ischemic stroke. *N Engl J Med* 1985; 313:1191–1200.
3. Fields WS, Lemak NA: Joint Study of Extracranial Arterial Occlusion. Internal carotid artery occlusion. *JAMA* 1976; 235:2734–2738.
4. Gertler JP, Cambria RP: The role of external carotid endarterectomy in the treatment of ipsilateral internal carotid occlusion: Collective review. *J Vasc Surg* 1987; 6:158–167.
5. Kistler JP, Ropper AH, Heros RC: Therapy of ischemic cerebral vascular disease due to atherothrombosis (part 1). *N Engl J Med* 1984; 311:27–34.
6. Kistler JP, Ropper AH, Heros RC: Therapy of ischemic cerebral vascular disease due to atherothrombosis (part 2). *N Engl J Med* 1984; 311:100–105.
7. Riles TS, Imparato AM, Kopelman I: Carotid artery stenosis with contralateral carotid occlusion: Long term results in 54 patients. *Surgery* 1980; 87:363–386.
8. Sachs SM, Fulenwider JT, Smith RB: Does contralateral carotid occlusion influence neurologic fate of carotid endarterectomy? *Surgery* 1984; 96:839–844.

PART TWO

Aneurysmal Disease

12   The Small Aortic Aneurysm

A 59-year-old dentist is referred for a 4.2-cm abdominal aortic aneurysm. This is asymptomatic and was an incidental finding on an intravenous pyelogram done to evaluate symptoms of moderate benign prostatic hypertrophy. He is otherwise in good health.

Consultant: James A. DeWeese, M.D.

Patients with small abdominal aneurysms frequently present in the surgeon's office with histories similar to that of this dentist. It is very rare that aneurysms are discovered by the patient even though they may have some medical background. The exception are the individuals who present with the complaint that they can "feel their heart in their stomach."

Aneurysms are also frequently missed during yearly physicals. I have suffered personal embarrassment by having a patient rupture an unsuspected aneurysm whom I had seen at six-month interval follow-ups of his femoropopliteal bypass graft. The reason for this failure to make an early diagnosis is not necessarily because of a lack of awareness nor of skillful palpation of the abdomen. The patients are, unfortunately, frequently obese and even large aneurysms may not be felt.

Historically flat plate X-rays of the abdomen were the earliest noninvasive tests used for the diagnosis of aneurysms. Aneurysms were identified by calcification in the wall or by soft tissue masses. The accuracy of diagnosis could be improved by obtaining oblique and lateral views. In a series of 123 patients we were able to identify over 90% of proven abdominal aortic aneurysms. Alert radiologists will recognize aneurysms during performance of many diagnostic studies including intravenous pyelogram, lumbar spine films, GI series, barium enemas, or biliary ultrasound examinations. Radiologist friends have been responsible for the referral of several patients with aneurysms to me. I am sure that many surgeons have similarly benefited, particularly in the 1950s and 1960s, when the education of physicians that aneurysmectomy was feasible, was so important.

SELECTION OF PATIENTS FOR OPERATION

The decision as to whether an operation should be advised has classically been based on the size of the aneurysm and the condition of the patient.

Size of the Aneurysm

Much attention has been directed toward the importance of aneurysm size, particularly in regard to the method of their measurement and the life history of untreated aneurysms of various sizes.

Physical examination may overestimate the size and provides only an estimation of the lateral diameter of the aneurysm. Radiographs taken obliquely or laterally are useful in identifying the presence of an aneurysm. However, an accurate measurement of the size is possible only in those aneurysms with abundant calcification in the wall (about 50%). In those with adequate calcification, however, radiographs can be used to serially follow such patients and is the cheapest noninvasive test to perform. Ultrasound may underestimate the size of the aneurysm unless gray scale units are used and the observer is experienced. It is also not reliable for the examination of the suprarenal aorta. Computerized axial tomography (CAT) is the most reliable of the techniques for the accurate measurement of both the infra- and suprarenal aorta. Unfortunately, it is also the most expensive and the other methods are preferred for serial examinations. Aortography is the most unreliable method for the measurement of the size of an aneurysm. Without calcification of the wall, the presence of intraluminal clot within the aneurysm sac often makes accurate measurement of size by angiography notoriously poor. Aortography is, of course, a valuable means of evaluating associated occlusive lesions in the aorta or iliac, renal, and visceral arteries, extent of aneurysmal disease, and other related vascular abnormalities.

I would obtain a CAT scan on our 59-year-old dentist to confirm the diagnosis of an aneurysm, to evaluate the suprarenal aorta, and to rule out a horseshoe kidney or an inflammatory aneurysm. Aortography would be performed only if further evaluation revealed possible extension of aneurysmal disease above the renal arteries, signs and symptoms of lower extremity arterial occlusive disease, recent onset of hypertension, abnormal renal function, or recent weight loss or postprandial pain, suggestive of possible mesenteric ischemia.

Many physicians have used the size of the aneurysm as the basis of their decision as to when even a healthy patient should be referred or advised to have an aneurysmectomy. There are several reports of the natural history of unoperated aneurysms of various sizes. Death due to rupture in patients with aneurysms greater than 7 cm in size occurs in approximately 75%. For aneurysms greater than 6 cm in size the incidence of rupture is approximately 40%; those greater than 5 cm in size, approximately 20%, and for less than 5 cm in size incidence is less than 5%. These figures have been used by many physicians to withhold operation from asymptomatic patients with relatively small aneurysms. On the other hand, in at least one autopsy series, the rupture rate was 18% for aneurysms less than 5 cm in size and 8% for those 4 cm and less in size. With small aneurysms, elective mortality rates have decreased to the 5% or lower range. The size at which operation is advised for healthy patients has also decreased progressively from 7 cm to 6 cm to 5 cm, and more recently to include aneurysms of any size by many surgeons. Justification for this more liberal approach is strengthened by the fact that it is estimated that only 50% of patients with ruptured aneurysms survive long enough to make it to the operating room, and the mortality rates for patients operated on for ruptured aneurysms is still greater than 50%. In addition, operative mortality rates for healthy patients are now approximately 2%. Therefore, even though our dentist's aneurysm is only 4.2 cm in diameter, operation will be advised unless a medical contraindication is found.

Condition of the Patient

Relative contraindications for elective surgery for small abdominal aneurysms include recent myocardial infarction, intractable congestive heart failure, severe pulmonary insufficiency, incapacitating residual from a stroke, renal failure, uncontrolled cancer, and advanced age (over 80). Most of these patients are best seen in the office at six-month intervals for examination and radiographs or ultrasounds. If there is a significant increase in the size of the aneurysm or the onset of symptoms such as unexplained back pain or abdominal pain and aneurysmal tenderness, operation may be advised at that point.

Myocardial infarction is the most frequent cause of operative mortality and also late deaths in most reported series of aneurysm resection. In hopes of decreasing this mortality rate, there is an increasing interest in a more aggressive cardiac evaluation of patients prior to aneurysm resection, with the performance of coronary artery bypass when appropriate. There is good evidence that this approach is indicated in patients with angina or previous myocardial infarction. It is less clear whether stress testing, multigated radionuclide scans, or coronary arteriography is routinely advisable in asymptomatic patients without previous myocardial infarctions.

I would therefore recommend that our patient have a careful history, physical examination, and standard electrocardiogram done, and also an evaluation of risk factors including smoking, hyperlipidemia, diabetes, hypertension, and family history of aneurysmal disease. If further evaluation seems indicated, a multigated radionuclide scan should be obtained. These scans are more sensitive than stress testing since they can identify ischemic wall motion abnormalities occurring with exercise. If ischemia is demonstrated, coronary arteriography should be performed and coronary bypass operation recommended if significant left main or three-vessel disease with suitable anatomy for operation is found. Balloon angioplasty should be recommended for an appropriate significant left anterior descending stenosis. Aneurysmectomy should then be performed three months after coronary artery bypass.

OPERATIVE MANAGEMENT

In addition to the usual preparations for abdominal surgery, the patient should have adequate intravenous hydration overnight and prophylactic antibiotics should be given the morning of the operation.

A long midline incision is used for routine operations. After a careful exploration, the small bowel is packed in a plastic bag and retracted to the right and outside of the abdomen. Heparin is administered. The iliac arteries are occluded following minimal dissection. The aorta is mobilized anteriorly and occluded. For small aneurysms this can almost always be performed below the renal arteries. The lumbar arteries, middle sacral, and inferior mesenteric arteries are much more frequently patent with small aneurysms. To avoid excessive blood loss, special care must be taken to occlude most of these vessels from outside of the aneurysm. In many instances this may be most easily accomplished by removal of the aneurysm. The aneurysm can be removed by proximal division of and elevation of the aneurysm with serial ligation of the lumbar vessels. It is very important that the iliac clamps are secure and that any debris is removed from the iliac vessels prior to reestablishing flow. Otherwise, "trash foot" is very likely to occur. Tube graft replacement is usually possible with small aneurysms. When a small aneurysm is removed it is not possible to use the aneurysm sac during closure of the posterior peritoneum and, special care must be taken to close the peritoneum and available retroperitoneal tissue over the entire graft, particularly at the site of the anastomoses. The anterior abdominal wall is closed with continuous monofilament suture, interrupted at least three times to approximate the fascia, absorbable suture to the subcutaneous tissues, and staples to the skin.

Postoperatively, the nasogastric tube is maintained to suction until gastrointestinal function returns. The patient is discharged from the hospital six to ten days postoperatively.

BIBLIOGRAPHY

1. Bernstein EF, Chan EL: Abdominal aortic aneurysm in high-risk patients. *Ann Surg* 1984; 200:255–263.
2. Brewster DC, Darling RC, Raines JK, et al: Assessment of abdominal aortic aneurysm size. *Circulation 56 [Suppl II]* 1977, 164–169.
3. Darling RC, Messina CR, Brewster DC, et al: Autopsy study of unoperated abdominal aortic aneurysms. A case for early resection. *Circulation 56 [Suppl II]* 1977, 161–164.
4. Hicks GL, Eastland MW, DeWeese, JA, et al: Survival improvement following aortic aneurysm resection. *Ann Surg* 1975; 181:863–869.
5. Hollier LH, Plate G, O'Brien PC, et al: Late survival after abdominal aortic aneurysm repair: Influence of coronary artery disease. *J Vasc Surg* 1984; 1:290–299.
6. May AG, DeWeese JA, Frank I, et al: Surgical treatment of abdominal aortic aneurysms. *Surgery* 1968; 68:711–721.
7. Pasch AR, Ricotta JJ, May AG, et al: Abdominal aortic aneurysm: The case for elective resection. *Circulation [Suppl I]* 1984, 1–4.

13 High-Risk Patient with Abdominal Aortic Aneurysm

A 67-year-old man is referred by his cardiologist with a 6 cm abdominal aortic aneurysm, detected on routine physical examination. The aneurysm is asymptomatic. He has had two previous myocardial infarctions and continues to experience angina. He has moderately severe chronic obstructive lung disease, hypertension, and a serum creatinine of 2.1 mg per 100 ml.

Consultant: L.H. Hollier, M.D.

Abdominal aortic aneurysm (AAA) is being seen with increasing frequency as the elderly population of the United States continues to increase. Since aneurysm is basically a degenerative disease of the arterial wall, there is no medical cure; as time goes on, the abdominal aortic aneurysm will generally continue to enlarge and ultimately will rupture. The definitive treatment of aneurysm is replacement with a prosthetic graft. In patients at good risk, this can be performed with a mortality rate of approximately 1% to 2%. Some patients, however, such as the case presented here, have associated medical problems that significantly increase the operative risk of aneurysm repair and complicate the perioperative management. When surgical treatment is considered, it is imperative that the physician attempt to stratify risks.

What is the risk of rupture of an untreated abdominal aortic aneurysm, and how large must an aneurysm be before surgery is recommended? Since the 1960s most physicians have recommended that abdominal aortic aneurysms larger than 6 cm be operated on and that aneurysms less than 6 cm be observed until they enlarge to a greater size. Szilagyi, et al, noted that rupture was the most common cause of death in unoperated aneurysms greater than 6 cm in size, whereas myocardial infarction was the most common cause of death in patients with aneurysms less than 6 cm in size. What has often been unappreciated, however, was the fact that, although myocardial infarction was the most common cause of death in patients with small aneurysms, rupture of the small unoperated aneurysm was still the cause of death in approximately 30% of patients with aneurysms smaller than 6 cm. Support for this concept is also provided by Darling, who noted in an autopsy series that 18.1% of 182 ruptured abdominal aortic aneurysms were less than 5 cm in diameter. Szilagyi and colleagues further documented that, even for small aneurysms, surgical treatment resulted in improved late survival. Thus, it seems evident that the *presence* of an abdominal aortic aneurysm, not the size, should be sufficient indication for surgical treatment.

Another question to be answered is: *Does the patient have such overwhelming medical problems that the risk of surgery is greater than the risk of aneurysm rupture?* This is not usually the case. In 1980, Flanigan, et al, reported the fate of 187 patients with asymptomatic abdominal aortic aneurysms who were denied operative repair at the time of initial evaluation because the aneurysm was thought to be "too small" or the surgeon believed them to be unacceptable operative risks. Despite this, however, 42 of these patients did ultimately undergo aneurysm repair because of rupture, improvement of the underlying risks, or increase in size or symptoms of the abdominal aortic aneurysm. Of the 153 patients who were managed expectantly, 34 patients (22.2%) developed aneurysm rupture or acute expansion necessitating operation; 56% of these patients died. Thus it is evident that abdominal aortic aneurysm is a lethal disease, even in a high-risk patient, and case selection should be liberal and recognize few operative contraindications. Attention should be turned instead to providing the patient with the safest method for aneurysm repair. If operative risk for elective aneurysm repair can be kept below 6% to 7%, overall survival will clearly be improved, even in high-risk patients.

We believe there are virtually no contraindications to aortic surgery for patients with acutely symptomatic, expanding, or ruptured abdominal aortic aneurysms. Similarly, we believe that patients with asymptomatic abdominal aortic aneurysms, even though they may have severe medical problems, should generally undergo elective repair of the aneurysm rather than waiting for the patient to get older and sicker waiting for the aneurysm to "grow-up," by which time the patient may be an even worse operative risk. Even though aneurysm repair in these patients may be associated with increased operative risk, this risk is generally less than that of nonoperative observation.

PREOPERATIVE ASSESSMENT

Evaluation of the routine patient with abdominal aortic aneurysm begins with a careful history and physical examination specifically attempting to identify any current history of chronic obstructive pulmonary disease or evidence of coronary artery disease such as angina or congestive heart failure. Standard tests for all patients prior to aneurysm surgery include chest roentgenogram, abdominal ultrasound, electrocardiogram, complete blood count and urinalysis, as well as a determination of serum creatinine, glucose, liver enzymes, and a coagulation profile. Intravenous pyelography is often obtained but is not mandatory if documentation of normal renal function is available. Aortography is not usually performed unless the patient has significant hypertension, elevated serum creatinine, reduction in femoral pulses, or symptoms of chronic intestinal ischemia.

Patients with severe hypertension and/or elevated serum creatinine may have associated renal artery stenosis that would be correctable prior to (by percutaneous transluminal angioplasty), or at the time of, aneurysm repair. Thus, preoperative angiography is mandatory in these patients. If high-grade renal artery stenosis is identified in a patient with severe hypertension or elevated creatinine and the renal artery stenosis is amenable to balloon angioplasty, this should be done prior to undertaking aneurysm repair. On the other hand, if this stenosis is a proximal orificial atherosclerotic stenosis contiguous with an aortic plaque, concomitant renal artery bypass would be done at the time of aneurysm repair, rather than by percutaneous transluminal angioplasty.

Chronic obstructive pulmonary disease is almost never, in my estimation, a contraindication to abdominal aortic aneurysm repair. Several techniques are currently available to minimize perioperative pulmonary risks. Intensive preoperative use of bronchodilators, antibiotics, and pulmonary toilet will help to improve the pulmonary risks in many patients. The perioperative placement of an epidural catheter and postoperative use of epidural morphine for pain relief allows the patient to continue to cough effectively without pain and the need for undue sedation. In some patients, the use of an extraperitoneal approach is possible and can minimize postoperative pulmonary dysfunction.

Coronary artery disease remains the most prevalent and worst risk factor in patients with abdominal aortic aneurysm. Although coronary artery disease alone does not preclude safe abdominal aortic aneurysm repair, proper preoperative evaluation and minimization of risks is highly desirable. Obviously, in those patients with significant coronary artery disease, coronary artery bypass grafting has been shown to lessen the risk of subsequent aneurysm repair.

Patients with abnormal ECG, angina, congestive heart failure, or history of prior myocardial infarction are usually given additional tests to further evaluate functional coronary artery disease. We prefer Dipyridamol-thallium scanning for this evaluation; if this radionuclide study is suggestive of significant functional coronary artery disease, coronary angiography is performed. Additionally, coronary angiography is routinely recommended in those patients who have angina at rest or with minimal exercise. On the other hand, if the patient is found to have stable coronary artery disease without specific areas of myocardium at risk, we would generally not recommend prophylactic myocardial revascularization. Figure 13–1 provides a schematic diagram of cardiac evaluation and management in patients with asymptomatic abdominal aortic aneurysm.

There are some aneurysm patients with coronary artery disease that are not suitable for revascularization because of diffuse multivessel disease, poor left ventricular function, or advanced age. Formerly, these patients were often denied elective abdominal aortic aneurysm repair, even though one third of these patients would be expected to die of rupture of their aneurysms. Currently, operative repair of abdominal aortic aneurysm, even in these high-risk patients, can be accomplished with low morbidity and mortality. Because of this, we will generally offer surgery to all patients with significant aneurysms, despite their coronary artery disease, but intensive perioperative cardiac management is mandatory.

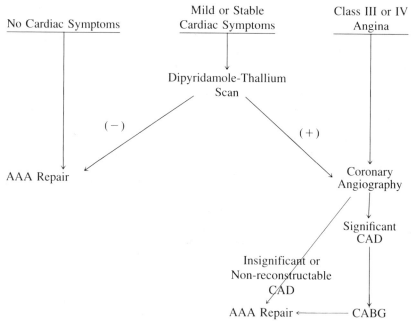

FIG 13–1.
Cardiac evaluation and management in patients with asymptomatic abdominal aortic aneurysm (AAA). (CAD = coronary artery disease; CABG = coronary artery bypass graft)

SPECIFIC MANAGEMENT OF THIS PATIENT

This 67 year old man has a large 6 cm abdominal aortic aneurysm that represents a specific threat of rupture. His two previous myocardial infarctions and continued angina indicate the need for preoperative coronary angiography. If significant coronary stenosis is found, the patient should undergo coronary artery bypass prior to aneurysm repair. If he has insignificant or nonreconstructable coronary lesions, I would plan to undertake aneurysm repair with additional cardiac support, as will be described shortly. His chronic obstructive coronary disease should be evaluated by pulmonary function studies with and without bronchodilators to determine if preoperative and postoperative bronchodilators would be helpful to him. Regardless of findings, he should be considered for aneurysm repair, but he may benefit from preoperative pulmonary preparation with bronchodilators and antibiotics. Because of his hypertension and elevated serum creatinine, I would perform aortography to determine the possible presence of renal artery stenosis. If no significant renal artery lesions were found, I would proceed with aneurysm repair making certain to maintain adequate hydration and provide intravenous mannitol and diuretics during the operative period. If renal artery stenosis were found and were suitable for balloon dilatation, I would consider doing this approximately two weeks prior to aneurysm repair. If this were unsuccessful, or if dilatation were not possible, I would plan revascularization of any high-grade stenosis, usually by Dacron bypass graft, at the time of aneurysm repair. If his pulmonary disease were severe and if he had no renal artery lesions, I would strongly consider undertaking the aneurysm repair through a left flank retroperitoneal approach. (If he had isolated left renal artery stenosis, I would similarly plan a left flank retroperitoneal approach for aneurysm repair and concomitant left renal artery revascularization.)

OPERATIVE MANAGEMENT OF CARDIAC DYSFUNCTION

This patient, and any other patient with significant cardiac disease, would undergo perioperative monitoring of cardiac hemodynamics with specific attempts to maintain optimum cardiac performance. During aneurysm surgery, Swan-Ganz monitoring is used routinely and fluid replacement is provided appropriately to keep the cardiac index above 2 L/minute/m^2. If the pulmonary capillary wedge pressure is low, additional fluid is given to keep the wedge pressure at an optimal level for that patient. If the wedge pressure is high or if peripheral resistance is elevated, intravenous nitroprusside is provided for systemic vasodilatation and reduction of left ventricular afterload. If these measures fail to correct low cardiac output, low-dose dopamine is given intravenously at a rate of about 2 to 3 mcg/kgm/minute. This will usually increase inotropic function of the heart and maintain satisfactory hemodynamics. The combined use of nitroprusside and dopamine is frequently used since this has been documented to increase left ventricular stroke work index and cardiac index while decreasing peripheral resistance and left ventricular end-diastolic pressure, thus improving subendocardial myocardial perfusion.

If cardiac function deteriorates despite these pharmacologic manipulations, and the cardiac index cannot be maintained above 2 L/minute/m^2, an intraaortic balloon is inserted percutaneously. The balloon is inserted by a puncture of the femoral artery in the groin and the balloon is guided up through the iliac vessels and through one limb of the bifurcated aortic graft that is being implanted. Actual insertion of the balloon is delayed until the aortic graft can be anastomosed to the aorta and the ipsilateral iliac artery. The aortic graft is then occluded manually and the intraaortic balloon is inserted from the groin up through the iliac artery and graft and advanced the measured distance into the descending thoracic aorta. Counterpulsation is instituted and the anastomosis of the remaining graft limb to the opposite iliac artery is then performed. The patient is maintained on 1:1 counterpulsation for about 48 hours or until hemodynamics are stabilized.

RESULTS

Abdominal aortic aneurysm repair in patients with no major risk factors can currently be achieved with an operative mortality rate of 1%. The particular patient presented in this case, however, has multiple risk factors that will significantly increase his perioperative risk. If coronary artery bypass grafting were indicated and could be successfully performed prior to aneurysm repair, I would still anticipate that the patient cited in this case problem could undergo aneurysm repair with a mortality rate of under 3%. If, however, his coronary disease were not reconstructable, aneurysm repair should still be undertaken and could be done with a much lower mortality than nonoperative management. We have previously reported our results of direct graft replacement of abdominal aortic aneurysm in patients who have exceptionally high-risk factors. Direct aneurysm repair in 106 of these patients was accomplished with an overall mortality of 5.7%. It is also important to recognize that these patients followed up to five years continue to show survival equal to that of regular aneurysm patients.

SUMMARY

Recent improvements in perioperative monitoring and pharmacologic management of cardiac dysfunction now allows graft replacement of abdominal aortic aneurysm even in high-risk patients. Indications for surgical repair of abdominal aortic aneurysm should be liberalized so that aneurysm repair can be undertaken electively before the development of rupture which would require emergency repair and the expectation of significantly poorer results.

BIBLIOGRAPHY

1. Brewster DC, Okada RD, Strauss HW, et al: Selection of patients for preoperative coronary angiography: Use of Dipyridamole-Stress-Thallium myocardial imaging. *J Vasc Surg* 1985; 2:504–510.
2. Brown OW, Hollier LH, Pairolero PC, et al: Abdominal aortic aneurysms and coronary artery disease. *Arch Surg* 1981; 116:1484–1488.
3. Darling RC: Ruptured arteriosclerotic abdominal aortic aneurysm. *Am J Surg* 1970; 119:397–401.
4. Flanigan DP, Quinn T, Kraft RO: Selective management of high risk patient with an abdominal aortic aneurysm. *Surg Gynecol Obstet* 1980; 150:171–176.
5. Hertzer NR: Myocardial ischemia. *Surgery* 1983; 93:97–101.
6. Hollier LH: The case against prophylactic coronary bypass. Advocates in vascular controversies, panel debate, part II. *Surgery* 1984; 96:78–87.
7. Hollier LH, Reigel MM, Kazmier FJ, et al: Conventional repair of AAA in the high-risk patient: A plea for abandonment of nonresective treatment. *J Vasc Surg* 1986; 3:712–717.
8. Hollier LH, Spittell JA, Puga FJ: Intra-aortic balloon counterpulsation as adjunct to aneurysmectomy in high-risk patients. *Mayo Clin Proc* 1981; 56(9):565–567.
9. Szilagyi DE, Elliott JP, Smith RF: Clinical fate of the patient with asymptomatic abdominal aortic aneurysm and unfit for surgical treatment. *Arch Surg* 1972; 104:600–606.

10. Szilagyi DF, Smith RF, DeRusso FJ, et al: Contribution of abdominal aortic aneurysmectomy to prolongation of life. *Ann Surg* 1966; 164:678–699.
11. Whittemore AD, Clowes AW, Hechtman HB, et al: Aortic aneurysm repair. Reduced operative mortality associated with maintenance of optimal cardiac performance. *Ann Surg* 1980; 192:414–421.

14 Thoracoabdominal Aneurysm

A 62-year-old man is transferred to your hospital with a 5 cm aortic aneurysm. This was noted as a prominent pulsation in the epigastrium by the patient himself. His internist obtained an ultrasound examination which suggested extension above the renal arteries.

Consultant: E. Stanley Crawford, M.D.

The limited information provided in this case is not unusual and I think fair enough because it should be up to the vascular surgeon to make the final judgments regarding management. These judgments result from an evaluation of all the facts regarding associated disease, location, extent, and size of the aneurysm. It is therefore proper that he direct the complete assessment of the patient, including selection of studies and consultants necessary to achieve this goal. The referring physician has thus really done his job, i.e., made the diagnosis of aneurysm and has recognized that the disease which threatens life expectancy in a relatively young patient may be successfully treated.

INDICATION FOR OPERATION BASED ON SIZE

Any patient with a symptomatic aortic aneurysm, regardless of size, location, and extent, should be considered for operative treatment because death from rupture or other complications is likely to occur in a short period of time. Conservative treatment is employed only in patients not likely to survive because of associated diseases that pose prohibitive operative risks or severely limit life expectancy as discussed in detail below.

Patients with asymptomatic aneurysms whose diameters are twice the size of the uninvolved aorta (5 to 6 cm) should be considered for elective operation regardless of location, provided that the operative risks are acceptable. The possibility of rupture appears to increase with size, the presence of hypertension, and chronic obstructive pulmonary disease. Elective operation becomes increasingly justified with these considerations.

The incidence of rupture in patients with asymptomatic abdominal aortic aneurysms 5 cm in diameter is estimated to be about 10% to 15% per year. The operative mortality rate in such patients with mild to moderate associated disease is 2% to 3%, even in patients requiring total abdominal aortic replacement. The incidence of paraplegia is about 1% to 2% in those patients requiring more extensive aortic replacement. The incidence of rupture of more extensive aneurysms involving both the descending thoracic and abdominal aorta appears to be about the same as that just described. The approach to elective operation in patients with aneurysms of the lower thoracic and abdominal aorta is similar since the risks of operation and its complications are only slightly more than that for abdominal operations. Elective operation that requires complete replacement of the descending thoracic and abdominal aorta is more clearly justified in patients with larger aneurysms, i.e., those aneurysms 6 cm or greater, due to the higher mortality (8% to 9%) and the higher incidence of neurologic disturbances of the lower extremities, i.e., paraplegia 10%, and paraparesis 10%. Our follow-up studies in 97 patients who were treated conservatively because of increased risks of operation or for staging of operation, were associated with 76% mortality in two years, with half of the deaths being due to rupture.

GENERAL CONSIDERATIONS

The common diseases or conditions that pose risk to aortic operation and postoperative management include diabetes, cancer, renal failure, chronic obstructive pulmonary disease (COPD), heart disease, liver disease, hypertension, peripheral vascular disease (brachiocephalic, visceral vessel, and aorto-iliofemoral artery obstruction), coagulation defects, and medications. These conditions are usually detected or suggested by the routine history and physical examination which is supplemented routinely by plain roentgenograms of the chest and abdomen, ECG, coagulation profile, blood gases, blood sugar, BUN, creatinine, and electrolytes. In fact, some conditions may be obvious and advanced from history and physical examination or review of preexisting data. Associated conditions posing extreme risk to operation or limiting life expectancy to less than two years constitute contraindication for aortic reconstruction, particularly in the patient with asymptomatic aneurysm. Definitive treatment in such cases is supportive therapy for the associated disease. Further concern with the aortic disease is unnecessary.

Pulmonary function studies are performed in the patient with COPD. Patients who do not retain CO_2 in arterial blood on room air and whose FEV_1 is greater than 1 are generally considered suitable for aneurysm operation at any level, particularly if improvement occurs with bronchial dilators. Regardless, cigarettes are withdrawn and operation postponed until bronchial secretions disappear. Elective operations that require chest incision and incision of the diaphragm are contraindicated in patients with more severe pulmonary dysfunction. Elective abdominal operation is usually well tolerated in patients whose FEV_1 is between 0.8 and 1 even with low arterial PO$_2$ values (<50), particularly if delayed for two to three months during which time the patients abstain from smoking, lose weight if obese, or gain weight if underweight, and participate in an exercise program. Pulmonary function does not change significantly in these cases, but the patients' ability to breathe without exhaustion often improves, allowing them to tolerate intra abdominal operation.

Patients with valvular heart disease, even with severe manifestations, and certain patients with ischemic heart disease are studied by heart catheterization and cineangiography. The latter patients include those with recent myocardial infarction, unstable angina, and recent onset of angina. Aortography may be combined with this study. Valve replacement and/or coronary artery reconstruction may be employed four to eight weeks before aneurysm operation for significant reduction in operative risk for aneurysm. Heart and distant aneurysm operation are rarely combined.

Mild disturbances of renal function manifested by blood creatinine levels up to 2 mg/dl are common and generally do not contraindicate elective operation. Contrast studies are, however, performed after good hydration which is maintained by intravenous fluids containing mannitol during the day of study. Moreover, digital subtraction angiography is frequently employed to reduce the amount of contrast needed. Hypotension is avoided during operation, and the period of suprarenal aortic clamping is minimized in these cases. Risks of operation increase with the degree of renal insufficiency. In fact, total renal failure requiring hemodialysis frequently occurs following thoracoabdominal aortic aneurysm operation in patients whose chronic creatinine levels are three or more. Death occurs in about 65% of these cases within two months from complications of renal failure and dialysis. An interesting observation has been survival in 85% of patients with renal failure when operation was employed months or several years after being well maintained on chronic hemodialysis. Assuming that patients with highly elevated creatinine levels (>4) are destined for dialysis within one to two years, we have successfully treated a small number of these cases with large asymptomatic aneurysm by first establishing a chronic dialysis program and performing aneurysm operation two to three months later. Thus, severe degrees of renal insufficiency may not always be a contraindication for operation because the life expectancy of a patient on dialysis may be extended for long periods, more than ten years. Finally, renal failure due to severe renal artery obstruction occasionally may either be improved or relieved by renal artery reconstruction. Aortography is performed in such patients in the search for such lesions after stabilization, hydration, and under conditions described above.

DETECTION AND EVALUATION OF AORTIC ANEURYSM

Abdominal aortic aneurysms are frequently not detected by physical examination, either because the abdomen is not carefully palpated or due to obesity. Fairly large aneurysms may not be detected in the large or overweight patient or in those patients with abdominal spasm or tenderness. This author finds it difficult to palpate an aneurysm in 10% to 15% of patients for such reasons. Indeed, over 70% of referred patients had the diagnosis suspected or made not by palpation but from abdominal calcifications in roentgenograms made for abdominal, back, flank, or hip pain, CT scans performed in search of abdominal, back, renal, and other abnormalities, or excretory pyelogram for genitorenal studies.

For some years, this author has recommended annual ultrasound examination of the aorta in patients > 55 years, just as routine electrocardiograms are done today. Regardless, the adequacy of this method is dependent on equipment employed and the skill of the operator. Other disadvantages include presence of intestinal air as is frequently present in the hospitalized patient and difficulties in determining the upper extent of aneurysm and associated branch vessel disease using generally available equipment. Its principal usefulness is screening and for following small aneurysms in patients with operative risks. CT scanning and MRI are much better methods of examination for diagnosis and determination of size and extent. Aortographic examination is best for detection of location and involvement of branch vessels by occlusive or aneurysmal disease. Studies employing contrast in patients with renal dysfunction must be carefully utilized as described above. MRI may be employed when the use of contrast media is not desired, but unfortunately, this method does not adequately evaluate the branch vessels for occlusive disease. Digital subtraction angiography using small quantities of contrast is frequently the preferred method.

The upper extent of aneurysm and presence of associated branch vessel disease cannot be determined by physical examination in many patients, and ultrasound examination does not help in the case presented here. This knowledge is crucial to operative management because extent and branch vessel involvement may be extremely difficult to determine by exploratory abdominal operation. This information should be determined before operation. Our increasing choice for the next step in evaluation of the type of patient presented here is CT scanning of the entire aorta with contrast enhancement because it would reveal the nature, location, extent, and size of aneurysm and certain associated diseases or conditions. This study would be adequate if it showed the aneurysm to be truly infrarenal in location, and operation would be performed in the standard fashion.

Aortography would be performed next, if visceral vessel involvement were suggested by CT scan, both to determine the presence of associated branch vessel disease if the aneurysm involved multiple visceral vessels, or to determine if the aneurysm was actually juxtarenal infrarenal in location when the CT scan suggested involvement limited to renal arteries.

JUXTARENAL INFRARENAL ANEURYSM

Juxtarenal infrarenal aneurysms are defined as those that involve the aorta up to and even including the lower edge of renal artery origins. Due to the fact that the involved aortic segment elongates as well as dilates during aneurysmal formation, the upper edge of the aneurysm may overlap the origins of the renal arteries and suggest renal artery origin involvement by CT scan, MRI, and aortography in AP position. Juxtarenal location is suggested by forward kinking of the aorta just below the level of the superior mesenteric artery on the lateral view of the aortogram.

Operation in these cases is performed through a midline incision. The aorta is clamped at the diaphragm and incised from the left renal vein superiorly to the aortic bifurcation inferiorly. The edges of the aneurysm are retracted and contained clot removed. Blood is aspirated with cell saver suction, the renal arteries identified, and the proximal anastomosis of the graft made just distal to the renal artery origins, including their lower margins when necessary. After completion of this proximal anastomosis, the graft is clamped distal to the anastomosis and blood flow restored into the visceral arteries by removing the upper clamp. Operation is completed in the standard fashion.

ANEURYSMS INVOLVING RENAL ARTERY ORIGINS

Upward extension of aneurysms limited to renal artery origin is rare except in patients in whom one or both renal arteries arise abnormally low from the aorta. In any case, when this form of limited involvement occurs, we usually perform operation using a modification of the technique just described. The aneurysms, including proximal segments of renal arteries and the uninvolved aorta, are exposed up to the superior mesenteric artery. This exposure is facilitated in most cases by mobilizing the left renal vein after ligating the adrenal, lumbar, and gonadal branches or, in those with large aneurysms, by simply interrupting the left renal vein proximal to these branches and retracting it to the left. The aorta is clamped above the celiac axis. The aneurysm is incised throughout its length and its edges retracted. The aorta is transsected above the aneurysm just distal to the superior mesenteric artery. A generous button of aortic tissue from which the renal artery arises is excised on each side and the corresponding renal artery mobilized. After the proximal aortic anastomosis is made to the aorta, an opening is made in the graft on each side and first one and then the other renal artery is attached to the graft with continuous suture using the button of aortic tissue. The aorta is flushed proximally, the graft clamped below the reattached arteries, and the proximal clamp removed to restore visceral arterial circulation while the graft-operation is completed.

The latter method of operation is relatively easy in thin and moderately built patients. This approach may be difficult in short, stocky, and obese patients. Thoracoabdominal retroperitoneal operation is recommended in such patients as employed in those with upward extension involving superior mesenteric and celiac arteries. The level of the thoracic incision varies from the eighth to fifth intercostal space depending on proximal extension of aneurysm. The chest incision is extended across the costal arch into a full-length midline abdominal incision. The abdominal aortic segment is exposed retroperitoneally by retracting descending colon, splenic flexure, spleen, left kidney, stomach, body, and tail of pancreas upward and to the right. The aorta is incised in the midline posteriorly, retracting the aneurysmal edges with stay sutures. Bleeding from celiac axis and superior mesenteric arteries is controlled with #4 balloon catheters, the renal arteries are perfused using biomedicus pump and special left atriorenal artery catheters. The proximal end of the graft is attached proximally, intercostal and lumbar arteries D8-L2 are reattached if possible, and finally the visceral vessels are reattached by the inclusion method. The distal end of the graft is attached appropriately to distal aorta, iliac, or femoral arteries. Proximal aortic pressure and cardiac hemodynamic dynamics may be controlled during aortic cross-clamping either using nitroprusside solution or by temporary atriofemoral bypass using Tygon tubing and centrifugal pump without heparin.

Bypass is not possible in about half the patients with thoracoabdominal aortic aneurysms or aneurysms involving the entire aorta. These patients are treated by simple proximal cross clamp. Proximal blood pressure and cardiac hemodynamics are controlled pharmacologically, monitoring these parameters using pulmonary artery balloon catheters, intraarterial blood pressure, ECG, blood gases, and electrolytes. Post-clamp acidosis is prevented by continuous administration of sodium bicarbonate solution during the period of aortic clamping. The solution is administered in a concentration of 1 mEq/cc. This solution is administered at a constant rate, the hourly volume calculated by multiplying the body weight in kilograms by three.

The risks of paraplegia vary with location, extent, and nature of the aneurysm and do not vary with the method of operation. The risks in patients with nondissecting aneurysms limited to the abdominal aorta, including its proximal segment, are 1% to 2%; 2% to 3% in patients in whom the aneurysm involves the abdominal aorta and the lower half of the descending thoracic aorta; and, 20% in patients in whom the aneurysm involves all or almost all of the abdominal aorta and descending thoracic aorta. The risk of paraplegia in patients with aneurysm formation secondary to chronic aortic dissection is about twice those observed in nondissections.

BIBLIOGRAPHY

1. Bernstein EF, Chan EL: Abdominal aortic aneurysm in high-risk patients. Outcome of selective management based on size and expansion rate. *Ann Surg* 1984; 200:255–263.
2. Crawford ES, Beckett WC, Greer MS: Juxtarenal infrarenal abdominal aortic aneurysm: Special diagnostic and therapeutic considerations. *Ann Surg* 1986; 203:661–670.
3. Crawford ES, DeNatale RW: Thoracoabdominal aortic aneurysm: Observations regarding the natural course of the disease. *J Vasc Surg* 1986; 2:578–582.
4. Crawford ES, Crawford JL: *Diseases of the Aorta including an Atlas of Angiographic Pathology and Surgical Technique,* Baltimore, Williams & Wilkins, 1984.
5. Cronenwett JL, Murphy TF, Zelenock GB, et al: Actuarial analysis of variables associated with rupture of small abdominal aortic aneurysms. *Surgery* 1985; 98:472–483.
6. Szilagyi DE, Elliott JP, Smith RF: Clinical fate of the patient with asymptomatic abdominal aortic aneurysm and unfit for surgical treatment. *Arch Surg* 1972; 104:600–606.

15 Ruptured Abdominal Aortic Aneurysms

A 72-year-old man is brought to the emergency room by ambulance after having collapsed at home. He is complaining of severe abdominal and back pain. Blood pressure is 100/50 mm Hg.

Consultants: John L. Ochsner, M.D. and Nelson Ancalmo, M.D.

No problem in vascular surgery requires more urgent care than a ruptured aortic aneurysm. Hence, a high index of suspicion and quick decisions are necessary if the patient is to have a successful outcome.

The case presented above typifies the difficulty in arriving at a correct diagnosis, since less than one half of the patients with a ruptured abdominal aneurysm have any knowledge of their condition. If the classical picture of severe excruciating abdominal and back pain with shock and a pulsatile abdominal mass is present, the diagnosis is simple and quick action can save the patient's life; when differential diagnoses are entertained, delay in surgical treatment has resulted in a higher mortality rate.

In most instances, the history and physical examination strongly suggest the diagnosis. At this moment, the surgeon should make immediate preparations to take the patient to the operating room. Any unnecessary delay, even when the patient is stable, can be detrimental to his or her survival.

The clinical picture is dependent on the containment of the rupture. Thus, two different scenarios may develop. Since the abdominal aorta lies retroperitoneally, the bleeding can initially be controlled within the retroperitoneum. The amount of blood loss is related to the size of the rupture site, the blood pressure, and the resistance of the retroperitoneal space. In the case presented herein, the rupture has been contained within the retroperitoneal space for the time being. The site of bleeding and whether the bleeding is continuous or intermittent affects the clinical picture. Once the retroperitoneal space is no longer able to contain the bleeding and/or when there is rupture into the peritoneal cavity, the clinical picture changes drastically to one of uncontrolled hemorrhage, i.e., shock and/or cardiac arrest secondary to hemorrhagic shock.

RESUSCITATION AND PREOPERATIVE MANAGEMENT

Since the risk of fatal hemorrhage is imminent in any patient with a diagnosis of ruptured aneurysm, we believe that no time should be wasted in obtaining confirmatory diagnostic and other preoperative studies. The patient should be immediately transferred to the operating room. In fact, if a referring physician calls and states he is referring a patient with a ruptured aneurysm, we have adopted a policy to bypass the emergency room and have the patient taken directly to the operating room. Confirmation of the diagnosis can be made in the OR, and at the same time a large bore central intravenous line can be inserted in the upper extremity for fluid replacement. Blood is drawn for blood typing and determination of blood chemistry values. However, Rh O negative blood can be used until type specific blood is available.

If the patient is stable, the operation should proceed as usual, but without delay. However, if the patient is in shock, resuscitation is performed by using a balanced salt solution which should be administered at the fastest flow possible until proximal aortic control is obtained.

We realize that some patients may be taken to the operating room only for the surgeon to recognize that they do not have a ruptured aneurysm. Except for the unnecessary cost of the operating room, no harm is done. When one compares this minor inconvenience to the catastrophe that can occur if uncontrolled hemorrhage develops during time expended in obtaining confirmatory diagnostic data or reviewing other symptoms, one realizes the importance of speed in treatment. We have experienced an unnecessary death when time was consumed during a preoperative chest roentgenogram.

INTRAOPERATIVE MANAGEMENT

Aortic aneurysms rupture in different manners and degrees. This variation will dictate the condition of the patient and hence the initial operative management. The most dramatic and urgent presentation is rupture into the free peritoneal cavity. Those who survive long enough to reach the operating room are in extreme shock without discernible blood pressure and are in a semiconscious or unconscious state. In these, the abdomen is immediately opened without preparing and draping or even administering anesthesia. The only hope for survival is to obtain proximal control of the aorta and replace the tremendous volume of intravascular fluids.

More commonly, patients with a ruptured aortic aneurysm who reach the hospital alive have had the bleeding controlled within the retroperitoneal space. In this circumstance, degree of rupture plays an important role. If the patient presents with a small rupture and the retroperitoneal hematoma has effectively tamponaded the leak, the patient will be stable and the operation can be performed in an orderly fashion as in an elective aneurysmectomy. On the other hand, if the rent in the aortic wall is large and actively bleeding, the patient may be in varying degrees of shock and the speed of aortic control is commensurate with the hemodynamic condition of the patient. The other two modalities of aortic rupture are enteric and inferior vena caval fistulae. They require a separate discussion since their presentation and management are totally different.

As we have mentioned repeatedly, the key to survival in a ruptured abdominal aortic aneurysm is to obtain proximal control. This requires adequate exposure and assistance during the operation. For a surgeon to embark on this kind of procedure through a limited abdominal incision, or with only a scrub nurse as his assistant, is to deny the patient a successful outcome. A midline incision from xiphoid to symphysis provides a fast and wide exposure, and the use of an upper hand retractor makes the infradiaphragmatic area more readily accessible. If the patient has no discernible blood pressure, an aortic compression clamp or one's fist is applied to the aorta at the level of the diaphragm and compresses the aorta against the vertebral bodies. The infrarenal aorta is then dissected and a vascular clamp placed about the aorta. If one is unable to control the bleeding with infradiaphragmatic compression, this portion of the aorta is exposed through the lesser omentum and clamped prior to infrarenal dissection.

During this control phase of the operation, the anesthesiologist should be resuscitating the patient with intratracheal intubation and administration of large volumes of intravenous fluids. The aneurysm is opened, care is taken not to enter the mesentery of the colon, and the surgeon can quickly place his index finger into the distal aorta to help control bleeding and also as a guide for location of the iliac arteries, which are clamped without encircling the arteries. In spite of the urgency to obtain vascular control, the presence of surrounding structures should always be kept in mind. A vascular clamp that includes the esophagus or perforates other structures becomes not only ineffective, but a potential source of contamination or continued bleeding.

Once the aorta is secured proximally and distally, all efforts should be directed toward resuscitation and proper preparation and draping if this has not been done before. Volume expanders, balanced salt solutions, blood, et cetera, should be given at this time to replace the intravascular volume lost. Antibiotics, arterial lines, Foley catheter, adequate level of anesthesia, proper draping of operative site, proper scrubbing by the surgeons, change of gowns, gloves, et cetera, and other routine preparations can now be taken care of while the patient's condition is stabilized.

Adequate heparinization should be obtained as soon as the aorta is cross-clamped. This will protect the viscera and extremities from clotting and assure proper reperfusion upon declamping. Aneurysmorrhaphy is then accomplished in the usual orderly fashion.

For the patient who is in a stable hemodynamic condition due to containment of the bleeding by the retroperitoneal space, anesthesia and the operation proceed as normal, except at an accelerated rate. No time is allowed for the luxury of a Swan-Ganz catheter, et cetera. The patient is hurriedly prepared and draped, and the abdomen opened in the usual manner. It is our opinion that one should control the proximal aorta at the immediate infrarenal area. The retroperitoneal space is opened high at the level of the renal vein, and the surgeon can, by blunt dissection with his index and middle finger, palpate both sides of the aorta and place a clamp at this level. Usually, blood has already dissected the necessary plane, allowing an easier approach to this blind dissection. We feel very comfortable with this avenue and prefer it to dissecting out the infradiaphragmatic aorta for proximal control. Once proximal control is obtained, the rest of the operation proceeds normally.

Since most of these cases do not allow time for preclotting of the graft, a woven Dacron graft with fairly small interstices such as the Ochsner 200* should be employed. This graft allows ease of handling with adequate control of bleeding and at the same time has normal ingrowth of tissue.

POSTOPERATIVE MANAGEMENT AND COMPLICATIONS

Since most of these patients develop prolonged paralytic ileus due to the extensive dissection caused by the retroperitoneal hematoma, the surgeon faces two problems: (1) prolonged gastric decompression and (2) the provision of adequate caloric intake. Although a nasogastric tube can provide adequate drainage, after a while it can become an inconvenience for the patient. An easy solution is to place a temporary gastrostomy by using one of the standard techniques. The second problem concerning nutritional support can be dealt with in different ways. One is by using total parenteral nutrition which conveys the potential complication of sepsis from a prolonged use of a central line. As an alternative, the surgeon may place, during surgery, a feeding jejunostomy tube that can be kept in place for as long as it is necessary. The placement of the gastrostomy tube and the feeding jejunostomy tube carries very little incidence of graft infection since these tubes are placed after the retroperitoneum has been properly closed.

All patients with ruptured abdominal aneurysms are taken to surgery without proper preoperative evaluation of all their associated disease. The most common and most serious complication seen after a ruptured abdominal aneurysm is myocardial infarction. The combination of coronary artery disease and hypotension results in ischemia of the myocardial muscle. The management of acute myocardial infarction after a ruptured abdominal aneurysm is basically the management of any other acute myocardial ischemia. Myocardial infarction is by far the most frequent cause of death after a ruptured abdominal aneurysm.

The second most common complication after repair of a ruptured abdominal aneurysm is acute renal failure. This is due to a combination of hypotension secondary to the loss of volume, low perfusion due to cross-clamping the aorta above the renal arteries, or embolization of debris from the aneurysmal contents. The use of hemodialysis usually allows these patients a better chance of survival, with restoration of some renal function.

A third major complication is respiratory failure. This may be the result of multiple blood transfusions, sometimes of unfiltered blood, and on several occa-

---

*Intervascular, Clearwater, Florida

sions excessive replacement of intravascular volume with secondary pulmonary edema.

Finally, several complications resulting in multiple organ failure are seen in patients who are subjected to severe stress and multiple trauma. The advanced age at which ruptured aneurysms are usually seen is a major contribution to the high incidence of complications and mortality in this group of patients.

SUMMARY

A ruptured abdominal aneurysm is a catastrophic event that requires from the surgeon the best skills in diagnosis and quick action in order to save these patients. No time should be wasted in obtaining routine tests or trying to confirm the suspected diagnosis. It must be stressed that the only chance the patient has of surviving is for the surgeon to obtain proximal control of the ruptured aorta and allow enough time for resuscitation after the aorta has been cross-clamped. In spite of all our efforts, the mortality rate is still around 40%, and this is directly related to the condition of the patient at the time of operation.

The ideal treatment for an aortic aneurysm is surgery on an elective basis, and that is why it is so important that surgery be contemplated without unnecessary delay, after all the preoperative evaluation is completed, for every patient in whom an aortic aneurysm is discovered, regardless of its size or location.

BIBLIOGRAPHY

1. Estes JE Jr: Abdominal aortic aneurysms: A study of 132 cases. *Circulation* 1950; 2:258–264.
2. Johnson G Jr, Schwartz JA: Ruptured infrarenal aortic aneurysm, in Ernst CB, Stanley JC (eds): *Current Therapy in Vascular Surgery*. Toronto, BC Decker Inc, 1987, pp 101–104.
3. Ochsner JL: Aneurysmal Disease, in Paul F. Nora (ed): *Operative Surgery*. Philadelphia, Lea & Febiger, 1977, pp 737–756.
4. Szilagyi DE, Smith RF, DeRusso FG, et al: Contribution of abdominal aortic aneurysms to prolongation of life. *Ann Surg* 1966; 164:678–699.

16 Associated Renal Artery Disease in Preoperative Aneurysm Patient

A 59-year-old man is admitted for operative repair of a 5.6-cm abdominal aortic aneurysm. He has a ten-year history of moderate hypertension, controlled by medication. Preoperative aortography is carried out, confirming an infrarenal aortic aneurysm and also revealing significant bilateral renal artery stenoses.

Consultants: Richard H. Dean, M.D. and
J. Benjamin Tribble, M.D.

The presentation of this patient is representative of a common situation in which an additional lesion or abnormality is uncovered during diagnostic evaluation of previously identified peripheral vascular disease.

The finding of unsuspected renal artery disease during angiographic delineation of either occlusive or aneurysmal disease of the aorto-iliac segment frequently produces a dilemma regarding both the obligation for further diagnostic study and the necessity of performing additional reconstructive vascular surgery. Although concern over leaving uncorrected anatomic disease in juxtaposition to an aortic reconstruction has led to an empiric and liberal approach to simultaneous renal reconstruction in many centers, exercise of clinical judgment and application of a selective approach to such combined procedures is more appropriate. With this in mind, examination of the currently available data and unproven biases that influence the decisions is integral to the exercise of such judgment. Information important to a reasoned approach may be obtained from an understanding of the natural history of renovascular disease and generalized atherosclerosis. Integration of this information then helps form a therapeutic plan appropriate to the individual patient.

EVALUATION

The specific problems requiring examination of the patient with an infrarenal aortic aneurysm and renal artery stenoses include the risk of rupture of the uncorrected aneurysm, the life expectancy of the patient unrelated to the presence of the aneurysm, the causative relationship between the renal artery stenosis and the hypertension, and the current and subsequent impact of the renovascular lesions on excretory renal function.

Since the information provided contains nothing about coexisting ischemic heart disease or other problems, further preoperative assessment is required before an informed operative strategy can be planned. The underlying reason for elective aneurysmal resection is to improve the long-term survival of this atherosclerotic patient, and thus the ultimate decision regarding the propriety of operation must be based on an understanding of the risk of the procedure itself and the probability that long-term survival will be enhanced by successful correction of the aneurysm. Our concept of a clinically important aneurysm in the usual atherosclerotic adult is one with at least a 4.0-cm cross-sectional diameter. In the patient with increasingly significant additional diseases and in the elderly patient, this defining size is increased in a correlative manner. Certainly this patient with a 5.6-cm aneurysm should be considered for operative correction.

Even in the absence of clinical symptoms of cardiac disease, we believe all patients should undergo preoperative assessment of myocardial function. Considering that as many as 50% of patients who undergo successful aneurysm replacement die over the succeeding ten years and that greater than 80% of those die of heart-related disease, we believe that efforts to identify patients at increased operative risk and those potentially at increased risk of early death from ischemic heart disease during the follow-up period after operation are of great importance. For this reason, this patient should undergo any one of the several screening stress tests for myocardial ischemia. If significant stress-induced ischemia or a strong clinical history of angina pectoris is uncovered, the patient should undergo coronary angiography, both to characterize his disease and to identify disease that requires operative correction.

Screening diagnostic studies should also be performed to exclude clinically silent yet severe cerebrovascular disease. Although multiple noninvasive techniques are available, we prefer the use of duplex scanning of the carotid arteries. When severe disease is uncovered, we believe carotid angiography is warranted to clarify further the severity of disease and its clinical implications.

Having considered associated vascular diseases, we turn to the most important issue of this case: Assessment of indications for concomitant renovascular reconstruction at the time of aneurysm repair. The first question to answer is whether or not the patient has either hypertension or azotemia. In the absence of either problem, the renovascular lesion is not functionally or clinically significant, and its correction will have no immediate impact on the patient's outcome. Frequently, however, the argument is forwarded that, because of the progressive nature of renovascular disease, correction of the renovascular lesion is important to prevent subsequent deterioration in function during follow-up. Nothing in the currently available literature supports this premise. In 1981 we published the results of follow-up studies in a group of 50 patients with proven renovascular disease randomized to continued drug therapy. The diagnosis of renovascular disease was made by positive renal vein renin ratios and/or positive split function studies—positive results of either that indicated functional significance of the renal artery disease. At the time of the report these patients had been followed for two to 114 months (mean, 44 months). Review of the data showed that 17 of the 41 patients (41%) with atherosclerotic lesions had progressive loss of some variable of renal function to a point beyond a predesignated acceptable limit. In 13 of these 17 patients the variable that had deteriorated beyond a "failure" limit was renal length, which had decreased by 10% or more of the length at the time the patient entered the study. Although this finding suggested that progressive loss of renal mass accompanied untreated renal artery lesions, it was documented only in patients who had significant lesions defined by either positive renal vein renin ratios or split renal function studies at the time they entered the study. It is important to restate that this study did not address the rate of deterioration in function of lesions that had not already progressed to the point of pathophysiologic importance. One must remember that a patient with diffuse atherosclerosis, as defined by the presence of both aortic and renovascular disease, surely has an increased risk of death from disease at other atherosclerotic sites. When one considers that death from such causes may occur before an anatomically significant yet pathophysiologically innocent renovascular lesion progresses to the point of clinical significance, then prophylactic renal revascularization has limited, if any, justification.

INDICATIONS FOR RENAL ARTERY REPAIR

A prerequisite for consideration of simultaneous renal revascularization is the presence of hypertension. If the patient is normotensive, then operation should be limited to aneurysm resection. If unilateral renal artery stenosis in a hypertensive patient is found, then simultaneous renal revascularization is undertaken only when functional significance is demonstrated by positive renal vein renin ratios or split renal function studies. The only exception to this approach is when hypertension that is poorly controlled is found and medications cannot be altered to obtain renin measurements. In this circumstance, renal revascularization is undertaken with the knowledge that the blood pressure benefit is less predictable.

When a patient—such as this patient—has bilateral renal artery stenoses and hypertension, the decision to correct the renovascular disease simultaneously with correction of the aneurysm is based on severity of both the hypertension and the renovascular lesions. When the renal artery lesions are not similarly severe, but instead there is severe disease on one side and only mild or moderate disease on the contralateral side, then the patient is treated as if only a unilateral lesion exists.

If both lesions are only moderately severe (65% to 80% stenosis), then renal revascularization is undertaken only if hypertension is severe. In contrast, if the lesions are both severe (greater than 80% stenosis) and the patient has drug-dependent hypertension, then bilateral simultaneous renal revascularization is undertaken without concern for the results of renal vein renin assays. Functional studies are not undertaken, because lack of lateralization does not exclude the presence of renovascular hypertension.

Renovascular hypertension secondary to severe bilateral renal artery stenoses is particularly difficult to control. Furthermore, at least mild azotemia is also often present. Since azotemia usually parallels the severity of hypertension, when a patient presents with severe azotemia yet only mild hypertension, the major cause of the azotemia is usually parenchymal disease. Characteristically, this variety of renovascular hypertension is associated with either total renal artery occlusions or extremely severe bilateral stenoses. When one contemplates simultaneous correction of incidentally identified bilateral renal artery stenoses with correction of an aortic aneurysm, one should compare the patient's status to that of this characteristic presentation. Clearly, the indications for renal revascularization increase as the patient's presentation more closely parallels this picture. In such situations, concomitant renal artery repair at the time of aneurysm surgery is indicated to preserve function, with improvement of hypertension a secondary goal. Such indications seem justified despite the acknowledged increased morbidity and mortality of combined operation.

BIBLIOGRAPHY

1. Dean RH: Renovascular hypertension, in Moore WS (ed): *Vascular Surgery: A Comprehensive Review.* New York, Grune & Stratton, 1983, pp 443–463.
2. Dean RH: Renovascular hypertension. *Curr Probl Surg* 1985; 22:6–67.
3. Dean RH, Keyser JE III, Dupont WD, et al: Aortic and renal vascular disease: Factors affecting the value of combined procedures. *Ann Surg* 1984; 200:336–344.
4. Dean RH, Kieffer RW, Smith BM, et al: Renovascular hypertension: Anatomic and renal function changes during drug therapy. *Arch Surg* 1981; 116:1408–1415.
5. Dean RH, Krueger TC, Whiteneck JM, et al: Operative management of renovascular hypertension: Results after a follow-up of fifteen to twenty-three years. *J Vasc Surg* 1984; 1:234–242.
6. Qvarfordt PG, Stoney RJ, Reilly LM, et al: Management of pararenal aneurysms of the abdominal aorta. *J Vasc Surg* 1986; 3:84–93.
7. Stoney RJ, Skioldebrand CG, Qvarfordt PG, et al: Juxtarenal aortic atherosclerosis. Surgical experience and functional result. *Ann Surg* 1984; 200:345–354.

17   Popliteal Artery Aneurysm

A 74-year-old man is seen for routine follow-up examination two years following successful repair of an abdominal aortic aneurysm. He has no vascular complaints. Examination is unremarkable except for a very prominent left popliteal
artery pulse.

Consultant: William M. Abbott, M.D.

The case describes a fairly common situation, but one which poses some dilemma
since, in this author's opinion, it is not entirely clear what the right course of action
is. Certainly, the finding of a prominent pulse in the popliteal space indicates the
possible presence of a popliteal artery aneurysm. It is also true that a popliteal
aneurysm poses some risk of limb loss. Exactly how serious that risk, however, is
not accurately known since there are no good studies of the natural history of popliteal artery aneurysms (i.e., left untreated) upon which to base informed decisions.
Furthermore, we do not know the best way to establish the diagnosis.
    Most published studies show that the results of treatment are better in patients
if they undergo elective operation prior to the advent of problems (symptoms or
complications). But, as just mentioned, it is not known with certainty what the
likelihood of the development of problems will be in patients when they present in
the still asymptomatic state. While data exists relating size to the risk of complications of an abdominal aortic aneurysm, there is no study that indicates a specific
size of a popliteal aneurysm that is more likely to be associated with problems. It
must also be mentioned that unlike abdominal aneurysms which usually rupture,
popliteal aneurysms are more prone to develop thromboembolic problems which
are often harder to detect or predict.
    The usual teaching, of course, is that once a popliteal artery aneurysm has
been diagnosed and has reached a certain size, surgical treatment is recommended.
However, it must be recognized that the surgical procedure is associated with definite complications. Actually, the morbidity from limb swelling in this author's experience can sometimes be especially incapacitating. Therefore, operations for popliteal artery aneurysm should not be undertaken lightly. This must be further
emphasized in the asymptomatic patient, as in the case described. Nevertheless, we

105

must come to grips with the fact that patients with popliteal artery aneurysm can have serious problems, and it is clearly appropriate to operate prophylactically on some of them.

DIAGNOSIS

The suspicion of popliteal artery aneurysm is almost always based on physical examination. The finding of a prominent pulse in the popliteal space calls attention to the possibility that such a lesion exists. However, a prominent pulse can also be due to arteriomegaly or generalized ectasia of the vessels common in patients with abdominal aortic aneurysm. Other mass lesions in the popliteal fossa also mimic aneurysm. Thus, some method is desirable to verify the diagnosis. Similarly, most surgeons would agree that it is reasonable to document the size of the aneurysm based on the premise that size probably does bear some relationship to the advent of symptoms or problems.

One method which clearly is not of great help in the diagnosis of popliteal artery aneurysm is contrast angiography, and it should not be used for this purpose. This is because an enlarged popliteal artery usually remolds its lumen with mural thrombus. Unless there is significant calcification in the wall, it is difficult to see anything other than a few "soft" signs such as luminal irregularity, loss of collateral branches, et cetera, which only imply the possible diagnosis. Angiography is indicated, as will be mentioned subsequently, in patients in whom an operation is to be performed, based on the need of seeing what the local anatomy is and defining the status of runoff vessels.

Probably the most commonly used modality for the diagnosis of popliteal artery aneurysm is ultrasound. In my experience, there is some question, however, about the accuracy of this method especially for estimating size. Clearly, if an aneurysm is imaged, it is likely to be there. However, the false negative rate is unknown and there are no well-documented studies about the accuracy of ultrasound for this diagnosis. Nevertheless, of the available methods, it remains the most useful based on the fact that it is easily obtained, gives a longitudinal view of the artery, and some information about mural thrombus.

It is my contention that the presence of mural thrombus is the key factor, not only in the identification of an aneurysm, but also is the best predictor of potential complications which are primarily thromboembolic. Mural thrombus is more thrombogenic than normal arterial intima, and thus when present, the possibilities of acute or chronic repetitive thromboembolic complications will be higher.

CT scanning is probably also useful in the diagnosis of popliteal aneurysm although it is somewhat more difficult to interpret because of the cross-sectional nature of the display. I, in particular, have not had a great deal of experience with it. Probably the most ideal method will ultimately prove to be magnetic resonance imaging (MRI). This produces scans in longitudinal (coronal or sagittal) orientation and provides the best detail regarding arterial wall anatomy yet developed. It will, in all likelihood, reliably discern mural thrombus better than ultrasound or any other extant method. Of course, it is currently very expensive and not widely available. At the Massachusetts General Hospital (MGH) we are just beginning a study in which we will prospectively compare all forms of imaging modalities for the diagnosis of popliteal artery aneurysm. Hopefully, this will give definite answers to the above-mentioned questions regarding diagnosis.

INDICATIONS FOR TREATMENT

Let us presume that we have made the diagnosis of a popliteal artery aneurysm by one method or another. For the purposes of definition, I believe that an aneurysm is a localized dilatation of a vessel 1.5 to 2 times the size of the proximal vessel, preferably in association with mural thrombus. In a popliteal artery normally 1 cm to 1.5 cm in size, a diagnosis of aneurysm would therefore be made when the popliteal artery becomes 2 cm to 3 cm in diameter. It must be emphasized, however, that the diagnosis is based on the size of the proximal artery. Although it would seem a little aggressive to operate on patients with popliteal artery dilatations of only 2 cm, nevertheless, if associated with mural thrombus, this probably does constitute significant aneurysmal disease. As a general rule, however, because of the difficulties in making the diagnosis and accurate sizing, I tend not to consider surgical intervention until the popliteal artery has reached at least 2.5 cm in size.

Probably the best indication for surgical intervention would be warning symptoms or silent signs of complications. The most common problems associated with popliteal aneurysms are thromboembolic complications, i.e., distal embolism occlusion of tibial vessels, and thrombosis of the aneurysm itself. However, since the clinical results are best if patients are treated before these occur, and since some are not reversible, this is not the best course of action. Rupture of a popliteal artery aneurysm does occur, although it is a fairly rare event. I have personally never seen a case. Local symptoms are probably more common than anticipated. These are caused by pressure on other structures in the popliteal space causing venous thrombosis and/or a nerve compression syndrome. Patients with local pain posterior to the knee and/or symptoms related to the posterior tibial nerve should have the diagnosis of aneurysm considered. If present, this warrants surgical intervention.

It is my general approach to take a patient, such as described, and perform ultrasound. If there is an aneurysm of greater than 2.5 or 3 cm, I usually recommend operation. If the size is less than that, I recommend continuing close observation. But I also usually have a frank discussion with the patient regarding the pros and cons of the two courses of action. I have seen instances in patients whom I have followed in which the aneurysm has increased in size. This I consider to be a probable indication for surgery. I have also seen the development of loose mural thrombus on ultrasound where such was not present in a previous examination. This, too, usually prompts a recommendation for operation.

Once a patient has been selected for surgical intervention, then contrast arteriography is usually performed to delineate local anatomy. Every so often one discovers that although the popliteal artery aneurysm is present with contrast filling the lumen, that all tibial vessels and identifiable outflow has been lost with the popliteal artery's patency being maintained by one of the genicular collaterals. The traditional view would be that this patient is not a surgical candidate since the likelihood of making his circulation measurably worse is significant. More recently, however, with the improvement in the results of distal tibial artery reconstruction, I have been operating on such patients, provided a reconstituted tibial vessel is seen on the angiogram. In actual fact, since this situation represents a complication (albeit silent), an even stronger case can be made for operating on such patients than those who are totally complication free.

CHOICE OF OPERATION

There are basically two types of surgical procedure that have been employed for popliteal aneurysm. The first is excision and interposition grafting and the second is exclusion with bypass grafting. There is no question in my mind that the second is preferable to the first in view of the significantly increased morbidity from the added dissection in the popliteal space required to remove a popliteal aneurysm. The problems associated with inadvertent entry into the popliteal vein with possible loss of continuity, and increased interruption of collateral artery vessels are both significant problems with the excisional operation. The desired result of the operation is the prevention of thromboembolic complications in the popliteal artery and distally, and the results with exclusion and bypass grafting are equivalent in achieving this.

The reconstruction which I prefer is illustrated in Figure 17–1. This involves suture ligation of a divided proximal popliteal artery with end-to-end proximal anastomosis and suture ligation without transection with end-to-side distal anastomosis (in essence, an end-to-end using end-to-side technique). This latter technique facilitates the anastomosis by stabilizing the distal popliteal artery. Occasionally, variations of this technique are used based on local factors, degree of disease, et cetera. In addition, there are occasions which, because of a very large aneurysm, some form of partial excision is indicated. When one does this, the control of collaterals is done from within the lumen of the aneurysm (endo-aneurysmorrhaphy). Also one should not try to dissect away too much of the aneurysm and certainly leave the back wall attached to the popliteal vein to avoid injury to it. In order to do this, however, greater exposure, with more mobilization of the artery, is required. In the usual instance (exclusion and bypass) it is not necessary to section the tendons on the medial side of the knee (hamstrings and gastrocnemius). However, with the excisional procedure it becomes necessary to do this. Although I was taught that one could take these tendons with impunity, it is my experience that the morbidity is greater and the recovery time longer in patients in whom this has been carried out.

One additional note involves the selection of graft material. Publications reflecting our own experience show that saphenous vein is clearly superior to a synthetic prosthesis. However, the prosthesis used in that series was knitted Dacron

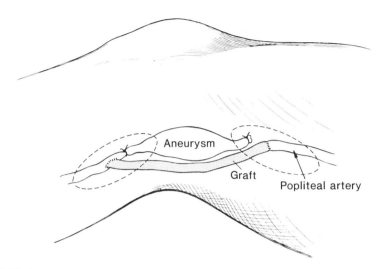

FIG 17–1
Schematic of the most commonly used surgical procedure for exclusion and bypass grafting for popliteal aneurysm.

since most of these patients had been treated prior to the availability of polytetrafluoroethylene (PTFE). I now have used PTFE in a significant number of patients with popliteal aneurysms and have not seen any complications with its use in such situations, in contrast to use of PTFE grafts for patients with occlusive disease requiring femoral-distal popliteal or tibial reconstructions. Thus, the higher flows usually present in grafts done for popliteal aneurysms, plus the shorter length of such grafts, must play a salutary role in the better performance of PTFE in this setting.

On the other hand, I think all things being equal, the saphenous vein will give superior results, and thus the operation that I perform preferentially begins with exploring the vein to assess its caliber. Unfortunately, as is often the case, the saphenous vein at the knee at least is not a very good size match to the rather enlarged vessels to which it is going to be attached. Thus, I am left with a dilemma as to whether to explore and use the vein from the thigh or whether to use a prosthetic. Although a clearcut answer is not apparent, my usual choice would be to use the vein from higher up the leg which is usually very satisfactory.

RESULTS

The results of the surgical treatment for popliteal artery aneurysm are excellent, especially if saphenous vein is used and the patient has been treated prior to the advent of symptoms or other complications. In a publication from the MGH involv-

TABLE 17-1
Early and Late Surgical Results for Popliteal Aneurysm

	EARLY GOOD RESULT	LATE GOOD RESULT
Asymptomatic	97%	89%
Complications	76%	76%
	$p < .01$	$p < .05$

ing 159 patients with 244 aneurysms, the patency of the reconstructions was excellent with an 80% patency at five years and a 65% patency at ten years. Early and late results were markedly superior in patients who were treated prior to development of complications, as shown in Table 17-1. Amputation in the asymptomatic group was 1% whereas in those with acute symptoms or complication, it was 18%. These results are similar to those in other published series.

In summary, although it must be reemphasized that good results are achieved with some morbidity, if a patient has a clearcut aneurysm of significant size, one can recommend operation with considerable confidence that potentially limb-threatening complications will be avoided and a surgical result will be achieved which is acceptable to both the surgeon and patient. The question, however, remains. Are we overtreating or undertreating this lesion? The answer to this important question awaits a randomized prospective study which after an accurate diagnosis will compare the natural history of asymptomatic lesions left untreated versus those operated on prophylactically.

BIBLIOGRAPHY

1. Evans WE, Vermilion BD: Popliteal and femoral aneurysms, in Rutherford RB (ed): *Vascular Surgery,* ed 2. Philadelphia, WB Saunders Co, 1984, pp 814–820.
2. Gooding GA, Effeney DJ: Ultrasound of femoral artery aneurysms. *AJR* 1980; 134:477–480.
3. Reilly MK, Abbott WM, Darling RC: Aggressive surgical management of popliteal artery aneurysms. *Am J Surg* 1983; 145:498–502.
4. Scott WW, Scott PP, Sanders RC: B-scan ultrasound in the diagnosis of popliteal aneurysms. *Surgery* 1977; 81:436–441.
5. Vermilion BD, Kimmins SA, Pace WG, Evans WE: A review of 147 popliteal aneurysms with long term follow-up. *Surgery* 1981; 90:1009–1014.

18 Femoral Anastomotic Aneurysm

A 65-year-old woman is referred for evaluation of intermittent discomfort in the right groin. She gives a history of an aorto-bifemoral graft procedure for occlusive disease performed at another hospital four years previously. Examination reveals a probable small pulsatile mass in the right groin.

Consultants: Christopher K. Zarins, M.D. and Hisham Bassiouny, M.D.

The case described is a typical presentation of a patient with a femoral anastomotic aneurysm. This complication occurs in 3% to 5% of patients undergoing aorto-femoral prosthetic reconstructive procedures. The average interval between the reconstructive procedure and the development of a sterile anastomotic aneurysm is about four years, as exemplified in this case presentation. If there is associated infection, pseudoaneurysms may appear as early as six months following the grafting procedure.

ETIOLOGY

Several etiologic factors have been proposed to explain the development of femoral anastomotic aneurysms. In one large series, arteriosclerotic degeneration of the host artery was incriminated as the predominant factor. Other factors that may play a role in anastomotic aneurysmal formation include prosthetic material deterioration and fatigue, overzealous endarterectomy at the anastomotic site and compliance mismatch between the graft and artery. In addition, excessive tension on the suture line or inadequate bites in the arterial wall or graft may lead to a ''serration effect,'' whereby the suture line separates with consequent hemorrhage that is contained within the surrounding fascial investment. Graft or suture line infection may also predispose to early pseudoaneurysm formation. Although some investigators have demonstrated an unexpectedly high yield of staphylococcus epidermidis after graft sonication and culture, further evidence is needed to support a cause and effect relationship. Arterial hypertension has been invoked as a systemic factor promoting aneurysmal degeneration; however, it is unlikely that it is the primary cause. Historically, braided silk sutures underwent fragmentation and degeneration, hence the current practice of using monofilament suture such as polypropylene or braided Dacron. In some cases, a history of trauma coincident with development of the aneurysm is present. Anastomotic aneurysms occur predominantly in the femoral location which may be related to undue mechanical shear or traction forces on the graft arterial junction resulting from extension of the hip.

DIAGNOSIS

Possible causes of a small pulsatile groin mass in the patient who has previously undergone aorto-femoral bypass include (1) a prominent femoral pulse secondary to prosthetic graft deterioration or due to fashioning of a wide hood at the time of anastomotic construction; (2) perigraft seroma or infection; (3) graft infection with pseudoaneurysmal formation; (4) true native arterial aneurysm degeneration; and (5) rarely, an overlying lymph node or hernia sac.

In the majority of cases these aneurysms are asymptomatic. However, chronic pain resulting from femoral nerve compression by the aneurysmal sac can be present in an intermittent or constant pattern. The presentation may be acute with a rapidly enlarging groin mass secondary to aneurysmal rupture and leakage and/or limb ischemia resulting from graft thrombosis or distal embolization. In most cases the diagnosis can be established by inspection and palpation of the groin due to the superficial location of the graft which may become quite prominent in thin patients and those with recent weight loss. Historical information concerning the size of the graft and whether an endarterectomy was performed during the initial procedure is helpful in estimating the width and quality of the femoral pulse. The presence of skin erythema, a sinus tract, or perigraft fluid collection should raise the suspicion of an existing graft infection.

In most cases it is difficult to discern between a pseudoaneurysm and a true aneurysmal degeneration of the common femoral artery. The distinction can be made pathologically by demonstrating the absence of the normal components of the arterial wall in a pseudoaneurysm. Patients who have undergone aorto-femoral bypass for aneurysmal disease may be at a higher risk for developing true femoral aneurysms at the anastomotic site. On examination, one should try to determine whether the pulse is transmitted through an enlarged lymph node or a hernial sac. A hernia can present as a groin mass but is usually medial to the vein and not pulsatile. In addition, it is unlikely that a hernia protrudes in the tunnel developed for the aorto-femoral graft limb. Physical examination should also include (1) abdominal palpation to detect any proximal anastomotic aneurysms; (2) careful examination of the ipsilateral extremity for any signs of ischemia or embolism; and (3) thorough inspection and palpation of the contralateral groin and lower extremity, as anastomotic aneurysms are frequently bilateral.

The next step in the diagnostic work is a duplex scan to confirm the presence of the aneurysm, visualize intraluminal clot, and investigate the outflow tract. Perigraft fluid collections can also be identified. An infusion CT scan is useful to rule out the possibility of a proximal anastomotic aneurysm which would increase the likelihood of infection, and to define the extent of paraprosthetic fluid collections. Conventional angiography is necessary to evaluate the proximal aortic anastomosis, visceral circulation, pelvic perfusion, and runoff vessels in order to safely plan extraanatomic bypass reconstruction if graft infection is established.

MANAGEMENT

Anastomotic aneurysms almost invariably enlarge and carry a significant risk of life and limb threatening complications. Rupture, thrombosis of the graft, or distal embolization can occur. Early diagnosis and elective management of these lesions is imperative. In general, operative repair of femoral anastomotic aneurysm should be undertaken in all patients except in a select few where the aneurysm is quite small (2 cms) or in high-risk patients with stable long-standing aneurysms. An urgent operation is indicated if recent increase in size is verified even if the patient is asymptomatic. Rupture and graft thromboses are obviously emergency situations that should be dealt with promptly.

TECHNIQUE

Most patients undergo repair of these aneurysms under epidural or spinal anesthesia. However, if extraanatomic reconstruction is anticipated, general anesthesia may be necessary. Prior to skin preparation, previous scars are marked to avoid ischemic skin flaps when the incisions are made. The field is generously prepped to encompass the abdomen, the involved extremity, and the contralateral groin. Proximal control can usually be accomplished through a groin incision directly over the pseudoaneurysm. Digital compression of the aorto-femoral bypass at the inguinal ligament gives prompt proximal control if the aneurysm is prematurely entered. In those instances when the aneurysm is located high in the femoral triangle extending under the inguinal ligament, digital compression may be difficult and a transverse suprainguinal retroperitoneal approach to gain proximal graft control separate from the pseudoaneurysm is advisable. Distal control is usually more difficult to achieve because of the dense scarring involving the femoral bifurcation. To preserve the integrity of the distal runoff and avoid iatrogenic injuries, the aneurysmal sac is incised and after evacuation of the mural thrombus, intraluminal back bleeding from the profunda femoris and superficial femoral artery can be controlled by 4 or 5F Fogarty balloon occlusion catheters. This technique is safe, expeditious, and avoids dissection of the distal runoff vessels.

Total excision of the aneurysmal sac is unnecessary and is associated with an increased risk of femoral nerve and femoral vein injuries. Following removal of the mural thrombus, the femoral bifurcation is inspected to determine if it is involved by the aneurysmal process. Proper reconstruction will depend on (1) distal runoff;

(2) common femoral artery patency and the presence or absence of retrograde pelvic perfusion; and (3) presence of graft infection. *De novo* reconstruction of the aneurysmal region is preferred to closure of suture line defects or aneurysmal plication. The use of a segment of common femoral arterial wall in the reconstruction is associated with frequent recurrence of the aneurysm and thus should be avoided. If the common femoral and external iliac arteries are occluded, a segment of new Dacron or PTFE prosthetic conduit is anastomosed end-to-end to the aorto-femoral graft limb. The distal anastomosis is performed to the femoral bifurcation, if preserved. If the superficial femoral artery is occluded, the distal anastomosis may be made directly to the profunda femoris artery or extended onto the profunda as a profundaplasty. Orificial outflow stenoses should be corrected with an endarterectomy or patch angioplasty, or both. If the superficial femoral artery is patent, flow to both the superficial femoral and profunda may be preserved by autogenous reconstruction of the femoral bifurcation. This can be achieved by a longitudinal incision of the medial wall of the superficial femoral and profunda femoris arteries and side-to-side anastomosis of the posterior walls. This creates a nondiseased more distal femoral bifurcation. The prosthetic graft is then anastomosed to the anterior wall of the new bifurcation in the standard fashion (Fig 18–1). This technique is preferable to a small bifurcation graft or side-limb branches.

When the common femoral artery is patent and retrograde flow to the pelvis

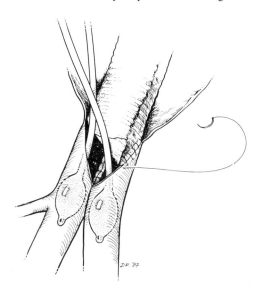

FIG 18–1.
Reconstruction of the common femoral bifurcation to provide outflow through both the superficial femoral and profunda arteries. Longitudinal incisions are made on the medial walls of the superficial femoral and profunda arteries and side-to-side anastomosis is performed posteriorly. The prosthetic bypass graft is anastomosed to the anterior wall of the newly reconstructed femoral bifurcation.

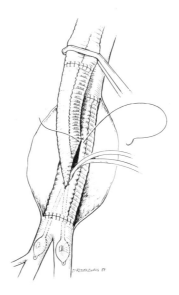

FIG 18–2.
Technique utilized to preserve retrograde pelvic arterial perfusion through the common femoral artery. The common femoral artery is replaced with an interposition graft and an end-to-side anastomosis of the aorto-femoral limb to the common femoral interposition graft is performed. A short segment interposition graft is usually necessary to provide length.

through the external iliac artery exists, a different reconstruction technique is utilized. The common femoral artery is replaced with an interposition graft from the external iliac artery to the profunda femoris and/or superficial femoral artery. The aorto-femoral bypass limb is then anastomosed end-to-side to the common femoral interposition graft. Usually there is insufficient length of the original aorto-femoral limb and an extension interposition graft must be used (Fig 18–2). Anastomoses are usually performed with 5/0 prolene. The wound is then thoroughly irrigated and after careful hemostasis, it is closed in layers to obliterate any potential dead space. The presence of infection established by a positive gram stain or preoperative cultures mandates excision of the infected graft, autogenous femoral artery reconstruction, and remote extraanatomic reconstruction, when necessary.

RESULTS

In the majority of cases, excellent results can be achieved following elective repair of femoral anastomotic aneurysms, with long-term patency in over 75% of cases, and a perioperative mortality, morbidity, and amputation rate of less than 5%. Complicated aneurysms repaired emergently, graft sepsis, or failure to correct the outflow tract portend a less favorable outcome.

SUMMARY

Femoral anastomotic aneurysms continue to challenge the vascular surgeon with an active clinical practice. Unfortunately, a measurable decline in the incidence of these lesions has not paralleled refinements in surgical technique, type of suture used, and improved quality of prosthetic conduits. Factors that may contribute to anastomotic aneurysmal formation include host arterial degeneration, infection, trauma, and excessive tension on the suture line. With careful follow-up, femoral anastomotic aneurysms can be identified early and appropriately investigated. Elective repair is favored and yields satisfactory results.

BIBLIOGRAPHY

1. Dennis JW, Littooy FN, Greisler HP, et al: Anastomotic pseudoaneurysms. A continuing late complication of vascular reconstructive procedures. *Arch Surg* 1986; 121:314–317.
2. Hollier LH, Batson RC, Cohn I Jr: Femoral anastomotic aneurysms. *Surgery* 1981; 191:715–720.
3. Satiani B, Kazmers M, Evans WE: Anastomotic arterial aneurysms. A continuing challenge. *Ann Surg* 1980; 192:674–682.
4. Schellack J, Salam A, Abouzeid MA, et al: Femoral anastomotic aneurysms: A continuing challenge. *J Vasc Surg* 1987; 6:308–317.
5. Smith RF: Anastomotic aneurysm. Current Therapy, in *Vasc Surg* 1987; pp 183–185.
6. Szilagyi DE, Smith RF, Elliott JP, et al: Anastomotic aneurysms after vascular reconstruction. *Surgery* 1975; 78:800–816.
7. Szilagyi DE, Elliott JP Jr, Smith RF, et al: A thirty-year survey of the reconstructive surgical treatment of aortoiliac occlusive disease. *J Vasc Surg* 1986; 3:421–436.
8. Tollefson ED, Bandyk DF, Kaebnick HW, et al: Surface biofilm disruption. Enhanced recovery of microorganisms from vascular prostheses. *Arch Surg* 1987; 122:38–43.

19 Incidental Colon Lesions Found at Operation for Abdominal Aortic Aneurysm

A 66-year-old man is admitted for elective repair of a 5.8-cm abdominal aortic aneurysm. At operation a firm mass is felt in the sigmoid colon in addition to the aneurysm.

Consultants: Willis H. Wagner, M.D. and
George Johnson, Jr., M.D.

INTRODUCTION

As life expectancy and the number of older patients requiring aneurysmorrhaphy increase, significant coincidental colonic disease will be more frequently encountered. A careful history and physical examination in these geriatric patients at high risk for concomitant disease may elicit signs and symptoms of previously unappreciated colonic pathology. A rectal examination with a specimen for occult blood is essential. The frequent use of CT scanning to investigate the size and extent of an abdominal aortic aneurysm (AAA) may also reveal an asymptomatic colon mass. In spite of these routine screening techniques, the dilemma in management of an unsuspected sigmoid lesion occasionally arises during aortic reconstruction.

Under these circumstances, optimal treatment of the aneurysm and the sigmoid colon will depend on many factors, including the size of the aneurysm and the presence of associated symptoms, the nature of the colon mass, evidence of metastatic disease, and the status of the patient. In most instances, replacement of the AAA should take precedence over colectomy. The issues to be considered will be addressed by a series of illustrative cases with different operative findings or clinical circumstances.

Case A: A 66-year-old man is admitted for elective repair of an abdominal aortic aneurysm. The patient is at good risk with no history of myocardial, pulmonary, or renal dysfunction. The physical examination reveals only a pulsatile abdominal mass which on ultrasound is a 5.8-cm abdominal aortic aneurysm. At the time of aneurysmorrhaphy, a firm, mobile mass is noted in the sigmoid colon. No adenopathy or intraperitoneal metastatic disease is evident.

Differentiation between benign or malignant disease may be difficult with a firm mass in the sigmoid. Thickened colon with foreshortened mesentery could represent quiescent diverticular or inflammatory bowel disease which would not warrant any intervention. Most villous or tubular adenomas may be removed endoscopically in the postoperative period, and this would be preferred to open excision at the time of aneurysm surgery.

The management of a concomitant obvious, localized sigmoid carcinoma is more problematic. Although Tilson has suggested a pathophysiologic or genetic association between AAA and carcinoma of all types, the simultaneous diagnosis of AAA and colon cancer is infrequent. This occurred once in his series of 69 patients with AAA diagnosed over a five-year period. In a classical study by Szilagyi on malignancy and AAA, malignant neoplasms of various types were diagnosed in 4% of 803 patients with AAA. However, in only four of these patients (0.5%) were the diagnoses of colorectal cancer and AAA made simultaneously in the preoperative period and in no case was an unsuspected colon cancer identified intraoperatively. Therefore, with careful attention to the history and physical examination, occult sigmoid cancer should rarely be encountered at aneurysm resection.

Our approach to coincidental AAA and colon carcinoma is determined by an assessment of which pathology poses the greatest risk to survival. Patients with large AAA (greater than 5 cm to 6 cm) have a 50% mortality at one year, and less than 10% survive for five years if treated nonoperatively according to Szilagyi's data. The behavior of such aneurysms is unpredictable, and rupture may occur at any time once they reach these proportions. In Szilagyi's series, excluding two patients with unresectable pancreatic carcinoma who died within three months of diagnosis, there were 14 patients with coincidental malignancy and large AAA who did not undergo aneurysm resection. Eight of these patients died from rupture of their aneurysms. Five ruptures occurred within six months of diagnosis, and all aneurysm-related deaths occurred within two years. Therefore, considering the current mortality rate of approximately 50% with aneurysm rupture, large aneurysms and aneurysms of any size with abdominal or back pain are considered an imminent threat to the patient's life, and early resection is indicated if survival is not drastically limited by malignancy.

Experience has been reported with simultaneous aortic reconstruction and gastrointestinal procedures, including abdomino-peroneal and sigmoid resection. However, most vascular surgeons consider creation of a colostomy a contraindication to simultaneous aortic replacement due to the grave concern for graft infection. Performance of an unanticipated colon procedure without adequate mechanical or antibiotic preparation would be expected to result in wound or peritoneal infection in more than one third of patients. A prosthetic graft has even greater risk of infection, with an attendant mortality in the range of 70%.

The intraoperative diagnosis of an asymptomatic, nonobstructing sigmoid carcinoma should not preempt resection of an aneurysm. Primary sigmoid resection in an unprepared colon would usually necessitate the use of a temporary colostomy. Because of increased risk of graft infection, colostomy closure (usually six to eight weeks later) should then precede aortic reconstruction. Even with delay of aneurysm resection until after closure of the colostomy, there can be low-grade contamination of the peritoneal cavity which may result in graft sepsis.

An additional consideration in the timing of operation is the theoretical risk of accelerated aneurysm rupture following abdominal surgical procedures. The underlying pathophysiology in AAA is believed by many to be a metabolic abnormality in the connective tissue matrix of the aortic media. Significantly increased elastase and collagenase enzymatic activity has been measured in the aortic wall of patients with AAA in comparison to patients with aortic occlusive disease, as reported by Busuttil, et al, and Cohen and associates. Since celiotomy is known in experimental animals to increase collagenolytic activity at local and remote sites, progressive weakening and dilatation of the aneurysm wall may occur after an operation. Swanson, et al, at UCSF reported an anecdoctal series of ten previously asymptomatic patients whose large abdominal aneurysms ruptured within 36 days of celiotomy. The presumed catabolism and collagen lysis which occurs in such patients prompted a policy of expeditious aneurysm resection after any recent celiotomy.

Therefore, when confronted with a firm, localized mass at the time of exploration for AAA, several factors would favor aneurysm resection: (1) uncertain diagnosis of the colon pathology; (2) the unpredictable nature of AAA rupture; (3) possible increase in the risk of rupture and aortic graft infection, if sigmoidectomy is performed primarily; (4) the usual need for colostomy and an additional procedure; and (5) the low probability of encountering an asymptomatic occult colon cancer. Even in the worse case where the mass is ultimately found to be a malignancy with nodal metastases, the five-year survival is in the range of 30% and the greatest risk to the patient's longevity may still be from an unresected aneurysm. If anticipated survival is limited by the finding of widely metastatic disease at exploration, no extirpative procedure of the aneurysm or colon would seem indicated. However, if the colon mass is bulky and obstruction appears imminent, a colectomy would be reasonable.

Case B: A 66-year-old man is admitted for elective repair of abdominal aortic aneurysm. At surgery a firm mass is felt in the sigmoid colon in addition to the aneurysm. This appears to be hyperemic and inflamed with a friable, thickened mesentery and several adhesions to small bowel in the area.

Evidence of active intraperitoneal inflammation is a contraindication to elective aneurysm resection. The only issue to consider is whether a sigmoidectomy is necessary. If a freely perforated or large contained pericolic abscess is identified, a Hartmann-type resection is appropriate. Otherwise, the prudent approach would be to close the abdomen, treat the inflammatory process, and establish a diagnosis.

The need for future sigmoid resection would depend on the underlying pathology and recurrence of symptoms.

Following resolution of clinical signs of peritoneal inflammation, the patient is still at increased risk for aortic graft infection with its extremely morbid consequences. Prosthetic graft sepsis has been reported by Casali and Read following aortic reconstruction as late as six months after apparently successful treatment of peritonitis. Bacteria cultured from the previous peritonitis and the infected graft were identical.

We consider a prior episode of peritoneal infection within six months of aortic reconstruction an indication for retroperitoneal approach. Although infected periaortic and iliac lymphatics may be encountered during this approach, we believe it is preferable to a transperitoneal exposure.

Case C: A 66-year-old man is admitted for elective repair of abdominal aortic aneurysm. On preoperative work-up, a history of hematochezia is elicited. His preoperative hematocrit is 28%. Flexible sigmoidoscopy reveals a polypoid mass at 20 cm and the pathologic diagnosis is adenocarcinoma. A CT scan demonstrates a 5.8-cm aneurysm, some thickening of the sigmoid colon wall, and no evidence of liver metastasis.

The preoperative diagnosis of sigmoid colon cancer alters our approach to these concomitant lesions from the previous recommendations when a malignancy is only suspected intraoperatively. In the case of established cancer, the size of the aneurysm assumes greater importance. While resection of a small aneurysm is reasonable in a healthy, low-risk patient with anticipated longevity, the short-term risk of rupture is sufficiently low that control of the malignancy becomes the first priority. However, if no hepatic or nodal metastases are found, the five-year survival after resection of a colon cancer may be as high as 85%. Careful postoperative surveillance of the aneurysm requires CT or ultrasound examination every six months. If symptoms related to the AAA develop or significant expansion is detected on serial examinations without evidence of recurrent malignancy, aneurysm resection should be performed.

Because of the low mortality rate for elective AAA resection and the improved accuracy of current imaging techniques, we consider an aneurysm to be large enough for routine replacement if greater than 5 cm by CT or ultrasound. In the absence of hepatic metastasis, aneurysms of this size still pose the greatest immediate threat to the patient's life. For this reason and for the lower risk of graft infection, AAA resection should precede sigmoidectomy. Standard colon preparation is performed as the findings at exploration may alter the preoperative plan and mandate a colon resection. Although we do not advocate it, some experts would perform simultaneous sigmoid resection after closure of the retroperitoneum at the time of aortic reconstruction in a patient at good risk.

A consensus among experts on the treatment of coexistent AAA and carcinoma of the colon is difficult to identify. A survey of 46 Professors of General and Vascular Surgery, published in 1985 by Lobbato, et al, showed that when the diagnosis is made preoperatively, approximately one third of the respondents favored primary colon resection, one third preferred primary aneurysm excision and one third reserved decision until the time of exploration. Only two of these surgeons recommended simultaneous operation.

Regardless of the staging of the aortic and colonic procedures, careful attention must be given to the blood supply of the left colon. Resection of a significant portion of the sigmoid mesentery may disrupt crucial collaterals from the pelvic and the superior mesenteric circulation. Therefore, if sigmoidectomy has been performed previously, or is anticipated in the future, we would routinely reimplant a patent inferior artery at the time of aortic reconstruction.

CONCLUSION

The concomitant findings of a colon mass and AAA pose a complex problem. Our recommendation for the staging of operations are given in Figure 19–1. In general, if the sigmoid mass is discovered intraoperatively and there is no acute inflammation or metastatic cancer, the surgeon should proceed with aneurysm resection. The

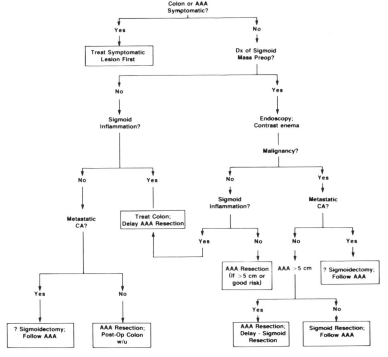

FIG 19–1.
Management of coincidental AAA and colon lesion.

treatment of sigmoid disease discovered preoperatively is determined by the colonic pathology and the size of the aneurysm.

BIBLIOGRAPHY

1. Busuttil RW, Abou-Zamzam AM, Machleder HI: Collagenase activity of the human aorta. *Arch Surg* 1980; 115:1373–1378.
2. Casali RE, Read RC: Abdominal aneurysmectomy following previous peritonitis. *Arch Surg* 1982; 117:1235–1236.
3. Cohen JR, Mandell C, Margolis I, et al: Altered aortic protease and antiprotease with ruptured abdominal aortic aneurysms. *Surg Gynecol Obstet* 1987; 164:355–358.
4. Lobbato VJ, Rothenberg RE, LaRaja RD, et al: Coexistence of abdominal aortic aneurysm and carcinoma of the colon: A dilemma. *J Vasc Surg* 1985; 2:724–726.
5. Ochsner JL, Cooley DA, DeBakey ME: Associated intra-abdominal lesions encountered during resection of aortic aneurysms surgical considerations. *Dis Colon Rectum* 1960; 3:489–490.
6. Swanson RJ, Littooy FN, Hunt TK, et al: Laparotomy as a precipitating factor in the rupture of intra-abdominal aneurysms. *Arch Surg* 1980; 115:299–304.
7. Szilagyi DE, Elliott JP, Berguer R: Coincidental malignancy and abdominal aortic aneurysm. *Arch Surg* 1967; 95:402–412.
8. Szilagyi DE, Smith RF, DeRusso FJ, et al: Contribution of abdominal aortic aneurysmectomy to prolongation of life. *Ann Surg* 1966; 164:679–699.
9. Tilson MD, Fieg EL, Harvey M: Malignant neoplasia in patients with abdominal aortic aneurysm. *Arch Surg* 1984; 119:792–794.
10. Tompkins WC, Chavez CM, Conn JH, et al: Combining intra-abdominal arterial grafting with gastrointestinal or biliary tract procedures. *Am J Surg* 1973; 126:598–600.

20 Colon Ischemia Following Aortic Surgery

You perform an uneventful abdominal aortic aneurysm repair on a 70-year-old man. Postoperatively, however, the patient remains in the intensive care unit with moderate tachycardia, marginal urine output, and progressive abdominal distension. Thirty-six hours postoperatively, he passes some blood-tinged liquid stool.

Consultants: Leslie W. Ottinger, M.D. and Jose P. Garcia, M.D.

This 70-year-old man has remained in the intensive care setting with nonspecific but worrisome symptoms of tachycardia, oliguria, and abdominal distension after uneventful repair of an abdominal aortic aneurysm. Now, 36 hours postoperatively, there has been the development of bloody diarrhea, a certain sign of an ischemic injury to the distal colon and perhaps a clue to the generally unsatisfactory course. On the way to evaluate the patient and develop a plan of management, what information might come to mind?

THOUGHTS ON THE WAY TO THE INTENSIVE CARE UNIT

First, is the sign of bloody diarrhea a reliable and typical one for colon injury? In fact, only perhaps a third of patients with an ischemic injury to the distal colon from sacrifice of the inferior mesenteric artery will have early bloody diarrhea. Another third will have simple diarrhea and the last third present systemic or local signs and symptoms of infarction or perforation without diarrhea of any sort. Still, bloody diarrhea at 36 hours almost surely makes the diagnosis: Diarrhea from spasm and irritability of the distal colon rather than the expected ileus following abdominal surgery; bleeding from infarction and slough of the mucosa.

Next, how common is the problem? In fact, it is so rare that the routine use of some effective preventative measures are generally felt unnecessary. These include preparation of the colon with orally administered nonabsorbable antibiotics, similar to those used prior to colon resection, and routine revascularization of the inferior mesenteric artery. Clinically important distal colon injuries due to ligation of the inferior mesenteric artery can be expected in perhaps 2% of elective operations and in twice that incidence in emergency operations, especially for ruptured aneurysms. In either event, intraoperative hypotension, trauma to the sigmoid colon and ligation of the inferior mesenteric vein will increase the likelihood of infarction.

Are there clues to subsequent development of intestinal infarction from the preoperative history and evaluation? Was there a history that suggests chronic episodic intestinal ischemia with weight loss, postprandial pain and intestinal dysfunction? In that event, the possibility of stenosis or occlusion of the superior mesenteric artery and celiac axis should be evaluated preoperatively, perhaps with the plan for reconstruction of the mesenteric vascular system at the time of aneurysm resection. Was a preoperative aortogram performed? Indeed, unsuspected mesenteric vascular disease is one of the primary indications for the routine use of preoperative angiography prior to aneurysm repair. Angiography would also have provided important information regarding the inferior mesenteric artery. Is it occluded, normal in appearance or unusually large? If occluded or normal, collateral inflow from the middle colic branch of the superior mesenteric artery and the hemorrhoidal branches of the hypogastric vessels must be preserved. Enlargement suggests the possible critical nature of the vessel as a collateral to the superior mesenteric artery, and the necessity to reimplant the inferior mesenteric artery, revascularize the superior mesenteric artery, or both at the time of aneurysm repair. Finally, has there been previous colon surgery which might interrupt collateral flow in marginal arteries to the sigmoid colon? In such circumstances, the dangers of colon ischemia will be increased, particularly if the inferior mesenteric artery is patent. Even if this vessel is occluded, extra efforts to preserve hypogastric system blood flow are warranted to preserve vital collateral flow, and excessive trauma or traction on the sigmoid mesentery avoided.

What about intraoperative management and clues? Was the inferior mesenteric artery carefully divided at its origin to preserve continuity of branches through the main trunk for collateral flow? Was there a hematoma in the sigmoid colon mesentery to suggest injury to mesenteric branch vessels, perhaps from retraction? Was inflow to at least one hypogastric artery preserved to enhance collateral flow to the left colon in case collateral flow from the superior mesenteric artery was deficient? Was the inferior mesenteric artery unusually large, in which case either reimplantation or revascularization by a small side graft would have been advisable? Finally, what did the left and sigmoid colon look like at the end of the procedure? Were there pulses in the peripheral branches of the superior mesenteric and hypogastric arteries? Since visual inspection of the colon itself is unrevealing in most cases of distal colon injury, should other measures to evaluate circulation have been used before completing the operation? These could have included demonstrating pulsatile mural flow with a Doppler device, examining the intestine under ultraviolet light after injection of fluorescein, or measuring the stump pressure. Of course there might be some consolation in not having used these, since most experienced vascular surgeons do not.

Last, in which of four clinical groups does this particular patient fall? Is this a case of superficial mucosal infarction, from which complete recovery after a few days or weeks of diarrhea will be observed? Or is this a case of partial thickness mural injury that will lead to a localized colitis and eventual stricture formation requiring resection after several weeks of diarrhea and partial obstruction? Of more concern is the possibility that our patient represents a case of localized full thickness infarction that will eventuate in local perforation and delayed abscess formation with resultant risk of prosthetic graft infection? In the worst scenario, is this a case of extensive colon and even small bowel infarction? In that event, unless the inferior mesenteric artery was also supplying the distribution of the superior mesenteric artery, one must wonder about the possibility of intraoperative embolization of a piece of atheroma to the main trunk of the superior mesenteric artery or of atherosclerotic debris to peripheral branches. Extensive infarction with fluid sequestration, metabolic acidosis and release of vasoactive factors resulting in hypotension and oliguria could give this clinical course. Emboli, large or small, to renal arteries might also account for oliguria.

SUBSEQUENT PATIENT MANAGEMENT

Although an ischemia injury to the distal colon can be presumed from the development of bloody diarrhea, diagnostic confirmation may be desired. In this event, rigid sigmoidoscopy at the bedside will suffice, since the injury extends into the upper rectum. Gentle visualization without preparation will characteristically show submucosal hemorrhage and marked friability. Infarction is not often seen. Later, mucosal slough with ulcers and patches of granulation tissue may be noted but are not seen in early stages. Flexible endoscopy is not needed and may risk perforation. Enema contrast studies also are not useful, often being normal at this early stage and also risking perforation.

In this particular patient, unless the tachycardia and decreased urine output can be otherwise explained, an extensive infarction must be suspected. The third sign, abdominal distension, is not specific enough to be helpful unless it reflects perforation and peritonitis, an unusual early event. Then, two immediate courses are available. One is angiography with selective visualization of the superior mesenteric artery. If it is normal, further observation might be elected. However, even a normal study would not exclude the possibility of colon ischemia, and if the diagnosis is seriously considered, immediate abdominal exploration is the best course. If infarction in the small bowel or colon proximal to the splenic flexure is found and there is occlusion of the main trunk of the superior mesenteric artery, restoration of flow by embolectomy or bypass graft is to be used. Then resection is carried out as needed, as in any case of acute occlusion of the superior mesenteric artery. If there is extensive infarction of only the left colon, resection with a transverse end colostomy and closure with drainage of the rectal stump is usually the best choice. The damage will have been done, and revascularization of the inferior mesenteric artery is not a useful alternative.

If there is no suspicion of extensive intestinal infarction, a more conservative approach is elected. Parenteral antibiotics are continued and close observation for evidence of local perforation is used. Persistence of fever and leukocytosis after a few days make this likely, as does increasing tenderness in the left abdomen. Ultrasound studies have little value, but a CT scan may show an early perforation and abscess. With perforation, drainage alone is seldom the best choice for management. Rather, resection of the involved colon and drainage with colostomy, with later restoration of colon continuity, is safer. Early diagnosis and management of perforation is to be stressed in order to avoid infection of the prosthetic graft.

The chance of direct contamination of the graft at the time of operation for perforation or infarction dictates careful management of the operative field. Packs are used to contain spillage during drainage of an abscess and transection of the bowel. The previous incision in the posterior peritoneum is carefully avoided. Dissection in the mesentery of the colon should be immediately adjacent to the colon itself.

The incidence of recovery with nonoperative management is high enough that most surgeons do not adopt the policy of early resection of ischemic colitis in every case. Persistence of symptoms of diarrhea and partial obstruction beyond a few weeks suggest stricturing of the colon and should be evaluated by barium enema and, in some cases, colonoscopy. Resection with primary anastomoses can usually be accomplished for this late complication.

Finally, the importance of precise management for the patient with a clinically apparent ischemic injury to the distal colon following elective aortic surgery should be stressed. Overall mortality rates for this diagnosis remain in the range of 50%. The colon injury itself is the cause or a major contributing cause in most of these fatal cases.

BIBLIOGRAPHY

1. Ernst CB: Intestinal ischemia following abdominal aortic reconstruction, in *Complications in Vascular Surgery*. Orlando, Grune & Stratton, 1985, pp 325–350.
2. Griffith JD: Extramural and intramural blood supply of the colon. *Br Med J* 1961; 1:323–326.
3. Mann A, Fazio VW, Lucas FV: A comparative study of the use of fluorescein and the Doppler device in the determination of intestinal viability. *Surg Gynecol Obstet* 1982; 154:53–64.
4. Marston A, Marcuson RW, Chapman M, et al: Experimental study of devascularization of the colon. *GUT* 1969; 10:121–130.
5. Ottinger LW, Darling RC, Nathan MJ, et al: Left colon ischemia complicating aorto-iliac reconstruction. *Arch Surg* 1972; 105:841–846.
6. Schroeder T, Christoffersen JK, Andersen J, et al: Ischemic colitis complicating reconstruction of the abdominal aorta. *Surg Gynecol Obstet* 1985; 160:299–303.

21　Aortoenteric Fistula

A 73-year-old man is brought to the emergency room with hematemesis and tarry stools. Two years ago he had undergone repair of an abdominal aortic aneurysm. One month previously he vomited some coffee grounds material but this was self-limited, and an upper gastrointestinal series obtained by his family physician was reported as negative.

Consultant: Calvin B. Ernst, M.D.

When encountering such a patient, one must recall the dictum that any patient with gastrointestinal bleeding and a history of aortic reconstruction must be assumed to have an aortoenteric fistula until proven otherwise. Although an aortoenteric fistula is a rare complication of aortic reconstruction and an unusual cause of gastrointestinal bleeding, assuming the worst helps focus attention on expeditious evaluation which is the key to successful management. Delay in diagnosis as a result of inappropriate diagnostic studies may preclude successful therapy because such delay may result in catastrophic hemorrhage requiring management under emergent circumstances with the inevitable fatal outcome. For these reasons, possible signs and symptoms of an aortoenteric fistula must be taken very seriously. Unfortunately, no currently available diagnostic test or combination of tests are sufficiently accurate to consistently identify aortoenteric communications. On occasion, the diagnosis can only be made by celiotomy.

CLASSIFICATION OF AORTOENTERIC FISTULAE

Aortoenteric fistulae may be primary or secondary. Secondary fistulae follow previous aortic reconstructive procedures, whereas the primary type arise *de novo,* usually from an aortic aneurysm.

　　Secondary fistulae, the subject of this discussion, are subdivided into graft anastomotic enteric fistulae, which are direct communications between aortic lumen and the bowel, and graft enteric erosions or paraprosthetic sinuses where a direct communication does not exist between aortic lumen and bowel. In the latter, gastrointestinal bleeding results from ulceration or erosion of the bowel wall. However, as the pathologic process evolves, gastrointestinal enzymes may dissect along the prosthesis to the aortic anastomosis which is digested, resulting in an aortoenteric fistula.

Over 80% of aortoenteric fistulae or paraprosthetic sinuses involve the third or fourth portions of the duodenum where it lies adjacent to the aortic prosthesis. Consequently, hematemesis may be one of the symptoms. However, when other segments of the gastrointestinal tract, well beyond the ligament Trietz are involved, hematemesis will never occur and rectal bleeding becomes a manifestation of such a complication.

The exact role of primary graft infection in the genesis of aortoenteric complications is impossible to determine because of the high incidence of positive cultures found at the time of repair of aortoenteric fistulae or sinuses. Undoubtedly, both mechanical and infectious factors play a role in the development of aortoenteric fistulae and most authors seem to favor a primary erosive process followed by secondary infection. Most important is the knowledge that infection is universally present; therefore, successful treatment requires management of both the gastrointestinal bleeding and the infected graft. Successful outcome hinges primarily on appropriate management of the graft complication, whereas the gastrointestinal problem assumes lesser importance.

CLINICAL PRESENTATION

The classic triad of abdominal pain, gastrointestinal bleeding, and sepsis is rarely found in any one patient. More commonly, patients present with a variety of symptoms including gastrointestinal bleeding, fever, malaise, septic emboli to the legs, and abdominal or back pain.

The magnitude of the bleeding depends on the type of fistula. A direct communication between the aorta and the bowel is manifest by intermittent massive gastrointestinal bleeding which may be accompanied by profound hypotension. Rarely, however, does the patient bleed to death even with a direct aortoenteric communication. Bleeding episodes are usually intermittent and occur over several days or weeks. On the other hand, bleeding from a graft enteric erosion or paraprosthetic sinus is characterized by low volume blood loss, usually manifest as occult lower gastrointestinal bleeding and leading to chronic anemia rather than hematemesis.

Signs of systemic sepsis are more common with graft enteric erosions or paraprosthetic sinuses than with fistulae. Therefore, symptoms related to either bleeding (for direct communications) or sepsis (for enteric erosions or paraprosthetic sinuses) may predominate.

Of note is that the average interval from aortic reconstruction to clinical recognition of an aortoenteric complication ranges widely from two days to 14 years with an average of three to five years. The interval between aortic surgery and bleeding in the current case is certainly compatible with a diagnosis of aortoenteric fistula.

DIAGNOSIS

Because of the vagarities in clinical presentation, a high index of suspicion must be maintained for diagnosis. Hence, the dictum that any patient with a history of aortic reconstruction who develops gastrointestinal bleeding should be considered to have an aortoenteric fistula until proven otherwise, should sensitize the clinician to aggressively investigate this possibility. Diagnostic evaluation of patients with suspected aortoenteric fistulae is dictated by their clinical presentations. Fortunately, most present with either nonexsanguinating hemorrhage or sepsis which permits deliberate but expeditious evaluation. Among patients with massive bleeding and profound hypotension, preoperative evaluation is not possible and diagnosis must be made at emergency celiotomy. Probably less than 20% of patients will present in this manner.

Numerous diagnostic studies have been proposed, but, individually, all have a low sensitivity, approximating only 50%. Gastroduodenal endoscopy appears to be the most reliable study and should be the first choice, yet diagnostic accuracy is only about 50%. It is important that the endoscopist thoroughly evaluate the third and fourth portions of the duodenum and not be misled by superficial erosions involving the proximal duodenum, stomach, or gastroesophageal junction. Hemodynamically unstable patients should be endoscoped in the operating room because, occasionally, such a patient may suddenly develop massive bleeding during the endoscopic examination.

Other diagnostic studies such as CT scanning, nuclear imaging techniques, barium contrast studies, and arteriography only indirectly suggest graft enteric fistulae by documenting paraprosthetic infection or anastomotic abnormalities. The specificity of such studies, however, is unacceptably low. In spite of the limited diagnostic potential, aortography is helpful in planning operation and I obtain it, if the patient's condition permits.

Recently, magnetic resonance imaging (MRI) has been suggested as a diagnostic modality for prosthetic infections. However, limited experience with MRI among patients with proven aortoenteric communications precludes a definitive statement regarding its accuracy. MRI does appear to be about 80% sensitive for aortic graft infection, however.

In summary, all hemodynamically stable patients should first undergo upper gastrointestinal endoscopy. In addition, CT scanning appears to be the most sensitive and readily available secondary diagnostic test which should be performed as well. Arteriography, although not mandatory, facilitates aortic reconstruction. If all diagnostic studies are negative, a period of cautious observation is justified. Should bleeding recur, or febrile symptoms not subside on antibiotic therapy, diagnostic celiotomy will be required to establish the diagnosis.

OPERATIVE MANAGEMENT

Operation represents the only treatment option for an aortoenteric fistula because, if left untreated, death is inevitable and universal. Objectives of operation are: (1) control of bleeding, (2) closure of the bowel defect, (3) eradication of associated infection, and (4) selective restoration of distal circulation.

The magnitude of the bleeding dictates urgency of operation. Massive bleeding mandates immediate operation. Most commonly, operation can be undertaken electively after appropriate preoperative evaluation, preparation, and planning.

After opening the abdomen, the bowel is dissected from the aortic graft. The most fortunate circumstance is to be able to control bleeding by infrarenal aortic clamping or by threading an aortic occlusion balloon catheter into the defect (Fig 21–1). Alternatively, aortic occlusion may be obtained at the diaphragmatic hiatus through the lesser space. After achieving control of bleeding, the aorta is further dissected and prepared for closure. Closure of the bowel defect may require only a few sutures or a segmental resection with a two layer end-to-end anastomosis.

After controlling hemorrhage and repairing the bowel defect, management of the aortic graft anastomosis provides the greatest challenge. Several treatment options exist including (1) the local repair of an anastomotic defect, (2) complete graft excision without revascularization, (3) partial or complete graft excision with *in situ* prosthetic graft replacement, (4) graft excision with autogenous tissue *in situ*

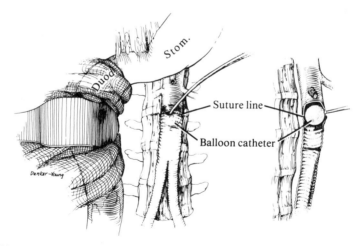

FIG 21–1.
Method of temporarily tamponading the aortic defect with a balloon-tipped catheter. The infrarenal aortic stump may then be precisely dissected and controlled in a standard manner. (From Ernst CB: Aortoenteric fistulas, in Haimovici H (ed): *Vascular Emergencies*. E Norwalk, CT, Appleton-Century-Crofts, 1982. Used with permission.)

replacement, and (5) complete graft excision with selective extraanatomic revascularization.

When analyzing published studies from centers most experienced in managing this complication, it is apparent that graft excision with restoration of distal circulation by selective extraanatomic reconstruction produces the best results. Certainly, any gross sepsis in the retroperitoneum mandates complete graft excision and secure aortic stump closure using viable healthy aortic tissue, and coverage of the aortic stump with a transposed pedicle of omentum (Fig 21–2). In unusual instances, however, with minimal or no retroperitoneal sepsis, repair of the bowel defect and graft excision and *in situ* replacement with a new prosthetic graft in the bed of the original graft has been successful in selected patients. Lesser procedures such as local suture repair are followed by a high incidence of fistula recurrence and death, and should be avoided.

Since aortic stump dehiscence may occur in up to one third of patients who undergo complete graft excision without replacement, partial or complete graft excision with replacement has possible merit because this dreaded complication is thereby prevented. Nonetheless, current practice still favors complete graft excision, repair of the bowel defect, and selective remote bypass. Accepting this approach, the timing and sequence of graft excision and extraanatomic reconstruction deserve comment.

Operation for exsanguinating hemorrhage precludes any preliminary remote bypass reconstructive procedure. Under these circumstances, a life-saving proce-

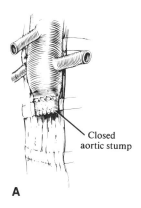
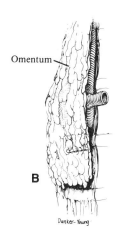

FIG 21–2.
Method of closing the infrarenal aorta following prosthesis excision. **A,** Proximal row of continuous horizontal mattress sutures is followed by a distal row of continuous over-and-over sutures. **B,** Omental graft, passed through the transverse mesicolon and sutured over the aortic stump, provides additional buttressing and protection.

dure is mandatory, necessitating graft excision followed by extraanatomic reconstruction, if required. Individuals most likely to require extraanatomic reconstruction, usually an axillobifemoral bypass, are those whose legs appear to be in jeopardy after excision of the aortic graft. These include individuals whose original aortic reconstruction was for aneurysmal disease, where collateral had not developed. Those in whom the original aortic procedure was for occlusive disease usually do not require immediate axillobifemoral bypass because of adequate preexisting collaterals. In either circumstance, if on examining the lower extremities in the operating room no Doppler sounds are audible at the ankles, immediate axillobifemoral bypass is necessary to prevent amputation. If, however, the patient's condition is so precarious that immediate extraanatomic reconstruction may prove fatal, then delayed amputation may be an acceptable alternative.

The majority of individuals may be operated on electively. Consequently, when anticipating need for extraanatomic reconstruction, such a procedure should be performed before aortic graft excision. Staging the two procedures with delay between remote bypass and aortic graft excision allows the patient to partially recover from the stress of the remote bypass. When possible, a three- to five-day interval appears optimal and justified.

A key technical point after removing the graft is to close the aortic stump with two layers of monofilament suture, being sure to use as healthy aortic tissue available as possible. I use a running horizontal mattress suture placed as proximal as necessary to secure healthy tissue, followed by a running over-and-over stitch distal to the mattress closure. This may require debridement of the aortic stump back to the renal arterial ostea in which case suprarenal aortic clamping is necessary. Rarely, aortic debridement must include the renal arteries. Under these circumstances, autogenous tissue reconstruction by means of bypass will be required to maintain function of at least one kidney. Use of healthy aorta minimizes aortic stump dehiscence which has been the Achilles' heel of graft excision and selective extraanatomic reconstruction. Such catastrophes have led to reassessment of *in situ* aortic regrafting after graft excision, feeling that recurrent graft infection is the lesser of two evils.

Whether the graft is completely excised and the aortic stump closed or a new prosthesis is placed in the bed of the old, another key technical maneuver is to suture a viable pedicle of omentum over the aortic stump or the newly placed graft to adequately isolate it in the retroperitoneum (Fig 21–2). Use of a pedicle of omentum provides infection resistant and possibly infection eradicating coverage of the retroperitoneal sepsis. The aortic stump should be biopsied and cultured for bacteria and long-term (six weeks to three months) antibiotic therapy should be given according to bacterial antibiotic sensitivity results.

In the event preoperative diagnosis cannot be made in a patient with chronic blood loss, anemia, and sepsis, diagnostic celiotomy has merit. Under such circumstances, it is mandatory that all bowel be dissected from the aortic graft as well as the aortic and distal iliac anastomoses. Only by separating all bowel segments from the graft can an aortoenteric fistula or paraprosthetic sinus be definitively excluded.

Simply palpating the retroperitoneum during diagnostic celiotomy does not suffice. Definitive treatment will then be dictated by operative findings.

RESULTS

Results depend on the clinical situation encountered. In general, staged preliminary extraanatomic reconstruction followed by graft excision results in a 25% mortality rate and an approximately 20% amputation rate. Recent reports suggest similar results with partial or complete graft excision and *in situ* regrafting. However, comparisons between treatment methods for this complex problem are not easy or justified, and validation of the latter "conservative" approach must be provided before it can be designated treatment of choice.

PREVENTION OF AORTOENTERIC FISTULA

Clearly, prevention of this catastrophic complication is more important than successful management. Many elements comprise the equation of prevention and in-

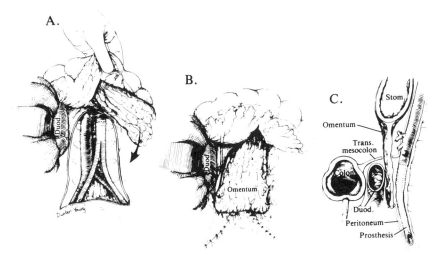

FIG 21–3.
A, Omentum passed through an incision in transverse mesocolon. **B,** Omentum sutured to the retroperitoneal tissues covers the prosthesis, separating the prosthesis from the duodenum. **C,** Sagittal view, showing omentum passed through the transverse mesocolon and interposed between the prosthesis and bowel. (From Ernst CB: Aortoenteric fistulas, in Haimovici H (ed): *Vascular Emergencies.* E Norwalk, CT, Appleton-Century-Crofts, 1982. Used with permission.)

clude gentle meticulous surgical technique when performing aortic reconstruction, use of synthetic suture, anastomosis to healthy aorta, end-to-end aortic anastomosis rather than end-to-side, and prophylactic antibiotics. The most important element is coverage of the aortic prosthesis with viable tissue. Following aneurysm repair, the debrided aneurysm sac must be closed over the prosthesis to isolate it from the bowel. Following reconstruction for occlusive disease, preaortic peritoneum should be imbricated over the prosthesis, interposing the left retroperitoneal flap to available tissue between the aortic graft and vena cava. Occasionally, in very thin individuals or in redo aortic operations, there is insufficient retroperitoneal tissue for adequate coverage. In this situation, a pedicle of omentum may be passed through the transverse mesicolon and sutured over the prosthesis (Fig 21–3). Adoption of these principles over the past three decades has probably been responsible for the steady decline in the incidence of secondary aortoenteric fistulae. Continued adherence to these practices may lead to the eventual eradication of this dreaded complication.

BIBLIOGRAPHY

1. Bunt TJ: Synthetic vascular graft infections. II. Graft-enteric erosions and graft-enteric fistulas. *Surgery* 1983; 94:1–9.
2. Champion MC, Sullivan SN, Coles JC, et al: Aortoenteric fistula. Incidence, presentation, recognition, and management. *Ann Surg* 1982; 195:314–317.
3. O'Donnell TF Jr, Scott G, Shepard A, et al: Improvements in the diagnosis and management of aortoenteric fistula. *Am J Surg* 1985; 149:481–486.
4. O'Hara PJ, Hertzer NR, Bevan EG, et al: Surgical management of infected abdominal aortic grafts: Review of a 25-year experience. *J Vasc Surg* 1986; 3:725–731.
5. O'Mara CS, Williams GM, Ernst CB: Secondary aortoenteric fistula. A 20 year experience. *Am J Surg* 1981; 142:203–209.
6. Reilly LM, Stoney RJ, Goldstone J, et al: Improved management of aortic graft infection: The influence of operation sequence and staging. *J Vasc Surg* 1987; 5:421–431.
7. Thomas WEG, Baird RN: Secondary aorto-enteric fistulae: Towards a more conservative approach. *Br J Surg* 1986; 73:875–878.
8. Trout HH III, Kozloff L, Giordano JM: Priority of revascularization in patients with graft enteric fistulas, infected arteries, or infected arterial prostheses. *Ann Surg* 1984; 199:669–683.
9. Walker WE, Cooley DA, Duncan JM, et al: The management of aortoduodenal fistula by *in situ* replacement of the infected abdominal aortic graft. *Ann Surg* 1987; 205:727–732.

22 Ischemic Foot Following Aneurysm Repair

A patient is admitted for elective repair of an abdominal aortic aneurysm. Peripheral pulses are present bilaterally preoperatively. At operation, aneurysmal disease involves the aortic bifurcation and both proximal common iliac arteries, and you insert an aortoiliac bifurcation graft. As the drapes are removed, it is noted that the right foot is cold, pale, and mottled.

Consultant: Fredric Jarrett, M.D.

Distal limb ischemia is one of the most feared complications in aortic surgery. Three major causes of arterial occlusion may be responsible: technical misadventures or clot in the iliac vessels, clot in the femoropopliteal system, or microemboli in the tibial and pedal vessels. As with many complications, the treatment is far more difficult than are planned measures to avoid their occurrence.

Preoperative evaluation should provide as much information as possible about the aortoiliac system and distal vessels from both the anatomic and functional viewpoint. I believe that all patients undergoing aortic aneurysm surgery should have noninvasive vascular laboratory evaluation including segmental Doppler pressures and waveforms before and after exercise. Even patients with palpable pedal pulses may have a measure of occlusive disease, and it is best to document any functional impairment prior to operation. It also is my practice to obtain biplanar aortography on all patients undergoing elective aortic aneurysm resection to define the extent and geographic limits of the aneurysm, and to identify renal artery stenoses and iliac and femoropopliteal occlusive disease. Such information is useful in planning certain intraoperative technical details and can also be of assistance if complications arise and secondary procedures become necessary.

PREVENTION

Distal thromboembolization during aneurysm resection can occur at three times during the operation: during dissection and mobilization of the aneurysm, at the time of clamp application, and during clamp release. The technical conduct of the aortic aneurysm resection is designed to minimize dissection and thereby prevent thromboemboli. Several points merit particular emphasis. The neck of the aneurysm need not be dissected circumferentially in most instances, since anterolateral dissection alone is sufficient to allow clamp application in the anteroposterior plane. The iliacs, likewise, need be dissected only enough to permit clamp application. The common iliacs are usually least diseased and adherent to the iliac veins at their bifurcation. Alternatively, control can be obtained of the external iliacs, or dissection obviated entirely by using intraluminal catheters for occlusion. Since complete excision of the aneurysm is only performed in cases of infected aneurysms, there is no reason to perform extensive dissection of the body of the aneurysm itself. Moreover, since the nerves controlling erectile function cross over the left side of the aorta and the left common iliac artery, particular care should be taken to perform only minimal dissection in these areas in sexually active men.

Adequate heparin should be given intravenously by the anesthetist just prior to cross-clamping; 100 units per kg is a more than adequate dose in almost all instances. Additional heparin may be given if clamp time exceeds one hour. The iliac vessels should be clamped before the neck of the aneurysm in an effort to prevent microembolization. After the aorta is opened, the intraluminal thrombus removed, and the lumbar vessels ligated, the neck of the aneurysm is forcefully irrigated with heparinized-saline solution to dislodge any adherent intraluminal thrombus which may be present. On some occasions, a limited endarterectomy of the neck of the aneurysm is necessary, just as it is with occlusive disease. After doing so, the graft is sewn in, working within the lumn of the aneurysm as much as possible. The iliac arteries should be palpated for evidence of occlusive disease prior to deciding on where to construct the distal anastomosis. If the common iliac artery is aneurysmal, the distal anastomosis may be performed at its bifurcation and an attempt made to fashion the hood of the graft so that both the hypogastric and external iliac are perfused. If the common iliac bifurcation is not adequate, the distal anastomosis can be constructed to the external iliac, or even to the common femoral, and the common iliac ligated just above the bifurcation or sewn closed from within the aneurysm. Construction of the distal anastomosis to the external iliac or femoral artery allows the surgeon to sew to a less diseased vessel, potentially avoiding dislodging atheromatous material, while at the same time allowing back perfusion of the hypogastrics. I prefer to remove the aortic clamp after completing the first iliac anastomosis. Before doing so, the graft can be flushed through the contralateral open limb which is then reclamped, and then the flow reestablished, first to the hypogastric and then to the external iliac. In this way, any small amount of clot present within the graft will be either flushed out or sent down the hypogastric system, hopefully with less sequelae. Next, the second iliac anastomosis is completed, and prior to tying the running suture, the graft is briefly flushed again and then the clamp removed from the hypogastric prior to establishing flow to the leg.

The iliac and femoral pulses should be palpated before closing the abdomen. A useful practice is to place the lower drapes so that the feet can be observed prior to closing the abdomen merely by walking to the foot of the table. In this way, occasional operative mishaps can be identified before the abdomen is closed.

RECOGNITION

A cold, pale, mottled foot observed after removal of the drapes suggests distal ischemia. It is important initially to distinguish true ischemia from the appearance of the feet in a hypothermic and vasoconstricted individual who has just undergone a major aortic procedure. Bilateral abnormalities make vasoconstriction and hypothermia more likely, while unilateral findings suggest ischemia due to thromboembolic occlusion of outflow vessels. It is equally important to distinguish large-vessel occlusion from small-vessel "trash." Femoral, popliteal, and pedal pulses should be checked. The absence of palpable pedal pulses initially is not necessarily indicative of ischemia, but a marked difference in the appearance and temperature of the two feet is, providing their circulation was approximately equal before operation. Doppler pulses are usually present even in the absence of palpable pedal pulses, although on several occasions Doppler pulses have not been initially audible in a patient who was hypothermic and whose operative procedure had been totally uneventful. Ankle pressures should be measured with the Doppler. Because our patient had intact pulses preoperatively, and presumably patent leg vessels and relatively normal circulation bilaterally, any significant Doppler systolic pressure difference would support a diagnosis of unilateral ischemia. Similarly, a marked reduction on both sides might suggest bilateral thromboembolic ischemia.

TREATMENT

If the femoral pulse is absent it is likely that a technical problem exists at the graft-to-iliac artery anastomosis, or clot is present in the iliofemoral system. The availability of additional cross-matched blood should be ascertained and the abdomen reprepped and draped. Since the legs may need to be explored as well, both legs should be prepped and draped in their entirety. Several technical options are available. One is to reopen the abdomen and reexplore the anastomosis between graft and iliac artery. Control of the graft limb may be obtained with a silastic loop, and control of the iliac vessel obtained at the site of its previous dissection. Additional systemic heparin should be given and the anastomosis taken down. Careful inspection of the inner aspect of the vessel should allow identification of a correctable technical problem (if one exists) such as an intimal flap, occlusive thrombus, or constriction of the iliac vessel due to application of a vascular clamp. The quality of the backbleeding should be noted, even though it is well understood that seemingly adequate backbleeding is no assurance of the patency of distal vessels. A Fogarty catheter can be passed distally through the open artery. This maneuver serves two purposes. The patency of the arterial system can be confirmed by passage of the catheter, and any distal thrombus may be retrieved by withdrawal of the catheter with the balloon inflated. If clot is retrieved, additional passes with the Fogarty catheter should be made until no further clot is obtained.

A second option, which is preferable if the external iliac is heavily diseased, is to explore the common femoral artery, which may be rapidly isolated through a longitudinal groin incision. This vessel will almost always be less diseased than the iliacs. Occasionally, the cause of the pulse deficit will be occluding clot which is found on opening the artery or on exploring its proximal inflow. Removal of this clot will restore inflow at systemic arterial pressure. Much more often, satisfactory inflow will not be obtained, but the common and superficial femoral will be open and free of clot. My preference in such circumstances is to construct a short graft to the common femoral. An additional segment of prosthetic graft can be rapidly sewn end-to-side to the involved aortoiliac graft limb, tunnelled retroperitoneally along the external iliac artery, and sewn end-to-side to the common femoral. The distal arterial tree should be explored with a Fogarty catheter prior to constructing the distal anastomosis. A completion arteriogram should be obtained to visualize the popliteal artery and its outflow. The circulatory status of the foot can then be reevaluated, and if the arteriogram is satisfactory, there is a good likelihood that the foot will improve.

If unilateral ischemia is observed with a normal femoral pulse, the problem is more difficult (Fig 22–1). Sometimes it is justified to return the patient to the intensive care unit for several hours of observation. If hypothermia and hypovolemia are present, they can be treated vigorously during this period. If findings of unilateral ischemia persist after several hours, they should be addressed by either performing an arteriogram or by exploring the femoropopliteal system operatively. If retrievable clot is present, its removal is the best method of reversing distal ischemia. My

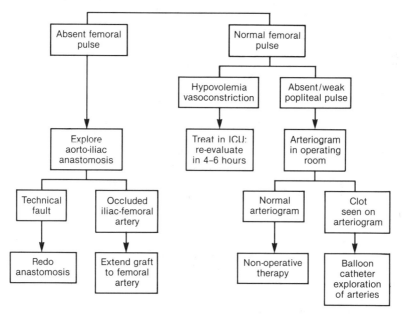

Fig 22-1
Algorithm for management of unilateral limb ischemia after aneurysm repair.

own perference is to deal with the problem in the operating room immediately. I believe an arteriogram should be obtained to attempt to demonstrate thromboembolic material in the popliteal and tibial vessels. If the popliteal pulse is absent, catheter embolectomy should be performed, and it is best attempted by a common femoral artery approach because of the size and easy accessibility of the common femoral. I obtain completion arteriograms after all embolectomies, since neither backbleeding nor passage of a balloon catheter is assurance of removal of all thromboembolic material. Most emboli in the popliteal artery can be removed by a catheter passed from the common femoral, but if femoral embolectomy is not completely successful, popliteal exploration should be undertaken. Dissection and control of the infragenicular popliteal, tibioperoneal trunk, and anterior tibial artery will allow an arteriotomy to be made in the popliteal artery, and a small balloon catheter to be directed selectively down the tibial vessels. If the popliteal artery is small it may require patching to allow closure without narrowing.

The least favorable situation therapeutically is one where clot is limited to distal tibial and foot arteries. Such clot is difficult or impossible to extract using balloon catheters, even if very small catheters and adjunctive techniques such as retrograde flushing with heparin saline are used. Nevertheless, such patients will do better if all retrievable clot is removed. If no clot is identified on the arteriogram, it is appropriate to return the patient to the intensive care unit. Further efforts should be aimed at support of the microcirculation by pharmacologic agents. Dextran may be used, giving a loading dose of 300 to 500 cc over five hours, then 25 cc per hour for several days, along with antiplatelet agents. If collateral circulation is adequate, limb salvage may be accomplished, although if perfusion pressures are low at ankle and transmetatarsal level, true rest pain or neuropathic pain may persist for long periods. Ischemic areas should be allowed to demarcate, and as long as the foot is viable and no infection is present, debridement or digital amputation can be delayed. It is difficult to judge the depth of areas of gangrene in this setting, and a philosophy of conservatism appears justified.

BIBLIOGRAPHY

1. Imparato AM, Berman IR, Bracco A, et al: Avoidance of shock and peripheral embolism during surgery of the abdominal aorta. *Surgery* 1973; 73:68–73.
2. Starr D, Laurie GM, Morris GC: Prevention of distal embolism during arterial reconstruction. *Am J Surg* 1979; 138:764–769.
3. Tchirkow G, Bevin E: Leg ischemia following surgery of abdominal aortic aneurysm. *Ann Surg* 1978; 188:166–170.
   Wylie EJ, Stoney RJ, Ehrenfeld WK: *Manual of Vascular Surgery,* vol I. New York, Springer-Verlag, 1980, pp 46–48.

PART THREE

Occlusive Disease

23 Multilevel Occlusive Disease

A 61-year-old construction worker is seen for rest pain and nonhealing ulceration over the lateral aspect of the right foot. Right ankle Doppler systolic pressure is 40 mm Hg. Femoral pulses are reduced and no pedal pulses can be felt. Angiography reveals diffuse aortoiliac disease and bilateral superficial femoral artery occlusions.

Consultant: Ronald J. Baird, M.D.

Atherosclerotic arterial obstruction rarely occurs at only one site. About half the patients with aortoiliac obstruction severe enough to require operation also have femoral artery narrowing or occlusion. This is known as "bi-level" or "tandem" obstruction. The usual surgical practice is to correct the upstream problem first and to repair the downstream obstruction at a later date. However, a few patients with severe tandem disease require concurrent repair of both the proximal and the distal lesions. The decision to perform a concurrent repair is usually made from the clinical and angiographic data: necrosis of tissue in the foot, a very low ankle systolic pressure, and complete superficial femoral artery obstruction combined with a poor collateral network from the deep femoral to the popliteal artery. There have been many attempts to use various preoperative or intraoperative measurements to quantify the relative importance of each level of obstruction. Few have achieved widespread clinical acceptance.

AORTOILIAC OBSTRUCTION

Clinically important narrowing in this area usually occurs in male cigarette smokers in their fifties and sixties. It is diagnosed by the symptoms of calf, thigh and buttock claudication and reduction of the amplitude of the common femoral pulse. Given time, it usually becomes bilateral.

It has been treated surgically by endarterectomy or arterial homograft bypass in the 1950s, by prosthetic aortoiliac bypass in the 1960s, and by prosthetic aorto-

143

bifemoral or cross-femoral bypass in the 1970s and 1980s. If relatively localized, it responds well to percutaneous transluminal dilation.

Both aortobifemoral and cross-femoral bypass allow the simultaneous correction of any narrowing in the proximal deep femoral artery. Both operations are currently performed in a relatively standardized fashion.

The main technical argument is whether or not the aortic anastomosis for an aortobifemoral bypass should be end-to-end or end-to-side. I prefer an end-to-end anastomosis about 4 cm above the origin of the inferior mesenteric artery with a short bifurcation, so that the left limb lies behind the inferior mesenteric arteries and veins. This technique keeps the prosthetic artery in the same anterior/posterior plane as the original arteries and thus reduces the danger of causing an aortointestinal fistula. The limbs of the graft should always be placed behind the ureters.

Of the patients who receive this operation, 2% to 3% die within 30 days. Half of these succumb to myocardial infarction, and the others to stroke, pulmonary embolus or multiple system failure.

Patients with severe aortoiliac disease face a ten-year decrease in expected lifespan, as compared with the general population. The ravages of increasing age and generalized atherosclerosis will cause death within five years of diagnosis for 25% and within ten years for 50% of these patients, according to Crawford's data.

Aortobifemoral bypass surgery provides a conduit with excellent long-term patency—85% still patent at five years after surgery, 70% at ten years, 60% at 15 years, and 55% at 20 years. This represents an attrition rate of 2% to 3% per year, compared to 5% to 6% per year with the reversed saphenous vein femoropopliteal bypass.

In simpler terms: Ten years after an aortofemoral bypass the expected patency is 70% and expected survival rate 50%; ten years after a femoropopliteal bypass with saphenous vein the expected patency is 50% and expected survival rate 30%.

If one iliac limb is relatively normal, a cross-femoral bypass is a shorter and safer operation, with only a moderately reduced long-term patency.

Percutaneous transluminal dilation provides a five-year patency rate of 60% for localized common iliac lesions and 50% for localized external iliac problems, according to an analysis of our experience with balloon angioplasty recently reported by Johnston.

FEMOROPOPLITEAL OBSTRUCTION

Clinically important femoropopliteal obstruction occurs about a decade later and is even more of a male problem. It also is usually bilateral.

From the 1950s to the late 1970s, it was treated by bypass with the reversed saphenous vein. Polytetrafluoroethylene (PTFE) grafts have been available for a decade and provide reasonable but less satisfactory patency. *In situ* saphenous vein bypass is currently popular and appears to provide the best results of any conduit in this area.

Patency is lost by the development of obstructive disease in the vein or by further upstream or downstream obstruction. With the reversed saphenous vein, the attrition rate was 5% to 6% per year. A useful working rule is to expect a ten-year patency of 50% and a ten-year survival of 30%.

Percutaneous transluminal dilation is useful for localized obstruction of the superficial femoral artery, but provides a five-year patency of only 40%.

COMBINED AORTOILIAC AND FEMOROPOPLITEAL OBSTRUCTIONS

Tandem disease is present in about half of the patients with clinically important symptoms. Usually either the upstream or the downstream problem is clearly the more important and is corrected at the initial procedure. If both appear to be of equal importance, the usual practice is to correct the upstream lesion and consider repair of the downstream lesion at a later date. This is rational, in view of the greater expectation of long-term patency from a proximal as compared to a distal bypass.

However, certain patients with severe tandem obstruction require concurrent repair of both the proximal and distal obstructions, and our patient would appear to be one of these.

Vascular surgeons have reported concurrent repair in 2% to 5% of their patients. The presence of necrosis in the foot, a very low ankle systolic pressure, and a poor collateral network from the deep femoral to the popliteal artery are factors favoring a concurrent operation.

Many attempts have been made to quantify, objectively, the hemodynamic data that justify an upstream, downstream, or concurrent repair. Measurement of the pressure/gradient across the aortoiliac obstruction is the only one which has achieved widespread clinical acceptance.

In the vascular laboratory one can measure the thigh pressure index, that is the thigh systolic pressure divided by the brachial systolic pressure. The difference between the systolic pressure in the thigh and in the ankle is the delta-P. The index of runoff resistance is delta-P divided by brachial systolic pressure. The lower the value of each of these calculations, the higher the likelihood of a satisfactory result from an isolated upstream repair, as shown in the reports of Bone, et al, Brewster and coworkers, and others. Unfortunately, no single laboratory value is an adequate predictor.

Measurement of the pressure gradient across the aortoiliac obstruction at aortography, in the blood flow laboratory, or on the operating table will quantify the degree of upstream obstruction. A gradient of 10 mm in the systolic pressure at rest is considered significant. It is also useful to measure the response of the femoral pressure to an intraarterial injection of 30 mg of papaverine. A fall of more than 15% is indicative of serious aortoiliac obstruction.

Hemodynamic measurements on completion of the aortofemoral bypass, such as flow rate through each limb of the bypass, duration from restoration of flow to return of a normal foot color, an audible Doppler ankle flow signal, or the ankle brachial pressure index achieved, have been interesting but not clearly predictive of the need for concurrent repair.

In practice, the surgeon is more comfortable in explaining the planned operation in detail to the patient, rather than asking for permission to vary the procedure depending on the results of intraoperative measurements. He will usually decide on the proper procedure from the preoperative clinical, angiographic and hemodynamic data available to him. Thus, the usual decision is to correct either the aortoiliac or the femoropopliteal problem according to which appears to be the most obstructive. If they appear to be of equal importance, then the upstream operation is usually performed and a decision on the downstream repair is delayed for three to six months. With the symptoms of claudication or rest pain, this is an easier course to follow than when there is a nonhealing ulcer or gangrene in part of the foot.

CONSIDERATION OF THIS SPECIFIC PATIENT

At age 61, the patient presents at the usual age for aortoiliac obstruction and slightly younger than that for femoropopliteal disease.

As a construction worker, he will be interested in treatment which allows as rapid a recovery as possible. He is probably a cigarette smoker who has smoked for over 40 years and will likely continue this habit, despite all advice to the contrary. His expectation of living to age 71 is about 30%.

The presence of rest pain, a nonhealing ulcer, and an ankle systolic pressure of 40 are indicative of severe ischemia that demands treatment. The reduction in both femoral pulses and the angiographic depiction of diffuse aortoiliac disease indicate that a cross-femoral bypass is not an appropriate option.

From the above, I believe he will eventually require correction of both the upstream and downstream problems and would be best treated by concurrent aortobifemoral and right femoropopliteal bypass.

SOME OF THE AVAILABLE OPTIONS

If the patient has symptoms of cardiac or cerebrovascular obstruction, the surgeon should explain that the risks of aortofemoral bypass would be higher than 3% and should consider initial percutaneous transluminal dilation (PTD). The results of the PTD are dependent on both the localization or diffuseness of the disease, and the skill and persistence of the interventional radiologist. I would arrange to review the films with the radiologist and would be influenced by his views.

If PTD of the iliac problem was successful, the patient should likely receive a right femoropopliteal bypass using an *in situ* saphenous vein. PTD of the complete femoral artery obstruction is unlikely to give a satisfactory long-term patency and would be considered only if the overall medical status was severe enough to prohibit any operative procedure.

If the below-knee outflow was excellent and the deep femoral-to-popliteal collaterals profuse, I would favor an initial aortobifemoral bypass and would expect healing of the ulcer. If not healed in a month or two, then femoropopliteal bypass would be done. I would follow this standard course only if I expected that the second operation would be necessary.

TECHNICAL DETAILS OF THE CONCURRENT AORTOFEMORAL AND FEMOROPOPLITEAL BYPASS OPERATION

The anesthetist should use a radial artery line and a Swan-Ganz catheter for proper hemodynamic control. Both feet are wrapped in clear plastic bags so that their color is visible. The surgical prep should include both legs.

The concurrent operation should only be considered or performed by an experienced surgeon, with sufficient help by well-trained residents or assistants to allow an expeditious operation in which the leg operation proceeds, at least in part, concurrently with the abdominal repair.

The groin arteries are exposed first. The status of the deep femoral arteries is determined by palpation and later by direct inspection of the ostea. The saphenous vein is exposed either while the abdomen is being opened or while it is being closed.

A midline incision and a Bookwalter Retractor are used. The aorta is exposed from the renal vein to the inferior mesenteric artery. Five thousand units of heparin are given and the aorta is clamped (from in front), just below the renal vein and 1 cm cephalad to the IMA. The aorta is transected 5 mm above the lower clamp and oversewn from back to front with 2–0 Prolene, knotted in front. The lower clamp is removed.

The aorta is opened by a 2-cm to 3-cm vertical anterior incision followed by a lateral extension. The incision does not cut the back of the aorta.

The Dacron graft should be of a low porosity, nonfraying design that does not require preclotting. It should be cut 2 cm to 2.5 cm above the bifurcation so that it fits easily into the area of opened aorta.

The aortic anastomosis is performed with 2–0 Prolene using a "parachute" stitch on the posterior wall and a one-knot technique anteriorly. The cut ends of the Prolene are tacked to the left so as to point away from the duodenum. The right limb should be brought down behind the right ureter to the groin. The left limb lies behind the inferior mesenteric vessels, as well as the ureter.

The common femoral anastomoses are performed concurrently with 4–0 or 5–0 Prolene. The surgeon should make sure that there is no deep femoral stenosis. If there is significant deep femoral stenosis, the toe of the graft should be carried down appropriately.

Air and clot are flushed from the prosthesis. The aortic clamp is removed slowly and with proper warning to the anesthetist. It is important at this stage of the operation for the surgeon to be able to see the arterial pressure read-out and avoid undue hypotension.

The posterior retroperitoneum is closed with an absorbable suture and the anterior abdominal wall with one layer of continuous 1–0 Prolene with a single knot at the bottom and one at the top. The ends of the Prolene are buried.

The saphenous vein will have been exposed from the groin to below the knee. No attempt is made to leave skin bridges. The side branches are tied or clipped.

A curved, partial occlusion clamp allows removal of the saphenous vein from the common femoral vein, which is then closed with 5–0 Prolene. The top 8 cm to 10 cm of the saphenous vein are freed up and the upper valve removed under direct vision.

The Leather valvulotome is attached to a cut Fogarty catheter that has been introduced via the cut end of the saphenous vein below the knee. A large "feeding tube" is sewn to the upper end of the valvulotome and perfused with Ringer's solution containing 1000 units of heparin at a pressure of 150 mm Hg. The valvulotome is drawn down with the cutting edge at right angles to the skin. Two or three passes are made until the distal flow is unimpeded.

The upper and lower anastomoses are standard. The heparin effect is reversed by protamine. Residual fistulae are looked for by listening to the Doppler signal and sequentially obstructing the vein. A completion arteriogram is rarely performed.

One would expect to complete the operation within four to five hours.

One would expect the ulcer to be healed within a month and the patient able to return to work in about six weeks.

A PTFE prosthesis would be used in place of the saphenous vein only if there were technical problems or if the vein was inadequate.

Conclusion

In a patient such as ours, with severe tandem obstruction and a nonhealing ulcer of the foot, the usual practice has been to perform an aortobifemoral bypass and wait for three months before considering a femoropopliteal bypass. However, in view of the incompleteness of the aortoiliac obstruction, the complete occlusion of the superficial femoral artery, the low ankle pressure, and the presence of a nonhealing ulcer, I would recommend a concurrent repair of both lesions.

BIBLIOGRAPHY

1. Baird RJ, Feldman P, Miles JT, et al: Subsequent downstream repair after aortoiliac and aortofemoral bypass operation. *Surgery* 1977; 82:785–793.
2. Baird RJ, Johnston KW, Walker PM, et al: Aortoiliofemoral disease, in Wilson SE, Veith FJ, Hobson RW II, et al (eds): *Vascular Surgery, Principles and Practice.* New York, McGraw-Hill Book Co, 1987, pp 344–352.

3. Baird RJ: Downstream revascularization after aortofemoral bypass grafting, in Bergan JJ, Yao JST (eds): *Reoperative Vascular Surgery*. Orlando, Grune & Stratton Inc, 1986, pp 223–230.
4. Bone GE, Hays AC, Slaymaker EE, et al: Value of segmental limb pressures in predicting results of aortofemoral bypass. *Am J Surg* 1976; 132:733–740.
5. Brewster DC, Perler BA, Robison JG, et al: Aortofemoral graft for multilevel occlusive disease. *Arch Surg* 1982; 177:1597–1601.
6. Crawford ES, Bomberger RA, Glasser DH, et al: Aortoiliac occlusive disease: Factors influencing survival and function following reconstructive operation over a 25-year period. *Surgery* 1981; 90:1055–1066.
7. Flanigan DP, Ryan TJ, Williams LR, et al: Aortofemoral or femoropopliteal revascularization? A prospective evaluation of the papaverine test. *J Vasc Surg* 1984; 1:215–223.
8. Johnston KW, Rae M, Hogg-Johnston SA, et al.: Five-year results of a prospective study of percutaneous transluminal angioplasty. *Ann Surg* 1987; 206:403–413.

24 High-Risk Patient with Aortoiliac Disease

A 69-year-old patient is admitted with rest pain in the right foot. There is a history of diabetes mellitus and hypertension. Four years ago, he sustained a small left hemispheric stroke, but eventually recovered with minimal residual deficit. He has had a prior myocardial infarct and continues to experience occasional angina and dyspnea on exertion. On examination, the right femoral pulse is absent and the left femoral pulse appears reduced.

Consultant: Robert B. Rutherford, M.D.

Even from this brief description, the patient can readily be identified as "high risk"—an elderly diabetic with hypertension and widespread arteriosclerosis already producing serious symptoms in three vascular beds: coronary, cerebral, and lower extremity. This is a patient who deserves careful and conservative care but clearly, if the rest pain is truly ischemic and persistent, some form of intervention is inevitable.

EVALUATION

The evaluation of such a patient requires objective characterization of the severity of ischemia and the occlusive arterial lesions responsible for it, as well as careful assessment of the nature and severity of concurrent clinical problems. This allows one to determine the need, feasibility, and risk of the various interventional options.

Assessment of Limb Ischemia

Evaluating chronic lower limb ischemia may be made more difficult in a diabetic by coexisting diabetic neuropathy and by calcific changes in the arterial wall. While the neuropathy may allow serious infections and even ulceration to go unrecognized and be neglected, it does *not* significantly decrease awareness of ischemic rest pain. The same pattern of severe forefoot pain occurring mainly with recumbency (i.e., nocturnal) and relieved by dependency but not analgesics, occurs in both diabetics and nondiabetics. However, in the early phases of diabetic neuropathy, before hypaesthia becomes apparent, patients can experience periods of pain at rest which are "neuritic" but not ischemic. However, this pain is usually more burning in character and not related to position or time of day.

Chronic ischemic rest pain is almost always due to multilevel disease, and in a diabetic presenting with an absent femoral pulse on the side of symptoms, one would presume the combination here will be iliac artery occlusion plus distal, infrapopliteal occlusive disease. The location and severity of the occlusive lesions may be confirmed by noninvasive studies, but again, the diabetic may have such calcified, incompressible arteries that segmental limb systolic pressure determinations will be artifactually elevated. Ordinarily, the presence of true ischemic rest pain can be confirmed by finding an ankle pressure below 40 mm Hg, but a diabetic with critical ischemia may register ankle pressures of over 200 mm Hg because of calcified arteries.

There are two possible solutions to this dilemma. Even with calcified arteries, toe pressures *are* reliable in the diabetic and normally the level runs about 10 mm Hg below ankle pressures (i.e., 30 mm Hg would correlate with critical ischemia). Second, plethysmographic tracings will also be reliable in such patients—they should have a barely "pulsatile" or flat contour at the ankle or transmetatarsal level if a critical level of forefoot ischemia exists.

In addition to detecting, localizing and gauging the severity of the arterial occlusive lesions (which the above combination does with 95% accuracy), these noninvasive studies may allow one to assess the hemodynamic significance of the contralateral iliac arterial disease suggested by the diminished left femoral pulse. This is important if a femorofemoral bypass is to be considered as an option. Flanigan, et al, have shown that a triphasic Doppler waveform recorded over the femoral artery offered the best correlation with functional patency of the donor iliac artery. Subsequently, he has also shown the value of a femoral:brachial pressure index before and after intraarterial papaverine injection for the same purpose.

Assessment of Operative Risk

Ordinarily this is done prior to arteriography. Almost all candidates for revascularization procedures require, in addition to the routine baseline studies, focused evaluation of vital organ function and circulation, as dictated by historical findings and preliminary tests. For example, in this patient, if the BUN and creatinine were elevated, creatinine clearance would be ordered. Noninvasive evaluation of carotid disease would be undertaken using duplex scanning. With a history of myocardial infarction, angina, and dyspnea on exertion, formal cardiac evaluation is advisable, including consultation by a cardiologist and, at minimum, an electrocardiogram, Persantine-Thallium study (since the patient cannot exercise on a treadmill), and a gated blood pool with the calculated ejection fraction. Without a history of smoking or respiratory complaints, pulmonary function in this patient would be screened only with a chest X-ray and arterial blood gases; but significant abnormalities here would dictate formal pulmonary function tests. While the baseline blood work and noninvasive studies would normally be carried out as an outpatient, particularly in younger, healthier patients, the remainder of the studies required in this patient justify inpatient evaluation and could be carried out in one day, following which, with good hydration, arteriography would be performed. The possible need for coronary arteriography might derail these plans, but they should be scheduled as outlined with the presumption that chronic stable angina will not interfere with pursuing most of the available therapeutic options.

Arteriography

Arteriography is normally done as the final preoperative study, *after* the need for intervention is firmly established and the patient's anesthetic risk has been assessed. It will provide an anatomic or, if you will, morphologic characterization of the responsible arterial occlusive lesions which, in turn, will determine the technical feasibility, if not advisability, of certain treatment options available. Such anatomic information will generally allow one to make a decision regarding the advisability of carrying out transluminal angioplasty at the same sitting. But this particular diabetic patient will need careful hydration and possibly even mannitol during the angiographic procedure, and it may be wiser to defer any dilation to a later time.

CHOICE OF INTERVENTIONAL THERAPY

From the finding of absent right femoral and reduced left femoral pulses in a patient with rest pain, it can be presumed that, in addition to the bilateral aortoiliac occlusive disease, there are additional occlusive lesions in the right leg. Without consideration of risk, the optimum procedure for the management of this patient's lower limb ischemia would be an aortobifemoral bypass. It offers the best long-term patency (85% to 90%) and hemodynamic result of any revascularization procedure applied to aortoiliac occlusive disease. And, in the face of poor runoff, better long-term results are obtained than with femorofemoral bypass when the iliac occlusive disease is hemodynamically significant on one side only.

However, one is not seeking long-term benefits here. This elderly hypertensive diabetic with symptomatic arteriosclerotic involvement in three different areas has a very limited life expectancy. Even without further details of the patient's evaluation, the risk can be presumed to be high enough that other options of revascularization should be considered. Malone and his colleagues, in reviewing the results of diabetics undergoing aortobifemoral bypass, found that *all* were dead within eight years and *all* had graft occlusions by 32 months!

Since there is no threatened tissue loss and the proximal lesion is presumably a complete iliac occlusion, one can probably ignore the distal disease and concentrate on bringing full inflow down to the femoral level. The remaining options, therefore, are (1) attempts to disobliterate the right iliac occlusion by a combination of thrombolytic therapy and transluminal angioplasty, (2) balloon dilation of the contralateral iliac artery followed by a femorofemoral bypass, (3) a right iliofemoral bypass, (4) a right axillounifemoral bypass, and (5) an axillobifemoral bypass.

The overall decision process followed by the author in choosing the appropriate treatment for symptomatic aortoiliac disease is outlined in Figure 24–1. Transluminal angioplasty is best applied to discrete (less than 5 cm), *partially* occlusive lesions of the common iliac artery where it may carry a close to 90% five-year patency rate. Although there are reports of management of total occlusions by balloon angioplasty, those beyond 2 cm in length are unlikely to be successful and may run a prohibitive risk of distal embolization which, in a patient with poor runoff, would be disastrous. If the patient *was truly a prohibitive risk* and a longer occlusion was encountered, but the history suggested that the occlusion was relatively recent (i.e., two to three weeks), a preliminary trial of thrombolytic therapy might be appropriate and, if it cleared the artery and revealed a stenosis, balloon dilation could then be performed.

If the left iliac is either not hemodynamically significantly stenosed or, even if it is but is amenable to balloon dilation, a femorofemoral bypass would become the procedure of choice. Without further information in the patient described, this would be the procedure I would most likely recommend. On the other hand, if a

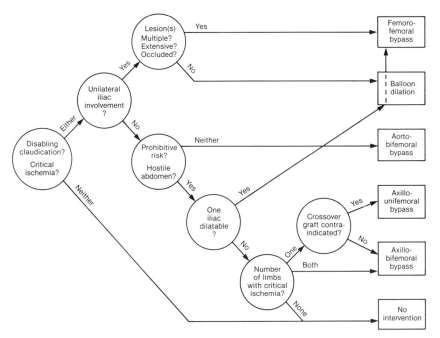

Fig 24-1
Algorithm depicting author's approach to aortoiliac occlusive disease.

right external iliac occlusion is seen on the preoperative arteriogram, and the common iliac proximal to this is not significantly involved, an iliofemoral bypass becomes a feasible option, particularly if the contralateral left iliac stenosis is not very favorable for dilation. When approached retroperitoneally through an oblique, lower quadrant incision, it presents a similar risk to femorofemoral bypass. However, the author has found that its long-term patency is clearly inferior to the latter. Both of these procedures can be performed under epidural anesthesia.

Only if the *contralateral* iliac disease is extensive, diffuse or multiple (i.e., unsuitable for dilation), or if the *ipsilateral* common iliac is unsuitable for proximal anastomosis, is one forced to fall back on axillofemoral bypass as the next best option. Patency rates with these bypasses are inferior to femorofemoral grafts which give better results as long as the donor iliac artery is or has been rendered functionally patent. In this regard, it is best to wait until after the results of the iliac dilation are clearly apparent and satisfactory before proceeding with a femorofemoral bypass. For the same reason, intraoperative dilation of the contralateral iliac artery with a Fogarty-Chin catheter is *not* recommended.

If the above options are found to be not feasible, one is left with a choice between an axillounifemoral and an axillobifemoral bypass in a patient in which the limb threatening ischemia exists only in one limb. Although some studies have found that the difference in patency between these two grafts is not statistically significant, even in these articles the mean difference favors axillobifemoral grafts. Other investigators, including the author, have found the difference to be quite significant in favor of the axillobifemoral bypass. In fact, we found that the five-year primary patencies favored axillobifemoral bypass over axillounifemoral bypass even when the cases were separated into good runoff (92% vs 54%) and poor runoff (41% vs 0%) groups. Thus, I would add a femorofemoral limb if the patient were stable under anesthesia *and* there was no sepsis, radiation or other hostile pathology in the path of the crossover. Our preference for configuration of the axillobifemoral is for the Blaisdell modification in which the femorofemoral limb is sewn to the mobilized and amputated stump of the common femoral artery. This avoids a double "piggy-back" anastomosis associated with the "inverted C" configuration, but gives the advantage of having increased flow throughout the length of the axillofemoral limb and improved patency (Fig 24–2). My choice of prosthesis is a knitted Dacron velour for the aortobifemoral bypass, but PTFE for the other bypasses mentioned. This is because the latter have a higher risk of thrombosis and are easier to thrombectomize if PTFE is used. I am not convinced that externally supported grafts are necessary in the latter setting.

Finally, I would mention two other options only to discourage their use. Sympathectomy can occasionally improve ischemic rest pain, but would not be indicated in this patient because most diabetics have already undergone autosympathectomy, and the procedure would entail the same anesthetic risk as all the other options other than aortobifemoral bypass. Primary amputation is also considered an option by some in such high-risk patients, but it would not be indicated for rest pain alone, i.e., without significant tissue loss. Even in the face of such ischemic lesions, BK amputation could not be condoned as a primary procedure when there are so many other low-risk options to choose from for achieving proximal inflow.

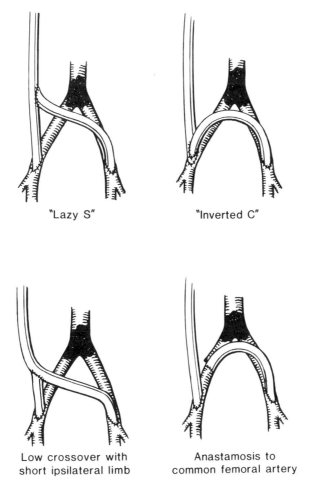

"Lazy S"   "Inverted C"

Low crossover with   Anastamosis to
short ipsilateral limb   common femoral artery

FIG 24-2.
Optional configurations in constructing an axillobifemoral bypass. Blaisdell's modification
is on the lower right.

BIBLIOGRAPHY

1. Blaisdell FW, Holcroft JW, Ward RE: Axillofemoral and femorofemoral bypass: History and evolution of technique, in Greenhalgh RM (ed): *Extra-anatomic and Secondary Arterial Reconstruction.* Pitman Brook Ltd, 1982.
2. Brewster DC, Darling RC: Optimal methods of aortoiliac reconstruction. *Surgery* 1978; 84:739–748.
3. Flanigan DP, Williams LR, Schwartz JA, et al: Hemodynamic evaluation of the aortoiliac system based on pharmacologic vasodilation. *Surgery* 1983; 93:709–714.
4. Johnston KW, Rae M, Hogg-Johnston SA, et al: 5-year results of a prospective study of percutaneous transluminal angioplasty. *Ann Surg* 1987; 206:403–413.

5. Malone JM, Moore WS, Goldstone J: The natural history of bilateral aortofemoral bypass grafts for ischemia of the lower extremities. *Arch Surg* 1975; 110:1300–1306.
6. Piotrowski J, Rutherford RB, Jones DN, et al: Aortobifemoral bypass: The operation of choice for unilateral iliac occlusion? Presented at the Western Vascular Society meeting, Monterey, CA, January 28-31, 1988. Submitted to Journal of Vascular Surgery.
7. Rutherford RB, Jones DN, Martin MS, et al: Serial hemodynamic assessment of aortobifemoral bypass. *J Vasc Surg* 1986; 4:429–435.
8. Rutherford RB, Lowenstein DH, Klein MF: Combining segmental systolic pressures and plethysmography to diagnose arterial occlusive disease of the legs. *Am J Surg* 1979; 138:211–219.
9. Rutherford RB, Patt A, Kumpe DA: Current role of percutaneous transluminal angioplasty, in Greenhalgh RM, Jamieson CW (eds): *Vascular Surgery; Issues in Current Practice*. London, Grune & Stratton, 1986, pp 229–244.
10. Rutherford RB, Patt A, Pearce WH: Extra-anatomic bypass: A closer view. *J Vasc Surg* 1987 in press.
11. Rutherford RB: Extra-anatomic bypass for aortoiliac occlusive disease, in Kempczinski RF (ed): *The Ischemic Leg*. Chicago, Yearbook Medical Publishers, 1985, p 327.

25 Unilateral Iliac Artery Occlusion

A 59-year-old man is seen with severe right leg claudication. He is otherwise in excellent health. The right femoral pulse is absent, but left femoral pulse appears intact. Angiography reveals total occlusion of the right common iliac artery. The left iliofemoral system shows scattered plaquing, but no significant lesion.

Consultant: Bruce J. Brener, M.D.

ASSESSMENT OF PATIENT IN THE OFFICE

This is a common clinical problem, but one would need more information before deciding whether or not the patient should have surgery. What is "severe" claudication? A comprehensive history should include details about the patient's occupation, family responsibilities, and leisure activities. Is he a construction foreman who climbs ladders, inspects buildings, supervises a large area of commercial construction? Is he an accountant who works at a desk? Does he go to the supermarket? Is tennis his main outlet? Is mountain climbing his hobby or does he divide his weekend between the garden and the television? To qualify for surgery the patient should be able to accomplish the activities which he thinks will be restored by the procedure. Some men are more upset about their image as young, fit and healthy and really have no true disability from their claudication.

Is there a history of coronary disease? We are told he is in excellent health. Symptoms suggestive of coronary disease would mandate a more extensive cardiac workup. It is pointless to operate on patients with angina and claudication. The angina would limit exercise once the claudication is alleviated. Is he a smoker? The patient would have to discontinue cigarettes. Does he have normal sexual function? Impotence might be relieved by surgery if the appropriate anatomic lesion were present. Are there symptoms in the opposite leg? Claudication might not be relieved by a unilateral procedure.

A more complete physical examination would be performed, of course. It would be useful to know if the patient has disease in the femoropopliteal segments as well as the aortoiliac vessels. The patient would be expected to have more disability if he has multisegmental disease. Furthermore, his symptoms may be only partly relieved by the inflow procedure if there are superficial femoral artery occlusions.

Finally, some clues may be obtained by history and physical examination about the etiology of the obstruction. Did the claudication begin suddenly? In the presence of cardiac disease or an aortic aneurysm, this acute onset might suggest an embolus to the right iliac artery. Did symptoms of claudication recently become more severe? This might mean an artery narrowed by an atherosclerotic plaque became totally occluded. Was there trauma from a diagnostic procedure? Was there a history of renal artery stenosis due to fibromuscular disease? Fibromuscular disease is a rare cause of iliac occlusion. Any symptoms of headache, blurred vision, arthritis? Arteritis is another unusual cause of iliac occlusion.

The patient should have segmental plethysmographic traces or segmental limb pressures and an exercise test in the office on the initial visit. This provides some documentation of the degree of disability. Some patients with an iliac occlusion can walk for over five minutes on the treadmill set at two miles per hour with a 10% grade. These patients often have minimal symptoms and may not require surgery. But most patients can walk for about two minutes. This condition would be disabling for an active man. The exercise test would give the surgeon the chance to observe the patient for signs of respiratory disease, cardiac symptoms, and arrhythmias.

ASSESSMENT OF PATIENT IN THE HOSPITAL

Assuming the patient is truly disabled and has undergone a trial of daily exercise, weight reduction if necessary, and cessation of smoking, he should undergo angiography. Traditionally, this has required admission to the hospital the day before the study, preangiographic intravenous hydration, perhaps a day of evaluation after angiography, and then surgery. With examination by peer review groups and increasing pressure to limit hospitalization, there is advancing initiative to perform angiography on an outpatient basis or to admit the patient to the hospital the day of angiography and eliminate the day between angiography and surgery. This may be acceptable in some patients, but not in others.

In this case angiography revealed an iliac occlusion and some plaques on the asymptomatic side. More details are required before the operation can be fully planned. The orifices of the profunda femoral and superficial femoral arteries should be visualized. This evaluation is important so that adequate runoff during surgery can be provided. Single plane evaluation of the iliac vessels can be misleading. Oblique views are more revealing; iliac stenosis and profunda stenosis seen in this projection may be hidden in the anterior-posterior view.

Unless the left iliac artery were perfectly normal on angiography, aortic, iliac, and femoral pressures should be measured through the angiography catheter. Intraarterial papaverine or cuff-induced ischemia can be used to increase flow through the left iliac artery. This would magnify any difference between aortic and femoral pressure by increasing the energy losses at the stenosis. We would not consider a young healthy individual to be a candidate for cross-femoral grafting if there were a pressure difference greater than 10% to 15% of the systemic pressure.

SURGICAL OPTIONS

There are at least eight "surgical options" for improving the circulation in a patient with unilateral iliac occlusive disease. These include transluminal angioplasty, transluminal angioplasty combined with femorofemoral bypass, aortobilateral iliac endarterectomy, aortobilateral femoral bypass, unilateral iliac endarterectomy, aortounilateral femoral bypass, iliofemoral bypass, and femorofemoral bypass.

Many radiologists will not perform angioplasty for complete iliac artery occlusion, as is present in our patient. Since the vessel may be tortuous but is not visible by angiography, the guide wire may perforate the wall. Perforation of the iliac artery would be more dangerous than perforation of the superficial femoral artery. Furthermore, one would not expect that splitting the atheroma and media by angioplasty would yield an adequate lumen, since the atherosclerotic lesion is large, and thrombus would occupy most of the vessel. However, angioplasty has been recommended for unilateral iliac stenosis. Many reports indicate that dilatation of iliac stenosis is more successful than similar procedures for superficial femoral artery lesions. However, several recent studies have documented a 30% incidence of significant recurrent or persistent disease within five years of the iliac dilatation. This result appears to be inferior to surgical intervention but is achieved at a lower risk. Clearly, the poorer long-term result may be less important in high-risk patients with limb threatening ischemia (although the results are even poorer in this group). Since surgery is not precluded by angioplasty, this radiological procedure may be recommended for short stenotic lesions in patients at good risk, but probably not for totally occlusive lesions.

In some high-risk patients with bilateral iliac disease, the lesser stenosis may be dilated by balloon angioplasty. A femorofemoral graft (see below) can be inserted if the dilatation results in restoration of the potential donor limb femoral pressure to normal. An interesting physiological question is posed by this procedure. Does increased flow through the dilated vessel have an effect on the natural history of this atherosclerotic lesion? Is the recurrence delayed or accelerated? Until more information is available, this must be considered a "compromise" procedure and be utilized for the poor risk patient.

Aortobilateral iliac endarterectomy is rarely carried out in current practice. Performance of this procedure may be a dying art form. Aortobilateral femoral bypass for bilateral iliac disease has overshadowed the more difficult and less durable endarterectomy, except in unusual circumstances. Aortobifemoral bypass would be a successful procedure in this patient. Presumably one would perform an end-to-end aortoprosthetic anastomosis in order to eliminate the division of flow between the graft limb and the normal iliac artery which would occur if the upper anastomosis were in an end-to-side configuration. Retrograde flow in the normal external iliac would preserve pelvic perfusion via the internal iliac vessels. Long-term patency can be expected to be high, approximately 80% to 90% at five years, particularly with patent femoral vessels. In good risk patients, this procedure has a low morbidity and mortality. The problems are: (1) Is this major abdominal procedure necessary or will a "lesser" procedure be equally successful? (2) Can the increased morbidity and mortality in the high-risk patient be avoided by a "lesser" procedure?

Unilateral bypass or endarterectomy via a retroperitoneal approach is favored by some surgeons. These procedures have a distinct advantage over aortobilateral femoral bypass in that they are of less magnitude and do not involve bypassing a relatively normal iliac vessel. Few surgeons perform iliac endarterectomy, but this may be a reasonable procedure for a localized lesion at the iliac bifurcation. Endarterectomy of the muscular external iliac artery is less successful than the common iliac. However, in this patient with common iliac occlusion the endarterectomy might include the distal aorta, the common iliac, and the iliac bifurcation. A bypass from the aorta to the femoral artery is a better approach. Unfortunately, the distal aorta is often calcified and atherosclerotic and contains thrombus. For bypass procedures the more proximal infrarenal aorta is preferred. An abdominal procedure to explore this level of aorta is more extensive; it is usually not carried out unless both iliac arteries are involved, particularly since other procedures are available (see below). Occasionally, the external iliac artery is occluded and the common iliac is patent. A bypass from the common iliac to the femoral is possible in some patients, but obviously not this one. However, in the older individual the common iliac is often severely calcified, making this operation more difficult.

In my opinion the best operation for unilateral iliac disease (particularly for total iliac occlusion) is a femorofemoral bypass. The requirements for this operation are adequate inflow via the donor iliac vessel and adequate runoff usually via the profunda femoris. In the highest risk patients one might accept mild iliac lesions in the donor artery or perform iliac angioplasty to correct any stenotic inflow lesions, as described above. These "compromise" procedures cannot be expected to have the same long-term patency as those with normal donor vessels. As with more extensive procedures, durability is also dependent on adequate femoral runoff. A number of techniques for ensuring outflow through the femoral vessels is noted in Figure 25–1,A–F. These maneuvers are applicable to aortofemoral grafting as well.

Femorofemoral bypass is a minimally traumatic procedure with approximately the same systemic effect as a bilateral inguinal herniorrhaphy. Avoiding the intraabdominal or retroperitoneal procedure lowers the risk and morbidity of this reconstruction. Sexual function is preserved because the pelvic periaortic plexus is undisturbed. Patency should approximate that of an aortofemoral procedure if the donor iliac artery remains normal. We have found that the donor iliac artery becomes progressively diseased in only 4.5% of properly selected patients followed for up to 15 years. Long-term patency is very close to that of aortofemoral reconstruction. Cummulative patency rates in 154 patients were 78.7% at five years, 68% at 10 years, and 60.2% at 15 years.

The main disadvantage of the femorofemoral bypass is the dissection of the

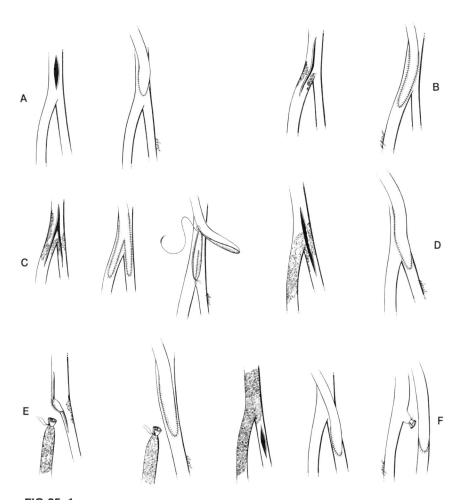

FIG 25–1.

Aortofemoral, iliofemoral, or femorofemoral bypass grafts are connected to the femoral vessels using techniques to ensure adequate flow beyond areas of stenosis. If the femoral bifurcation is free of disease, an unusual circumstance, the anastomosis may be performed at this level **A.** If there is a plaque at the origin of the superficial femoral artery the incision in the common femoral can be extended through the diseased area **B.**

If the origins of both the superficial and deep arteries are stenotic, the incision can be extended through the lesion in one artery and the orifice of the other endarterectomized through this opening or, a Y-shaped incision can be made and repaired with a double patch or by suturing the adjacent walls together **C.**

Commonly, the superficial femoral artery is occluded and the profunda orifice is stenotic. The incision can be extended through the stenosis without **D** or with **E** transection of the superficial femoral artery. When the common femoral and superficial femoral arteries are occluded the anastomosis is performed either end-to-side or end-to-end to the profunda vessel **F.**

"normal" femoral artery on the donor side. This exposes the uninvolved artery to the risk of damage. This should occur very infrequently if the procedure is performed by experienced vascular surgeons. Because of the infrequent morbidity and acceptable long-term patency, I prefer this procedure over the others for arterial reconstruction for unilateral iliac occlusion.

SUMMARY

Patients with an absent femoral pulse and claudication should have a complete history and physical examination. Inquiries about the severity of claudication, sexual function, and associated diseases should be made. An exercise test would be helpful in evaluating the degree of disability, extent of cardiopulmonary disease, and to some extent the circulatory status of the better leg. Angiography would be particularly helpful if it included oblique views and pressure measurements. Although many procedures are available for patients with unilateral iliac occlusion, femorofemoral bypass has remained a low-risk, durable reconstruction, and is my procedure of choice.

BIBLIOGRAPHY

1. Brener B, Raines JK, Darling RC, et al: Measurement of systolic femoral artery pressure during reactive hyperemia: An estimate of aortoiliac disease. *Circulation (Suppl II)* 1974; 50:259–267.
2. Brewster DC, Darling RC: Optimal methods of aorto-iliac reconstruction. *Surgery* 1978; 84:739–740.
3. Dick L, Brief DK, Alpert J: A twelve-year experience with femorofemoral crossover grafts. *Arch Surg* 1980; 115:1359–1365.
4. Johnston KW, Rae M, Hogg-Johnston SA, et al: Five year results of a prospective study of percutaneous transluminal angioplasty. *Ann Surg* 1987; 206:403–413.

26 Total Juxtarenal Aortic Occlusion

A 67-year-old woman is admitted with a three-month history of severe recurrent lower extremity ischemia. Six years previously she had undergone aortoiliac grafting for occlusive disease. Currently, neither femoral pulse is palpable. Aortography reveals total occlusion of the abdominal aorta and prior graft, extending to the level of the renal arteries.

Consultants: Ronald J. Stoney, M.D., and Kimberley J. Hansen, M.D.

The case described represents a classic example of secondary aortic occlusion resulting from failure of a prosthetic infrarenal aortic reconstruction. Primary aortic occlusion occurs spontaneously when localized aortoiliac atherosclerosis progresses to occlusion of the native aortic outflow. The process is gradual, allowing time for collateral circulation to develop in most cases of primary occlusion. Secondary aortic occlusions may be more abrupt and presentation more emergently.

Both types of aortic occlusion rely on blood flow through patent aortic branches to halt the cephalad propagation of aortic thrombosis. Aortic occlusion is most frequently in the terminal aorta initially, with patent lumbar arteries and the inferior mesenteric artery providing aortic runoff. As thrombus layers within the aorta, gradual obliteration of these branch ostia occurs and the thrombus propagates proximally, eventually halted by blood flowing into the renal arteries. Although the collateral flow through the infrarenal aortic branches ceases, proximal afferent sources are numerous: intercostal, mesenteric, and internal mammary arteries. Rich interconnections with arteries within the pelvis and hip region ensure limb perfusion.

Clinical Presentation

The level of aortic occlusion and the effective collateral blood flow determine the degree of limb ischemia present. For most patients, it is surprisingly mild, with claudication the most prominent symptom. Rest pain, tissue necrosis, or gangrene are rare, at least initially, but can occur in the later phases of this disorder when the level of occlusion has ascended to the juxtarenal aorta and there is significant coexisting femoropopliteal occlusive disease.

Evaluation

The physical examination is the key evaluation in initially defining this lesion. Absent femoral pulses are highly suggestive of this entity, and when coupled with absence of aortic pulsation the clinical diagnosis is verified. Aortography will be necessary to accurately define the level of occlusion, collateral pathways, status of the proximal aorta, and the condition of the lower extremity vasculature.

The translumbar approach for aortography was preferred here at UCSF for many years. Excellent definition of the level of occlusion and the status of the renal arteries and the proximal abdominal aorta was regularly obtained. However, biplane and oblique views were not feasible with this technique and visualization of the distal circulation was incomplete or inadequate in nearly half of the patients undergoing this form of aortography. The superiority of the Seldinger approach for aortography became apparent with this lesion as soon as we had the benefit of radiologists experienced in this technique. Using the transaxillary route, a catheter can be placed in the proximal abdominal aorta and biplane and selective views may be obtained to evaluate the occlusive process. The level and configuration of the aortic thrombus can be clearly identified, as well as the status of the major aortic branches. Visualization of collateral pathways to the iliofemoral arteries can frequently be achieved using delayed filming following contrast injection. If the presence of nonopacified blood in proximal collateral sources of the internal mammary epigastric system does not allow adequate distal femoral artery opacification, the arterial catheter can be repositioned for arch and/or subclavian injection, with filming over the femoral arteries, which then will be satisfactorily imaged by contrast passing through this collateral route.

OPERATIVE INTERVENTION

Goals of Operation

Improvement in limb perfusion is one objective of operative intervention for patients with aortic occlusion. This dramatically improves or relieves their symptoms. Perhaps a more important consideration for patients with juxtarenal occlusion, however, is the potential for cephalad propagation of their aortic thrombus. This can be removed and the aorta reopened or replaced with a prosthetic graft. This method of revascularization ensures limb revascularization and of more importance is the complete removal of the unstable aortic thrombus that, eventually, may lead to renal or visceral artery ischemia.

The natural history of aortic occlusion is variable, and the patient's outcome depends on whether the occlusion remains stable or progresses in a cephalad direction. In a series of unoperated patients reported from UCSF, more than one third succumbed to renal and/or visceral infarction that resulted from the cephalad propagation of the aortic thrombus. This observation is scarcely new, for Leriche pointed it out 30 years earlier. Thrombotic and embolic occlusion of renal and visceral aortic branches are obvious mechanisms of interrupting flow in these major aortic vascular beds, further promoting ascending aortic thrombosis. The presence of pararenal aortic atherosclerosis with renal and visceral ostial stenosis appear to favor a progressive aortic thrombosis rather than a stable one. The undiseased juxtarenal aorta and branches are more likely to remain patent, and evidence in our own patients show no change in the level of the aortic occlusion. At the present time, no clinical or experimental data have been reported evaluating the natural history of aortic occlusion based on the status of the pararenal aorta and its branches.

Direct Reoperation

The patient with an occluded aortic graft is not a candidate for graft thrombectomy when the juxtarenal aorta is occluded by thrombus. Catheter passage and balloon manipulation of the fragile thrombus could easily result in renal artery embolization. Furthermore, thrombectomy catheters are ineffective at removing the layers of thrombus in the large aortic portion of a bifurcation graft. Inadequate graft thrombectomy usually results in rethrombosis.

Direct reoperation for a failed aortic graft is feasible and safe. Exposure of the supra-renal aorta and renal arteries is usually easy since the previous infrarenal aortic procedure which has failed rarely involve such proximal aortic exposure; thus, the dissection is carried out in undissected tissues. On the other hand, the incorporated perigraft scar can be incised down to the level of the graft which is most easily mobilized in this plane. The application of temporary suprarenal aortic and bilateral renal artery clamps provides control for graft removal, aortic thrombectomy, and reattachment of a new graft. Depending on the length of the infrarenal aortic cuff, clamps can usually be repositioned so as to restore renal bloodflow following the thrombectomy. The iliac limbs of the graft are prepared for distal anastomosis, usually to the common femoral arteries, but this will depend on their status and the level of the previous graft's distal anastomosis.

When direct operation is selected for primary aortic occlusion, the dissection proceeds as previously described and involves the perirenal aorta. When the extent of the occlusive disease is known to involve the femoral arteries, then aortofemoral grafting is carried out. If, however, the aortic occlusion is confined to the terminal aorta and proximal iliac arteries, aortoiliac thromboendarterectomy is feasible.

A longitudinal anterior aortotomy facilitates the juxtarenal aortic thrombus removal after which the aortotomy is closed to permit infrarenal aortic reclamping with restoration of renal perfusion. The remainder of the aortic endarterectomy employs the open technique while the common iliac arteries are endarterectomized with loop strippers using the semiclosed technique.

These two methods of aortoiliac reconstruction emphasize temporary suprarenal aortic and renal branch clamp control to allow precise removal of the aortic thrombus, and avoidance of renal embolization with minimal renal ischemia (average 15 minutes). Increased cardiac strain resulting from supra-renal aortic clamping can be assessed during operation using systemic and pulmonary artery pressures or the two dimensional transesophageal echocardiograph. Real time beat-to-beat cardiac performance is observed during the latter technique, and changes in cardiac volume, contractility, and wall motion can be ascertained and rapidly treated to reverse disturbing trends or minimize damage. These measures are necessary to reduce myocardial dysfunction and subsequent morbidity and mortality from this procedure to the 2% to 3% range which can be consistently achieved. Such results justify direct operative intervention rather than indirect bypass procedures which ignore the intraluminal aortic thrombosis and its potential fatal consequences.

EXTRA ANATOMIC RECONSTRUCTION

We have not utilized extraanatomic reconstructions for either primary or secondary aortic occlusion or any other form of occlusive or aneurysmal disease of the aortoiliac segment in the absence of primary aortic or prosthetic graft sepsis. A particular concern has been the unstable juxtarenal aortic thrombus. In fact, progressive thrombosis has occurred in a number of our patients with oversewn aortic stump following treatment of chronic perigraft infection. In such instances, we have reoperated on patients, reopened the infrarenal aortic stump, and reconstructed the distal aorta with a new graft one year or more following successful treatment of the primary retroperitoneal graft infection.

Axillofemoral and cross-femoral bypass would seem to be, at first glance, a satisfactory method for bypassing the chronically occluded aorta. However, disappointing late patency rates of these subcutaneous small diameter bypasses have been repeatedly observed by many experienced surgeons. For these reasons, we prefer bypass from the thoracic aorta for extraanatomic bypass of the aortoiliac segment. The thoracic aorta has two attractive sites for origination of a bypass graft. Both offer access for the attachment of an aortic prosthesis of adequate size (16 mm to 22 mm). These sites are the ascending aorta exposed through a median sternotomy, and the supraceliac (distal thoracic) aorta usually approached through a high midline laparotomy and transcrural exposure. Recently, we have begun to reassess Buscaglia and Blaisdells' approach to the upper abdominal aorta. They reported reflecting of the descending colon, spleen, pancreas, and stomach from left to right. They described exposure of the upper half of the abdominal aorta and we have confirmed their observation as well. Thorough access to the peridiaphragmatic aorta is achieved, and this segment is usually undiseased, thereby allowing easy control for prosthetic aortic graft attachment.

Grafts of adequate size for aortic bypass can be established either on the ascending aorta or perhaps more easily the supraceliac (distal descending thoracic aorta) and can be arranged for iliac or femoral distal graft anastomosis depending on the extremity vasculature. These grafts have patency rates that compare favorably with infrarenal aortic replacements and would, predictably, be a reliable and durable alternative method of limb revascularization *if the surgeon wishes to avoid direct reoperation* in the region of the occluded infrarenal aorta.

CONCLUSION

This discussion has focused on the features of primary and secondary aortic occlusion. Although limb ischemia is usually the primary problem, a significant clinical concern is the natural history of aortic thrombosis itself. Proximal extension of aortic thrombus is halted only by blood flow in the aortic branches. The thrombus progressing cephalad may encroach on one or both renal arterial branch orifices. Embolic or thrombotic branch artery occlusion are organ or life-threatening. Treatment is aimed primarily at preventing the problem of aortic thrombus propagation rather than the treatment of extremity ischemia itself. Although both primary and secondary aortic occlusion are effectively treated by pararenal aortic control, thrombectomy, and distal aortic reconstructions, many surgeons utilize extraanatomic methods of aortic bypass. When the pararenal aorta and renal and visceral branches are undiseased, then extraanatomic bypass from the distal thoracic aorta may be a satisfactory alternative to direct pararenal aortic reconstruction. The vascular surgeon's own management of aortic occlusion will be determined in part by his or her familiarity with operations on the pararenal aorta and the status of the intraaortic thrombus itself.

BIBLIOGRAPHY

1. Bergan JJ, Trippel OH: Management of juxtarenal aortic occlusions. *Arch Surg* 1963; 87:230–238.
2. Buscaglia LC, Blaisdell FW, Lim RC: Penetrating abdominal vascular injuries. *Arch Surg* 1969; 99:764–769.
3. DeBakey ME: Basic concepts of therapy in arterial disease. *Bull NY Acad Med* 1963; 39:707–749.
4. Frantz SL, Kaplitt JJ, Beil AR, et al: Ascending aorto-bilateral femoral artery bypass for the totally occluded infrarenal abdominal aorta. *Surgery* 1974; 75:471–475.
5. Froysaker T, Skagseth E, Dundas P, et al: Bypass procedures in the treatment of obstructions of the abdominal aorta. *J Cardiovasc Surg* 1973; 14:317–321.
6. Gomes MMR, Bernatz PE: Aortoiliac occlusive disease. Extension cephalad to origin of renal arteries with surgical considerations and results. *Arch Surg* 1970; 101:161–166.
7. Johnson JK: Ascending thrombosis of abdominal aorta as fatal complication of Leriche's syndrome. *Arch Surg* 1954; 69:663–668.
8. Nunn DB, Kamal MA: Bypass grafting from the thoracic aorta to femoral arteries for high aortoiliac occlusive disease. *Surgery* 1972; 72:749–755.
9. Starer F, Sutton D: Aortic thrombosis. *Br Med J* 1958; 1:1255–1263.
10. Wyatt GM, Felson B: Aortic thrombosis as a cause of hypertension: An arteriographic study. *Radiology* 1957; 69:676–683.

27 Small Aorta Syndrome

A 51-year-old woman is admitted with severe bilateral lower extremity claudication. Only faint femoral pulses can be felt on either side. Angiography reveals small aortic, iliac, and femoral vessels. There is high-grade stenosis of the distal abdominal aorta and proximal common iliac arteries. The iliac arteries measure approximately 6 mm and the common femoral arteries approximately 4 mm; runoff is open bilaterally.

Consultant: Dominic A. DeLaurentis, M.D.

A hypoplastic aortoiliac system or "Small Aorta Syndrome" is a fairly common variant of atherosclerosis, and is most likely to occur in women under 50 years of age. Although not mentioned in the example case, it is not unusual for older patients with Small Aorta Syndrome to give a claudication history which often spans five to ten years. These patients are heavy cigarette smokers, nondiabetic, and usually nonhypertensive. In my practice, hypoplastic aortoiliac atherosclerotic occlusive disease is present in approximately 20% of women undergoing aortoiliac reconstruction.

DEFINITION

Although the various names given to this disease implicate only the aorta or iliac arteries, it is important to note that the *femoral, popliteal,* and *tibial* arteries are also involved in the hypoplastic process. Whether this entity should be considered a separate syndrome may be questioned, but the problems and hazards encountered during surgical reconstruction (especially to the uninitiated) cannot be, and this was our original reason for reporting this group of patients. In a recent review of the literature, I found that major amputations following failed vascular reconstruction still occur in this group of patients. Amputation represents a catastrophic complication, since the indication for surgery is usually claudication in a young woman. The claudication in these individuals is more symptomatic and dramatic than in the typical older patients with aortoiliac disease, because it occurs at a life period when the patient is physically quite active.

What diameters make an aorto-iliac-femoral system hypoplastic is not known. We compared arteriograms documenting this syndrome to normal arteriograms, and concluded that to be considered hypoplastic the diameter of the infrarenal aorta should measure less than 15 mm, the common iliac artery less than 8 mm, and the external iliac and common femorals less than 4 mm. Although the Small Aorta Syndrome can occur in males, the incidence in males undergoing aortoiliac reconstruction in my series of patients between 1965 and 1985 was only 1%. Therefore, an active vascular surgeon should expect to encounter this lesion in one out of five women undergoing aortoiliac reconstruction and rarely in a male. Occasionally, a patient may be confused with the rare entity of coarctation of the abdominal aorta; however, the lack of renal artery disease and systemic hypertension in patients with Small Aorta Syndrome should rule this out.

The etiology of this hypoplasia is not known. The most likely explanation is that this represents a congenital over fusion of the distal aortae, producing a small aortoiliac system. Symptoms then occur early in life because of normally occurring atherosclerosis in the infrarenal aorta.

MANAGEMENT

In elderly patients, with minimal ischemic symptoms consisting only of mild claudication, no operative management is recommended. Instead, cessation of smoking, weight loss, exercise, and dietary change is insisted upon. If on the other hand, the ischemia is severe, or the patient is young and insists on relief of claudication, operative arterial reconstruction is the method of choice. Percutaneous arterial angioplasty is not recommended because of the diffuse nature of the disease and the technical problems of introducing catheters in small femoral and axillary arteries. Indeed, because of arterial thrombosis that occurred with retrograde femoral and axillary arteriography in some early patients, I prefer to use translumbar aortography to outline the aorta, iliac, and femoral arteries in these patients. High (T-12) translumbar aortography is safe, gives good visualization, and is especially helpful in this group of patients.

I have found that approximately two thirds of these patients have coexisting brachiocephalic occlusive disease. Consequently, these patients should be carefully evaluated by physical examination, duplex scanning, and OPG testing. Brachiocephalic intraarterial digital angiography should be done if any of the lesions are judged significant by noninvasive testing or if they are causing symptoms.

SURGICAL APPROACH

I prefer aortic bypass techniques since endarterectomy is not easily accomplished in these small fibrotic vessels in which a satisfactory plane for endarterectomy is often difficult to establish. Aortography will often show a lesion that looks very localized to the aortic bifurcation and which should, but often does not, lend itself to endarterectomy (Fig 27–1). In the management of 35 patients with hypoplastic aortoiliac systems, I was able to carry out a successful endarterectomy in only one patient. Several times endarterectomy was started but had to be abandoned in favor of a bypass. Occasionally, with very limited stenosis of the aorta, a patch technique can be used; however, patching usually has to be carried down to both common iliac arteries. I use knitted Dacron for the patch, although there is no reason why Polytetrafluorethylene (PTFE) cannot be used.

When the aorta is not completely occluded, I believe end-to-side anastomosis of the graft at the aortic site is the procedure of choice. This should be carried out just below the renal vessels where the aorta is widest and the wall least calcified. This end-to-side anastomosis of the bifurcation graft should be of an onlay-type so that maximum diameters are obtained. If the aorta is completely occluded distally,

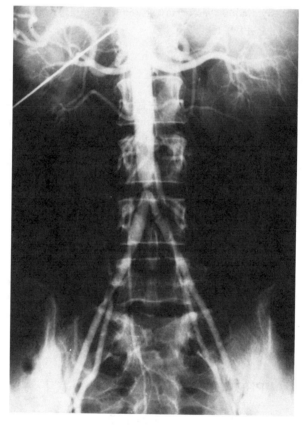

FIG 27–1.
Typical preoperative translumbar aortogram in a 39-year-old woman with severe bilateral claudication, illustrative of the Small Aorta Syndrome.

I transect and spatulate the aorta and do an end-to-end anastomosis to the proximal infrarenal aorta. When the occlusion in the aorta extends to the renal level, control of the aorta above the renals is mandatory in order to carry out a thromboendarterectomy of the juxtarenal aorta. The aorta below the renal is then transected and an end-to-end anastomosis done. Before any surgical procedure is carried out, it is important that small bifurcated grafts be available. I usually use a 12 × 7 mm knitted Dacron graft manufactured by Meadox Medicals, Inc. A 12 × 6 mm bifurcation graft is made by a number of graft manufacturers, while a 10 × 5 knitted bifurcation graft is available from Golaski Laboratories.

Full heparinization is carried out prior to aortic clamping. However, before heparinization and prior to carrying out the bypass, a bilateral lumbar sympathectomy is usually performed. Although there are no data to support this procedure as a method of increasing long-term patency rates, I feel that peripheral resistance is decreased by sympathectomy and, consequently, early patency rates may be improved. Also, these patients often complain of cold feet and the sympathectomy reverses this complaint. *A warning:* Under no circumstances should bilateral lumbar sympathectomy be relied on to keep open a vascular reconstruction which is not done in a most meticulous manner!

After the proximal anastomosis is completed, attention is turned to the distal anastomosis and this is either to the external iliac or the common femoral artery in the groin. The common iliac in these patients is usually short, has a definite posterior atherosclerotic plaque, and usually does not lend itself well to a long anastomosis. I prefer to use the intraabdominal external iliac when the runoff into the femoropopliteal tree is open, as in the above described patient. When the external iliac is used, the advantages are fewer incisions, all of the graft is kept in the abdomen, ambulation is easier, and there is a decreased incidence of infection and false aneurysm.

When the superficial femoral artery is occluded, the bypass *must* be brought down to the common femoral artery and profunda orifice and a decision *must* be made with regard to a synchronous femoropopliteal bypass. Unless there are some unusual contraindications, I practically always carry out a femoropopliteal bypass in these patients. If this is not performed, the small profunda may be unable to accept all of the flow and could lead to early thrombosis. If at all possible, the femoropopliteal bypass should be performed using reversed saphenous vein because the popliteal arteries are extremely small. In patients with occluded superficial femoral arteries and tissue necrosis or rest pain, I always perform a synchronous femoropopliteal bypass. All distal anastomoses are long and end-to-side, and at least five interrupted sutures at the toe of the anastomosis are inserted to prevent outflow stricture. The small iliac and femoral vessels are often soft and can be gently dilated up to 4 mm with coronary artery dilators prior to performing the anastomosis. After the graft is opened and flow established, these small vessels will often dilate dramatically within a period of minutes. The diameter can increase 50% to 60%. This is usually an excellent indication that the bypass will be successful. I use a loop with 2.5× magnification to construct the distal anastomosis with either 5–0, 6–0, or 7–0 polypropylene sutures.

Other approaches that can be used when the standard aortoiliac or aortofemoral bypass is not feasible are the axillofemoral or the descending thoracic aorta to femoral artery bypass. Often, the axillofemoral bypass is not possible in these patients because of concomitant brachiocephalic occlusive disease. Therefore, if one contemplates this operation, it is imperative that good axillary inflow be assured before this alternative is used. I personally do not like to use axillofemoral bypass in this young group of patients and have not done so. When I find, for whatever reason, that a standard aortoiliac or aortofemoral bypass is not possible, I perform a descending thoracic aorta to femoral artery bypass. The details of this operation have been previously described. (See Bibliography.)

Although these patients occasionally may present with only one occluded or stenotic iliac artery, a standard femorofemoral bypass is not recommended because the disease involves the aorta and both iliacs and a femorofemoral bypass tends to thrombose. If a femorofemoral bypass is used, I would caution against a prosthesis and try to use autogenous vein for the graft.

Complications we have encountered following reconstruction for Small Aorta Syndrome include bleeding, thrombosis, and postsympathectomy neuralgia. Anastomotic aneurysms have not as yet been detected. Because of the younger age and less extensive generalized atherosclerosis in these patients, the mortality rate in our series has been zero.

FOLLOW-UP

In follow-up I have noticed that the patients who stopped smoking have the best prognosis; those that continue to smoke usually develop coronary artery disease, strokes, and progression of atherosclerosis in the lower extremities. Thus, long-term patency rates are good only if the patient stops smoking, loses weight, and controls serum lipids. In the follow-up, late deaths were due to coronary artery disease, strokes, and carcinoma of the lung. Thus, the most common long-term atherosclerotic problems are coronary artery disease and cerebrovascular disease, and the most common nonvascular cause of late death has been carcinoma of the lung. Postoperatively, I prescribe aspirin 300 mgs a day and dipyridamole 50 mgs three times a day, although these medications have never been shown to be of any direct benefit. Patients should be examined at least every six months, at which time Doppler ankle pressures and other noninvasive studies should be carried out. Superficial femoral artery stenosis or occlusion can be detected early by these measures, and when found, should be corrected promptly to prevent thrombosis of the ipsilateral limb of the aortoiliac or aortofemoral graft. I have had no experience with Pentoxifylline in this particular group of patients.

In addition to the routine lower extremity vascular follow-up, these patients, especially if still smoking, should have routine chest X-rays. At follow-up they should be carefully evaluated for brachiocephalic atherosclerotic occlusive problems and angina.

BIBLIOGRAPHY

1. Ameli FM, Hoy, F: Preoperative diagnosis and management of the hypoplastic vessels system. *J Cardiovasc Surg* 1983; 24:654–657.
2. Dale WA: The small aorta syndrome, in Dale WA (ed): *Management of Vascular Surgical Problems*. New York, McGraw-Hill Book Co, 1985, pp 270–276.
3. DeLaurentis DA, Friedmann P, Wolferth CC Jr, et al: Atherosclerosis and the hypoplastic aortoiliac system. *Surgery* 1978; 83:27–37.
4. DeLaurentis DA: The hypoplastic aortoiliac syndrome, in Veith FA (ed): *Critical Problems in Vascular Surgery*. New York, Appleton-Century-Crofts, 1982, pp 411–428.
5. DeLaurentis DA: Aortoiliac hypoplasia, in Ernst CB, Stanley JC (eds): *Current Therapy in Vascular Surgery*. Burlington, Ontario, Canada, BC, Decker, Inc, 1987, pp 156–157.
6. Rosenfeld JC, Savarese RP, DeLaurentis DA: Distal thoracic aorta to femoral artery bypass: A surgical alternative. *J Vasc Surg* 1987; 2:747–750.

28 Aortofemoral Graft Limb Occlusion

A 68-year-old plumber is seen in the emergency room for the sudden onset of a cold left leg. Three years ago he underwent aortobifemoral bypass grafting for severe claudication, with marked improvement in walking distance. On the morning of admission, he suddenly developed recurrent left leg ischemia. Examination reveals an absent left femoral pulse, and a good right femoral pulse. The left foot is cool, with slightly diminished sensation but intact motion.

Consultant: Victor M. Bernhard, M.D.

AORTOFEMORAL GRAFT OCCLUSION

The described case is a typical presentation of acute occlusion of one limb of a previously well-functioning aortofemoral graft. This will occur in 10% to 25% of patients over a five- to ten-year follow-up period and, as in this patient, most commonly appears within three years after the original operation. Characteristically, the limb with the thrombosed graft was more ischemic than prior to the initial procedure. A bolus of heparin should be administered during initial evaluation to prevent propagating thrombus since the occlusion has occurred acutely. Although the limb at initial presentation was marginally viable, the severity of ischemia should be continually assessed by repeated clinical and Doppler examination of the extremity to determine the urgency of revascularization while investigations preliminary to revascularization are in progress. Immediate intervention to restore circulation will be required if motor and sensory function are significantly reduced and Doppler flow is absent in the pedal vessels. In most instances, however, there will be sufficient time to evaluate the quality and character of the outflow, determine the status of the opposite femoral and the aortic anastomoses, and assess risk factors.

PATHOGENESIS

The most common cause of aortofemoral graft limb occlusion following a period of successful graft function is obstruction in the runoff bed. In 50% to 75% of cases, the superficial femoral artery was occluded at the time of the initial surgery or was severely diseased and has gone on to complete obstruction. The remaining outflow tract is generally the profunda femoris, which has become compromised due to fibrointimal hyperplasia or atherosclerosis at and just distal to the femoral anastomosis. Since the obstructing process occurs over months, sufficient collaterals will generally develop to maintain at least marginal limb viability. In the majority of patients with progressive loss of outflow, the deep femoral artery beyond the area of obstruction is relatively normal and has large geniculate connections to the popliteal-tibial runoff vessels.

Although this scenario occurs in 60% to 80% of patients, other causes must be considered. Anastomotic false aneurysm may promote either acute embolic or thrombotic occlusion and is suggested when a mass can be felt in the groin or if there is a pulsatile widening at the opposite femoral anastomosis. A source of embolism from the heart or aorta proximal to the aortic anastomosis should be searched for if a perianastomotic problem is not identified at surgery. Rarely, a hypercoagulable state or a defect in the graft wall may be implicated. Graft limb thrombosis which occurs in the immediate postoperative period after the original operation is usually due to technical misadventures during the performance of the distal anastomosis, failure to appreciate severity of profunda stenosis, graft kinking or twisting, or external compression. Bilateral simultaneous graft limb occlusion usually indicates a mechanical problem at the aortic anastomosis or in the proximal aorta, or severe cardiac dysfunction.

MANAGEMENT OPTIONS

Historically, replacement of the thrombosed limb or the entire graft was the recommended procedure. This is a relatively formidable undertaking with increased morbidity and mortality. The feasibility of graft thrombectomy and a runoff procedure, usually profundaplasty, was first suggested by Lyons and Weismann as a simpler method for resolving the problem. This technique has evolved into the most commonly employed method for reestablishing function in an occluded graft limb. A reasonable alternative which can be used when thrombectomy cannot be accomplished is a femorofemoral bypass from the opposite patent graft limb or axillofemoral bypass if this is not feasible. A more recent innovation is the application of lytic therapy to clear thrombus from the occluded graft, followed by surgical intervention or balloon dilatation to repair the outflow tract. Replacement of the aortofemoral graft is now reserved for those individuals who have progressing obstructive disease in the infrarenal aorta at and above the proximal anastomosis, aortic anastomotic false aneurysm, or significant graft dilatation or degeneration.

PREOPERATIVE EVALUATION

Arteriography, although not essential, should be obtained shortly after admission since it provides valuable information for patient management. The quality of the aorta above the graft and aortic anastomosis can be assessed. The appearance of the patent portion of the graft and the opposite femoral anastomosis can be determined to look for anastomotic false aneurysm or progressing outflow disease which may lead to occlusion in the opposite extremity. The quality of the runoff in the obstructed limb can usually be defined since collateral development in most instances will permit contrast filling of the profunda and the popliteal-tibial runoff vessels. If the outflow cannot be visualized, but the patient had a viable and functional extremity prior to graft occlusion, profunda patency can usually be established beyond the point of stenosis or the popliteal-tibial vessels will generally be available for infrainguinal bypass. Arteriography rarely identifies the cause of limb occlusion since this is usually buried in fresh clot and will be revealed at the time of surgical intervention.

A CT scan should be obtained to rule out an anastomotic aortic aneurysm whenever there is clinical or angiographic evidence of anastomotic aneurysm in the contralateral femoral artery or if an unexpected aneurysm is identified at surgery.

Preoperative evaluation can be accomplished within a very short period of time in most patients and should not materially delay intervention to relieve severe ischemia. As long as limb viability is not in question, the operative procedure can be safely delayed until cardiac, pulmonary, renal or other problems can be resolved or improved. However, if the extremity is clearly in jeopardy, preliminary investigation should be aborted and the patient brought directly to the operating room for prompt revascularization. In this circumstance, intraoperative arteriography is employed as needed to evaluate runoff potential.

OPERATIVE TECHNIQUE

The most commonly employed procedure is graft limb thrombectomy and profundaplasty (Fig 28–1). Occasionally, bypass to the popliteal or tibial vessels may be necessary when profunda runoff cannot be established or is inadequate.

The operative procedure is usually performed under general anesthesia. However, in a high-risk patient, local infiltration or continuous caudal can be employed. The field should be prepped widely so that the aorta, the opposite groin, and the vessels down to the foot can be approached, if necessary. The previous groin incision is opened to expose the distal end of the thrombosed graft, the anastomosis, and the common femoral artery and its branches. The lateral circumflex femoral vein overlying the proximal portion of the deep femoral artery should usually be divided in order to obtain easy access to this vessel. If groin scarring is very dense, extensive dissection at the common femoral anastomosis can be abandoned and the profunda femoris artery exposed by extending the incision distally so that dissection can proceed through normal tissue beyond the scar from the previous operative procedure. As an alternative, the midprofunda can be exposed through an intermuscular plane developed lateral to the upper portion of the sartorius muscle which is displaced medially.

The graft is disconnected from its former femoral anastomosis and the anasto-

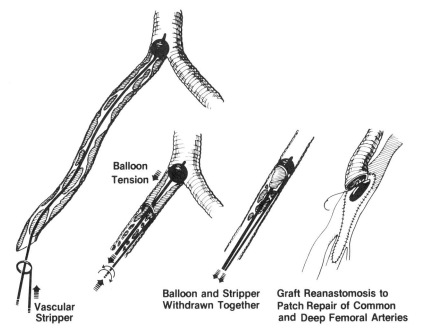

Balloon
Tension

Vascular
Stripper

Balloon and Stripper
Withdrawn Together

Graft Reanastomosis to
Patch Repair of Common
and Deep Femoral Arteries

FIG 28–1.
Technique of graft limb thrombectomy employing balloon catheter and an endarterectomy loop stripper. Subsequent reanastomosis following profunda femoris patch angioplasty.

motic area inspected to identify the obstructing problem. Inflow is established most frequently by thrombectomy of the occluded limb of the aortofemoral graft. This is performed after full systemic heparinization has been established by intravenous administration of 150 u per kgm. A No. 5 or No. 6 Fogarty balloon catheter is passed cephalad through the clot into the patent proximal aortic portion of the graft. This should be done slowly and gently to avoid inadvertent cross-embolization from the proximal end of the thrombus into the contralateral patent limb. The balloon is fully distended and the catheter withdrawn to extract the obstructing thrombus. This maneuver is performed several times until the quality of flow which is reestablished through the obstructed limb has the vigorous, pulsatile, unobstructed characteristics of a normal graft at the time of original insertion. This simple technique may be sufficient if thrombosis is very recent. However, when thrombosis has been present for more than a few days or when satisfactory flow cannot be obtained, an arterial endarterectomy ring stripper can be employed to remove the residual thrombus and pseudointima which remain adherent to the arterial wall. The technique, originally described by Ernst, et al, requires that the Fogarty catheter be passed first through the ring of the stripper and then up the limb of the graft. The balloon is inflated in the aortic portion of the prosthesis and pulled down tightly to obstruct the orifice of the graft limb. The ring of the stripper, which should fit comfortably, but not too tightly in the graft, is then passed proximally through the limb with an oscillating motion. The stripper is advanced until it reaches the inflated balloon which is held tightly in place to avoid embolization to the opposite extremity. The balloon is then deflated just enough so that the balloon and stripper can be withdrawn *en masse* to remove any residual thrombotic material. A chronic thrombotic plug is frequently dislodged by this technique following which there is an unobstructed gush of blood through the limb.

The completeness of thrombectomy can be confirmed by retrograde arteriography through the distal limb of the thrombectomized graft, as described by Hyde and Brewster, or by arterial endoscopy. The latter requires replacement of the balloon catheter to temporarily occlude the inflow orifice of the graft limb. While the lumen is being vigorously irrigated with saline to clear blood from the field, the inner graft surface is inspected with a vascular endoscope.

During thrombectomy maneuvers, the opposite femoral pulse should be continuously monitored. Direct compression of the femoral pulse should be maintained temporarily while the catheter is being passed through the upper end of the clot so that preferential flow will not be down the open extremity during these manipulations. After completion of the procedure, it is important to directly inspect the circulation, not only in the revascularized limb, but in the contralateral extremity to look for possible cross-embolization. Direct exposure of the opposite groin will be required if that femoral pulse has diminished or disappeared. If the femoral pulse is present but the distal pulses have disappeared, or if the previously normal extremity now appears to be ischemic, intraoperative arteriography should be performed to define the approach for contralateral embolectomy.

Although effective restoration of flow is most readily accomplished when thrombosis has been recent, graft thrombectomy has been successfully performed more than six months after thrombosis has occurred. Therefore, attempted thrombectomy is always an appropriate initial step. Occasionally, the presence of thrombus in the aortic portion of the graft, which may extend up into the patient's normal aorta, may preclude the use of catheter thrombectomy since extraction may be incomplete or balloon catheter manipulation may promote embolism to the opposite extremity. Femorofemoral bypass from the patent contralateral limb is the commonly employed alternative when thrombectomy is unsuccessful or is contraindicated.

The adequacy of the profunda femoris and the superficial femoral arteries as outflow tracts may be apparent on the preoperative arteriogram. However, if outflow vessels were not demonstrated or an arteriogram was not done, the quality of the profunda and the superficial femoral beyond the point of obstruction can be assessed by direct inspection after these vessels are exposed and the previous anastomosis disconnected. Incision is made through the area of stenosis into the patent distal vessel. As an alternative, an arteriotomy can be made directly into the profunda below the obstruction and beyond the area of scarring at a point where the vessel appears to be relatively soft and not involved with atherosclerosis. Any thrombus present is removed directly with a Fogarty catheter. If the profunda can be easily probed with the balloon catheter to a distance of 20 cm to 25 cm, it is probably a satisfactory vessel for outflow. This can be confirmed by completion arteriography after restoration of circulation.

Any one of a variety of strategies may be employed at the level of the occluded femoral anastomosis to restore runoff into the profunda or SFA, depending on the local pathology and anatomy. Most commonly, a simple patch profundaplasty with or without local endarterectomy will provide widely patent runoff beyond the obstruction into a relatively normal profunda. Occasionally, extended profundaplasty several centimeters beyond the vessel origin will be necessary. In some patients, the superficial femoral may also be opened beyond the point of obstruction into a reasonably patent vessel so that outflow through both vessels can be restored. Autogenous tissue should be used for the patch angioplasty and is readily obtained from the saphenous vein or may be constructed from an endarterectomized segment of the adjacent occluded superficial femoral artery. In the event that the profunda or proximal superficial femoral are inadequate, a more distal bypass may be necessary. Operative arteriography may be required to define the appropriate distal vessel to be exposed for this anastomosis. The precise bypass technique to be employed will depend on the available outflow vessel and the presence or absence of a satisfactory vein. After the outflow obstruction is corrected, circulation is restored by anastomosis of the reopened graft limb to the repaired femoral artery or to a bypass graft to the popliteal or tibial vessels.

On occasion, no mechanical obstruction to flow will be identified and simple thrombectomy alone will suffice to restore circulation. Under these circumstances, however, it is appropriate, during the immediate postoperative period, to search for a more proximal embolic source and thoroughly evaluate the coagulation system to identify a potential hypercoagulable state.

Intraarterial lytic therapy may be used to clear the thrombosed limb of the graft and balloon dilatation angioplasty may then successfully relieve the obstruction in the outflow tract. This nonsurgical approach has advantages for the extremely high-risk patient. However, the use of lytic agents is contraindicated when immediate revascularization is required or if potential bleeding problems are present. Since a surgical procedure to establish outflow is almost invariably required and mechanical thrombectomy is quickly and reliably accomplished through the same incision, there seems to be little advantage to the use of thrombolysis. Furthermore, lytic therapy has its own complications, poses a delay in limb revascularization, and is very costly in terms of additional usage of radiology and the intensive care unit.

RESULTS

Restoration of circulation and limb salvage by any combination of the above-described methods can be accomplished in more than 90% of patients.

Thrombectomy using current techniques will successfully clear the limb in at least 80% of patients so that femorofemoral bypass or some other procedure will be infrequently required. Profundaplasty alone will also provide satisfactory outflow for the majority of limbs so that bypass to the popliteal or tibial vessels will be necessary in no more than 25% to 30%.

Long-term graft patency is achieved in 60% to 75% of limbs after initial thrombectomy and graft function may be further improved by repeated operations if rethrombosis occurs. In the event that adequate distal circulation cannot be achieved to save an ischemic foot, it is nevertheless important to restore flow to the profunda whenever possible to support healing of a below-knee amputation. Failure to do so under these circumstances will usually result in amputation at the above-knee or high-thigh level.

Unless there are major contraindications, an aggressive approach to aortofemoral graft limb thrombosis is warranted in all patients. Thrombectomy or femorofemoral bypass and appropriate repair of the outflow tract can be accomplished with a high likelihood of success, very low morbidity, and an operative mortality of 2%.

BIBLIOGRAPHY

1. Bernhard VM, Ray LI, Towne JB: The reoperation of choice for aortofemoral graft occlusion. *Surgery* 1977; 82:867–874.
2. Brewster DC, Meier GH III, Darling RC, et al: Reoperation for aortofemoral graft limb occlusion: Optimal methods and long-term results. *J Vasc Surg* 1987; 5:363–372.
3. Cohn LH, Moore WS, Hall AD: Extra-abdominal management of late aortofemoral graft thrombosis. *Surgery* 1970; 67:775–779.
4. Crawford ES, Manning LG, Kelly TF: "Redo" surgery after operations for aneurysm and occlusion of the abdominal aorta. *Surgery* 1977; 81:41–52.
5. Ernst CB, Daugherty ME: Removal of a thrombotic plug from an occluded limb of an aortofemoral graft. *Arch Surg* 1978; 113:301–302.
6. Hyde GL, McCready RA, Schwartz RW: Durability of thrombectomy of occluded aortofemoral graft limbs. *Surgery* 1983; 94:748–751.
7. LeGrand DR, Vermilion BD, Hayes JP, et al: Management of the occluded aortofemoral graft limb. *Surgery* 1983; 93:818–821.
8. Lyons JH Jr, Weismann RE: Surgical management of late closure of aortofemoral reconstruction grafts. *N Engl J Med* 1968; 278:1035–1037.
9. Towne JB, Bernhard VM: Technique of intraoperative endoscopic evaluation of occluded aortofemoral grafts following thrombectomy. *Surg Gynecol Obstet* 1979; 148:87–89.
10. Van Breda A, Robison JC, Feldman L, et al: Local thrombolysis in the treatment of arterial graft occlusions. *J Vasc Surg* 1984; 1:103–112.

29 Aortofemoral Graft with Groin Infection

Aortobifemoral grafting is carried out electively for severe claudication in a 58-year-old lawyer. Recovery appears uneventful and a good result is obtained with complete relief of claudication. Three months postoperatively, he returns with drainage from the right groin. Examination reveals a draining sinus in the midportion of the prior groin incision. Femoral and distal pulses are present.

Consultant: Jerry Goldstone, M.D.

The presentation of this case is typical for early onset of infection involving at least one limb of a bilateral aortofemoral bypass graft. The presenting manifestation in this case, namely a draining sinus in the groin, is rather typical since groin wound complications are by far the most common presenting manifestations of infected aortofemoral arterial grafts. Management and treatment priorities are: first, to establish the diagnosis of graft infection; second, to establish the extent of involvement of the graft in the infectious process; third, to determine the anatomic and physiologic status of both the native and reconstructed arterial circulation; fourth, preparation of the patient for major surgery; and fifth, staged arterial revascularization and infected graft removal.

ESTABLISHMENT OF THE PRESENCE OF PROSTHETIC GRAFT INFECTION

Whenever a complication such as a false aneurysm, draining sinus, wound infection, et cetera, occurs at an incision overlying a prosthetic arterial graft, the possibility of infection involving the underlying graft must be seriously considered. In the patient described above, a draining sinus involves the right groin incision, and the surgeon should be alerted to the possibility of infection of the underlying graft. Cultures of the draining material should be obtained, although it should be recognized that there is a poor correlation between the culture results obtained from this source and the results of intraoperative cultures obtained from infected grafts when they are removed. Therefore, one cannot base the selection of antibiotic therapy entirely on these culture results, but the antibiotic spectrum should at least cover whatever organisms are cultured preoperatively.

Perhaps the easiest and quickest means of establishing the presence of infection in this case is by performing a sinogram. Water-soluble contrast material can be injected through a small rubber catheter placed into the sinus tract. This should establish communication of the sinus tract with the graft itself. Any portion of the graft outlined by the sinogram is not incorporated by surrounding fibrous tissue and can be assumed to be infected. Routine laboratory tests such as leukocyte count and erythrocyte sedimentation rate are frequently normal in the presence of a graft infection and therefore, are not helpful in establishing the diagnosis, although sometimes an elevated sedimentation rate is the only hint of an unsuspected graft infection. Isotope labelled white cell scans can be helpful if they indicate a focal "hot spot." However, Indium-111 labelled leukocyte scans are commonly positive for about three months following graft implantation and therefore, in this case, would be of questionable diagnostic value.

ESTABLISHMENT OF THE EXTENT OF INFECTION

It is important to establish the extent of involvement of the graft by the infectious process. If infection is limited to one groin, as in this case the right side, it is possible to treat the patient by partial graft removal.

The sinogram and occasionally the indium-labelled white cell scan may document involvement of the contralateral femoral limb or the main body of the graft. However, the most useful methods for determining this have been either computerized tomographic (CT) or magnetic resonance (MR) scans. At three months post-implantation, there should be no fluid around a graft and therefore, the presence of fluid or air bubbles should be considered as presumptive evidence of perigraft infection. This may be manifested on the magnetic resonance image as inflammation involving the adjacent psoas muscles. Ultrasonography is probably not as accurate in identifying perigraft fluid as are CT and MR scanning. None of the tests, however, are absolutely reliable, especially when they are negative. That is, grafts may be infected and surrounded by fluid but not identified as such by either CT or MR scans. Therefore, surgical exploration and direct inspection of the graft itself is often required to establish not only the presence of infection but its extent.

ARTERIOGRAPHIC AND PHYSIOLOGIC EVALUATION

This patient has intact femoral and distal pulses and it can therefore be assumed that the superficial femoral, popliteal and infrapopliteal vessels have no significant obstructing lesions. Nevertheless, a thorough noninvasive evaluation should be performed to obtain objective physiologic data. A thorough angiographic evaluation of the aorta and runoff vessels is also important in order to identify the prosthetic as well as native anatomy. This will greatly facilitate the planning of the reconstructive procedure that will be required to provide blood flow to the legs on removal of the infected graft. Of particular importance are the status of the internal iliac and the superficial femoral arteries; the former because of concern about pelvic blood flow after graft removal, and the latter for selection of the distal anastomotic site of an axillofemoral bypass graft.

PREPARATION OF THE PATIENT FOR MAJOR SURGERY

Control of hemorrhage is an obvious treatment priority in patients with either anastomotic disruption or bleeding from an aortoenteric fistula. Similarly, control of the infection itself may be urgent if there is an abscess with frank sepsis. Incision and drainage of a groin abscess can sometimes be an important early maneuver. This patient, fortunately, has neither of these problems. He is relatively young and not chronically ill, therefore, preoperative preparation should be fairly simple and straightforward. Appropriate broad-spectrum antibiotics should be administered and prompt surgical treatment undertaken. Many patients, however, are older and debilitated and may benefit from a few days of cardiac, pulmonary, and nutritional evaluation and support. One should, however, avoid unnecessary delays since they are frequently associated with the development of additional infection-related complications.

SURGICAL TREATMENT

Even though graft infection is highly probable in this patient, if all of the diagnostic studies, including sinography and the various scans, do not indicate communication of the draining sinus with the graft itself, exploration of the sinus tract should be considered. This must, of course, be done carefully so that if the graft is truly uninfected, it does not get contaminated by the exploration. If wound exploration identifies the presence of prosthetic graft in the base of the wound, and the area of contamination appears to be limited and does not involve an anastomosis, some surgeons would attempt to treat this localized infection by local antibiotic or povidone iodine (Betadine) irrigation and dressing changes. This form of local treatment for very circumscribed prosthetic graft infections is occasionally successful, but even eventual closure of the draining wound does not ensure permanent solution to the infectious problem and long-term follow-up is mandatory.

A small percentage of patients similar to the one discussed herein can be expected to have infection limited to one graft limb. Partial graft excision may successfully treat the problem. The most important step in this approach is exploration of the ipsilateral graft limb, in this case the right limb, through a suprainguinal retroperitoneal incision. If exposure of the graft limb at this level reveals a well-incorporated graft with no surrounding fluid, it can be assumed that the infection does not involve the remainder of the graft. In this situation, the graft can be divided at this point and oversewn as far proximally and distally as possible and the retroperitoneal tunnel obliterated with soft tissues. Revascularization of the ipsilateral lower extremity can be accomplished using an obturator bypass to the superficial femoral or deep femoral artery, followed by closure of the fresh surgical wounds and then removal of the distal portion of the infected graft by opening the infected groin wound. Alternatively, a prosthetic or autogenous (saphenous vein) femorofemoral bypass can be constructed, originating in the uninfected left groin and terminating in the right superficial femoral artery employing a course away from the infected right groin.

Much more common is the extent of involvement of the right graft limb that precludes partial graft excision, or there will be evidence indicating that the body and/or left limb of the graft are also infected. In either of these situations, the entire graft must be removed. This is best accomplished in a staged fashion with preliminary lower extremity revascularization being performed as the first stage. The preferred method employs axillofemoral bypass with prosthetic material. Externally supported Dacron or PTFE graft material, usually 8 mm to 10 mm in diameter, should be used. A number of factors influence the selection of the donor axillary artery including the upper extremity blood pressures, and the status of the superficial femoral arteries. If possible, the right axillary artery is chosen so that should a subsequent thoracic aorta to femoral reconstruction become necessary, the axillofemoral graft will not need to be divided preliminarily. In addition, when there is a blood pressure difference between the arms, the left side is often much lower than the right. If there is a patent superficial femoral artery on only one side, it is preferable to use it as the distal axillofemoral anastomotic site because of its relative ease of exposure in the proximal thigh.

This is accomplished through a longitudinal incision along the lateral border of the sartorius muscle. After closure of the axillary and thigh wounds, femorofemoral bypass to revascularize the other leg must be performed. I prefer to use an autogenous graft for this portion of the procedure, either saphenous vein or endarterectomized superficial femoral artery if it was occluded. In this case, both superficial femoral arteries are patent and therefore the saphenous vein would be employed. Since autogenous grafts can be expected to heal even in the presence of infection, the femorofemoral bypass can be inserted through the original groin incisions. The aortofemoral graft limbs can be detached and oversewn at this point and pushed back up under the inguinal ligament for later removal. The cross-femoral anastomoses can be either end-to-end or end-to-side to the femoral arteries, but efforts should be made to ensure retrograde perfusion of the pelvic arteries on at least one side in order to avoid colonic ischemia.

Five to seven days after revascularization of the lower extremities, the entire aortic bifurcation graft should be removed through a transabdominal or retroperitoneal approach. If the original aortic anastomosis was end-to-end, temporary suprarenal or supraceliac cross-clamping may be necessary to ensure adequate debridement and closure of the aortic stump. The most important part of this stage is the closure of the aortic stump which must be accomplished in healthy tissue and without tension. A double layered closure employing monofilament sutures is preferable. Debridement of the aortic stump to reach healthy appearing tissues is important since one of the most common causes of death in these patients is dehisence of the aortic stump closure. A sample of the debrided aorta should be submitted for microbiological analysis since we have found that those patients who suffered dehisence of their aortic stumps invariably had infection involving the aorta itself in contrast to those who had infection involving only the prosthetic graft. If there is a significant amount of necrotic material in the retroperitoneum, it should also be carefully and thoroughly debrided. Retroperitoneal drains can be employed when frank pus is present. Removal of the limbs of the graft can frequently be difficult, especially if the graft is of Dacron velour construction and special care must be paid to avoid injury to the ureters. This portion of the procedure is often associated with considerable bleeding because of the dissection in the inflamed tissue beds.

If the proximal aortic anastomosis had been performed in an end-to-side fashion, primary closure of the anastomotic defect can sometimes be accomplished or an autogenous patch may be used to maintain patency in the distal aorta. In some situations the entire arterial reconstruction is preferably autogenous. This requires extensive use of endarterectomy and/or saphenous veins and endarterectomized SFA.

Intravenous antibiotics should be maintained for seven to ten days after infected graft removal. The antibiotic used may need to be changed depending on the results of the microbiologic studies on the removed specimens. If the aortic stump is culture positive, six weeks of culture-specific intravenous antibiotics followed by an additional six weeks of oral antibiotics are indicated. Antiplatelet but not anticoagulant drugs are prescribed postoperatively. The patient can be discharged from the hospital when all of the incisions are satisfactorily healed. Careful long-term follow-up is necessary to monitor the function of the new reconstruction and to detect new graft infection which has occurred in 15% to 20% of patients treated in this manner.

Neither the first nor the second stage can be considered to be the "easy" operation. This is because the first stage revascularization is usually difficult and complicated due to anatomic and pathologic features in the runoff arteries. Nevertheless, the stress on the patient, as well as the surgical team is less when two relatively short operations are performed instead of a single extensive and prolonged one. Our studies indicate that the metabolic stresses, the intravenous fluid requirements, as well as the blood loss are reduced when this type of staged approach is used. More important, the morbidity (including limb loss) and mortality are also reduced.

BIBLIOGRAPHY

1. Bandyk DF, Berni GA, Thiele BL, et al: Aortofemoral graft infection due to Staphylococcus epidermidis. *Arch Surg* 1984; 119:102–108.

2. Goldstone J, Effeney DJ: Prevention of arterial graft infections, in Bernhárd VM, Towne JB (eds): *Complications in Vascular Surgery* 2. New York, Grune & Stratton, 1985, pp 487–498.

3. Lawrence PF, Dries DJ, Alazraki N, et al: Indium-III-labelled leukocyte scanning for detection of prosthetic vascular graft infection. *J Vasc Surg* 1985; 2:165–173.

4. Liekweg WJ Jr, Greenfield LJ: Vascular prosthetic infections: Collected experience and results of treatment. *Surgery* 1977; 81:335–342.

5. MacBeth GA, Rubin JR, McIntyre KE Jr, et al: The relevance of arterial wall microbiology to the treatment of prosthetic graft infections: Graft infection vs. arterial infection. *J Vasc Surg* 1984; 1:750–756.

6. Mark A, Moss AA, Lusby R, et al: CT evaluation of complications of abdominal aortic surgery. *Radiology* 1982; 145:409–414.

7. Reilly LM, Altman H, Lusby RJ, et al: Late results following surgical management of vascular graft infection. *J Vasc Surg* 1984; 1:36–44.

8. Reilly LM, Goldstone J, Ehrenfeld WK, et al: Gastrointestinal tract involvement by prosthetic graft infection: The significance of gastrointestinal hemorrhage. *Ann Surg* 1985; 202:342–348.

9. Reilly LM, Goldstone J: The infected aortic graft, in Bergan JJ, Yao JST (eds): *Reoperative Arterial Surgery*. Orlando, Grune and Stratton, 1986, pp 231–253.

10. Reilly LM, Stoney RJ, Goldstone J: Improved management of aortic graft infection: The influence of operation sequence and staging. *J Vasc Surg* 1987; 5:412–431.

11. Rubin JR, Malone JM, Goldstone J: The role of the lymphatic system in acute arterial prosthetic graft infections. *J Vasc Surg* 1985; 2:92–98.

12. Trout HH III, Kozloff L, Giordano JM: Priority of revascularization in patients with graft enteric fistulas, infected arteries, or infected arterial prostheses. *Ann Surg* 1984; 199:669–683.

30 Renal Artery Stenosis and Hypertension

A 54-year-old nurse is seen for a four-year history of increasingly difficult-to-control hypertension. Intravenous pyelography has been performed by her internist, showing some delay in function on the right. The right kidney measures 2 cm less than the left. An abdominal bruit is heard. She is otherwise in good health, and the remainder of her physical examination is normal.

Consultant: James C. Stanley, M.D.

The presentation of this case is rather typical of renovascular hypertension secondary to unilateral renal artery stenotic disease. Uncontrolled hypertension, such as that which affects this patient, represents a significant threat to an individual's health. Unfortunately, hypertension often remains inadequately treated until serious end-organ complications occur, including stroke, heart failure, and renal insufficiency. Stenotic renal artery disease is the cause of elevated blood pressure in approximately 1% of all hypertensive patients, and may account for approximately 5% of patients exhibiting severe hypertension.

The major issues confronting clinicians in managing cases of suspected renovascular hypertension include: (1) recognition of the type of underlying renal artery disease; (2) establishment of the fact that the stenotic lesion is indeed contributing to secondary hypertension; and (3) the choice of an appropriate form of treatment, be it modification of an existing drug program, percutaneous transluminal angioplasty, or operative intervention. Each of these topics will be addressed independently, with attention directed to renovascular hypertension in general, as well as this case in particular.

ETIOLOGY

Atherosclerosis is the most common type of renal artery occlusive disease, occurring in 60% to 70% of renovascular hypertensives. Nearly half of these patients have coexisting clinically overt arteriosclerotic occlusive disease. Hypertension most often becomes evident in the latter part of the sixth decade of life with men affected twice as often as women. Atherosclerotic occlusive disease affecting the proximal renal artery is an unlikely cause of this patient's hypertension, although such cannot be excluded on the basis of history and physical findings alone.

Arterial fibrodysplasia, which is the second most common cause of renovascular hypertension, is a more likely etiology of hypertension in the case presented. This type of renal artery stenotic disease encompasses a heterogenic group of lesions including intimal fibroplasia, medial fibrodysplasia, and perimedial dysplasia. Intimal fibroplasia accounts for 5% of this group and tends to occur in younger adults and children, whereas medial fibrodysplasia, accounting for nearly 85% of dysplastic lesions, invariably affects women during their fourth and fifth decades of life. Although bilateral stenoses exist in approximately 60% of patients, only 15% to 20% actually have functionally important bilateral disease. Medial fibrodysplasia typically has a string-of-beads appearance, caused by a series of stenoses with intervening true aneurysms. Perimedial dysplasia, the last in this group of stenoses, accounts for approximately 10% of dysplastic renal arteries. Perimedial dysplasia, like medial fibrodysplasia, invariably affects women, primarily during their fifth decade of life. It is usually manifest by multiple constrictions in the midrenal artery, but unlike medial dysplasia there are no mural aneurysms.

Excessive release of renin from the juxtaglomerular apparatus of the kidney occurs once a pressure gradient of approximately 10 mm Hg develops across a renal artery stenosis, regardless of the etiology of the stenosis. Renin acts on renin substrate, an alpha$_2$ globulin produced in the liver, to form the dectapeptide angiotensin I. This latter substance is cleaved of two amino acids by angiotensin converting enzyme (ACE) to produce angiotensin II, which is a potent vasopressor responsible for the vasoconstrictive element of renovascular hypertension. Indirectly, angiotensin II also acts to increase production of aldosterone with subsequent retention of sodium, the latter representing the volume element of renovascular hypertension.

DIAGNOSIS

Unfortunately, clinical manifestations of renovascular hypertension are not pathognomonic of this disease entity. Certain sorting strategies, although far from perfect, offer the best means of identifying patients with renovascular hypertension (Fig 30–1). Clinical clues supporting further investigative studies include: systolic-diastolic upper abdominal bruits; patients presenting initially with diastolic blood pressures greater than 115 mm Hg or exhibiting a sudden worsening of what was thought to be preexisting essential hypertension; elevated blood pressure in pediatric-age patients, or female patients under the age of 50; as well as any patient in whom high blood pressure develops *de novo* after age 50. Patients with drug-resistant hypertension and malignant hypertension are also more apt to have this secondary form of hypertension. In particular, patients who demonstrate deterioration of renal function while receiving multiple antihypertensive drugs, including ACE inhibitors, must be suspect for underlying renal artery stenotic disease and renovascular hypertension.

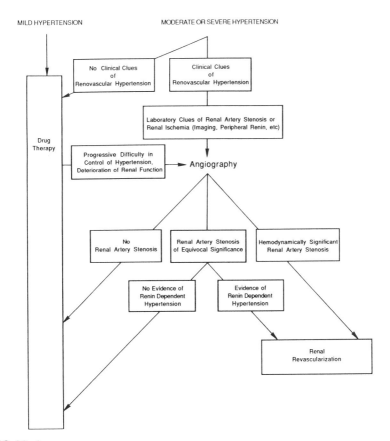

FIG 30–1.
Algorithm for management of renovascular hypertension.

Multiple clinical clues strongly indicative of renovascular hypertension justify early arteriographic studies. With less obvious clinical clues, certain laboratory studies may provide further evidence of renal artery stenosis and renal ischemia. Such studies include hypertensive urography, split renal function studies, renograms, renal scans, and peripheral renin determinations. None of these tests is sensitive or specific enough to be entirely reliable for screening purposes. The most common of these studies is hypertensive urography in the form of rapid sequence excretory pyelograms. Urograms are suggestive of renal artery stenosis when: (1) unilateral delays occur in the calyceal appearance of contrast; (2) differences in renal length exist, with the right kidney being 2.0 cm smaller than the left or the left being 1.5 cm smaller than the right; (3) hyperconcentration of contrast is evident on delayed films; and (4) ureteral notching due to tortuous collateral vessels is apparent. Because of bilateral disease or unilateral segmental lesions, hypertensive urograms are often not helpful. Indeed, in the presence of proven renovascular hypertension at the University of Michigan, abnormal urograms were noted in only 24% of pediatric patients, 47% of adults with arterial fibrodysplasia and 72% of adults having atherosclerotic disease.

Conventional arteriography is an important means of assessing the anatomic presence and morphologic character of renal artery disease. Furthermore, the presence of collateral vessels circumventing a stenotic lesion substantiates the functional importance of the renal artery disease. A pressure gradient of 10 mm Hg, or greater, results in collateral development and abnormal renin production. Intravenous digital subtraction arteriography (DSA) is inadequate for anything other than demonstrating the most obvious of main renal artery lesions. Collateral and segmental vessels are poorly depicted by intravenous DSA. Such is not the case with intraarterial DSA which often provides high enough resolution of small vessel anatomy so as to be comparable to the accuracy of conventional angiography.

If arteriography demonstrates collateral vessels circumventing a stenotic renal artery lesion, further studies are not necessary. However, if the importance of the stenosis appears equivocal or if bilateral stenoses are present, and the question arises as to whether one or both sides are contributing to the high blood pressure, then renin assays should be performed.

Assessment of renin activity in renal vein blood and peripheral blood provides useful information regarding hypertension secondary to renal artery stenotic disease. Renal vein renin ratios, RVRR, comparing renin activity from the effluent of the suspected ischemic kidney to that of the contralateral kidney, is diagnostic when the RVRR is > 1.48. Renin production may be excessively high from both kidneys, and if equally high from each side, RVRR data will not reveal abnormal renin release. This occurs in approximately 15% of cases. The renal:systemic renin index, RSRI, documents the contribution of each kidney to the total circulating renin. The RSRI is calculated by subtracting systemic renin activity from that of the renal vein, and dividing the remainder by the systemic renin activity. Hypersecretion occurs with an individual RSRI > 0.48, and suppression occurs when the RSRI approaches 0. The specificity of the RSRI is approximately twice that of RVRR, although false negatives do occur. RSRI evidence of ipsilateral hypersecretion and contralateral suppression is an accurate indicator of curable unilateral renovascular hypertension.

TREATMENT

Newer antihypertensive drugs have markedly improved the medical management of patients with renovascular hypertension. The use of calcium channel blockers and beta blocking agents such as propanolol or atenolol are commonly used first-line drugs. In instances of more refractory hypertension, especially due to bilateral disease or unilateral lesions with contralateral parenchymal disease, addition of a thiazide or similar diuretic is recommended, although with impaired renal function use of a loop diuretic such as furosemide would be more effective. ACE inhibitors, such as captopril and enalapril, appear to be the most effective drugs in treating renovascular hypertension. However, because of their potential deleterious effect on renal function by decreasing systemic blood pressure and altering intrarenal autoregulation, the use of ACE inhibitors should be avoided when the entire renal parenchymal mass is at risk, as is the case with bilateral disease or with a solitary kidney. Certain patients having mild or even moderate renovascular hypertension may be adequately treated with drug therapy alone. However, stenotic disease of the renal artery often progresses with a potential for loss of renal mass and function. Thus, definitive means of restoring normal renal blood flow may be a more logical therapy once a diagnosis of renovascular hypertension has been established.

Percutaneous transluminal angioplasty (PTA) of renal artery stenotic disease has important patient benefits compared to operative intervention, although accompanying risks and long-term results are less well defined than is the case with surgical treatment. Intimal and medial dysplastic stenoses not involving segmental vessels are the lesions most amenable to PTA. Conversely, ostial lesions associated with developmental aortic anomalies or aortic spill-over atherosclerosis are less amenable to PTA.

Initial benefits following PTA in carefully selected patients with fibrodysplastic lesions approach 90%, and 50% to 60% with arteriosclerotic stenoses. Recurrences with the former are uncommon but follow PTA of atherosclerotic lesions in 30% to 50% of cases. PTA might be appropriate in the patient currently presented if a short main renal artery dysplastic lesion was noted. However, segmental vessel involvement exists in 20% of these cases, and in such a setting PTA would be inappropriate in that intimal flaps and medial dissections in smaller segmental vessels are relatively common and likely to result in arterial occlusion and renal infarction. Significant complications occur in 5% to 10% of renal PTA procedures.

Operative intervention has been the standard therapy of renovascular hypertension for both atherosclerotic and fibrodysplastic disease. Autogenous saphenous vein aortorenal bypass is the most commonly performed procedure in adults, and a similar revascularization with internal iliac artery is the most common type of reconstruction undertaken in pediatric-age patients. In the case of left-sided lesions a splenorenal bypass offers an attractive alternative to aortorenal bypass in adults. However, before undertaking the latter, one should document that the proximal celiac artery is not involved with an occlusive lesion which might perpetuate the hypertensive state following a splenorenal bypass. Other alternative bypass procedures are occasionally useful, such as using a saphenous vein bypass from the hepatic or gastroduodenal arteries for right-sided disease. Use of prosthetic grafts when autologous vessels are not available is also appropriate. Similarly, surgeons should be prepared to perform *ex vivo* repairs with bench reconstruction of diseased vessels when complex segmental renal artery disease exists. Although it is unlikely that the patient presented here has a proximal ostial atherosclerotic stenosis, a transaortic endarterectomy would be favored should such a lesion exist. Renal arteriotomy and local endarterectomy patch graft closure of the renal artery would be an

TABLE 30-1.

Surgical Treatment of Renovascular Hypertension* Comparative Overall Results

INSTITUTION	TIME PERIOD	NUMBER OF PATIENTS	RATIO OF ARTERIOSCLEROTIC TO NONARTERIOSCLEROTIC DISEASE	OPERATIVE OUTCOME			SURGICAL MORTALITY
				CURED	IMPROVED	FAILURE	
University of California, Los Angeles†	1958–1977	503	1.0/2.0	64%	23%	13%	2.1%
Baylor College of Medicine	1959–1979	489	3.2/1.0	36%	29%	35%	1.8%
University of Michigan	1961–1980	313	1.0/1.5	47%	42%	11%	1.9%
Cleveland Clinic‡	1962–1978	225	1.5/1.0	50%	34%	16%	3.1%
University of Rome, L'Aguila§	1960–1977	219	4.1/1.0	53%	28%	19%	3.2%
University of California, San Francisco‡	1958–1977	128	2.0/1.0	39%	34%	27%	1.6%
University of Lund Malmo, Sweden	1971–1977	125	1.1/1.0	55%	25%	20%	0.9%
Vanderbilt University	1961–1972	122	1.8/1.0	59%	31%	10%	5.4%||
Columbia University**	1962–1976	116	1.3/1.0	66%	19%	15%	1.0%
Hospital Alguelongue Montpellier, France	1965–1976	110	2.3/1.0	55%	34%	11%	1.8%
St. Mary's Hospital London, England	Unstated	110	2.4/1.0	37%	54%	9%	Unstated

*From Stanley JC, Ernst CB, Fry WJ: *Renovascular Hypertension*, WB Saunders, 1984, p 365. Used by permission.
†Series includes 230 primary, secondary or partial nephrectomies; Stated mortality is that from 1972–77 experience (142 cases).
‡Data from overlapping publications, not inclusive of entire experience.
§Series includes 61 nephrectomies.
||Mortality from more recent experience was 0.5% among 200 reconstructions, excluding those associated with aortic surgery.
**Series includes 42 nephrectomies.

TABLE 30–2.
Surgical Treatment of Renovascular Hypertension* Results in Specific Patient Subgroups† University of Michigan Experience, 1961–1980

| SUBGROUP | NUMBER OF PATIENTS | PRIMARY OPERATIVE PROCEDURES | | OPERATIVE OUTCOME‡ | | | SURGICAL MORTALITY§ |
		ARTERIAL RECONSTRUCTION	NEPHRECTOMY	CURED	IMPROVED	FAILURE	
Fibrodysplasia, Pediatric	34	39	2	85%	12%	3%	0%
Fibrodysplasia, Adult	144	160	6	55%	39%	6%	0%
Arteriosclerosis, Focal Renal Artery Disease	64	63	3	33%	58%	9%	0%
Arteriosclerosis, Overt Generalized Disease	71	70	6	25%	47%	28%	8.5%‖

*From Stanley JC, Ernst CB, Fry WJ: *Renovascular Hypertension*, WB Saunders, 1984, p 369. Used by permission.
†Represents results of 415 operations (356 primary, 59 secondary).
‡Effect of operation on blood pressure defined as *Cured* if blood pressures were 150/90 mm Hg or less for a minimum of six months, during which no antihypertensive medications were administered (lower pressure levels were utilized in evaluating pediatric patients). *Improved* if normotensive while on drug therapy, or if diastolic blood pressures ranged between 90 and 100 mm Hg, but were at least 15% lower than preoperative levels. None of the improved patients were receiving converting enzyme inhibitors. *Failure* if diastolic blood pressures were greater than 90 mm Hg but less than 15% lower than preoperative levels, or if they were greater than 110 mm Hg.
§Surgical mortality includes all deaths within 30 days of operation.
‖Four of six deaths in this series associated with concomitant aortic reconstructive surgery.

appropriate alternative in this situation. It is unacceptable to incur greater than a 5% primary nephrectomy rate because of technical difficulties in the surgical management of either atherosclerotic or fibrodysplastic renal artery disease.

Contemporary surgical treatment of renovascular hypertension has provided very satisfactory results (Table 30–1). Differences among individual experiences usually reflect the most prevalent disease entity causing the secondary hypertension being treated. Pediatric patients are most likely to be cured after restoration of renal blood flow. Adults, such as in the case currently presented, with arterial fibrodysplasia benefit from operation more often than those with atherosclerotic disease. This is in part a reflection of the relatively infrequent coexistence of essential hypertension or nephrosclerosis in younger patients. Atherosclerotic renovascular hypertension has often been considered a homogenous disease entity, although there would appear to be at least two clinical subgroups of patients with these lesions, including: (1) those having focal renal artery disease with their only clinical manifestation of atherosclerosis being secondary hypertension; and (2) a group having clinically overt extrarenal arteriosclerosis such as extracranial cerebrovascular disease manifest by stroke or transient ischemic attacks, coronary artery disease with angina or prior myocardial infarction, aneurysmal disease of the abdominal aorta or its branches, and symptomatic peripheral arterial occlusive disease.

The surgical management of renovascular hypertensives may be best assessed by reviewing the results at an individual institution (Table 30–2), where patients were categorized into the four distinct subgroups: (1) pediatric patients, up to 17 years of age, (2) adults with fibrodysplastic disease, (3) adults having arteriosclerotic renal artery lesions *without*, or (4) *with* overt extrarenal arteriosclerotic cardiovascular disease. Operative therapy appeared to be most beneficial with pediatric and adult fibrodysplastic categories, where 97% and 94% of patients, respectively, were cured or improved. Outcomes were also satisfactory in adults with focal atherosclerotic disease, where 91% were cured or improved. Adults exhibiting clinically overt generalized arteriosclerosis had a 72% salutory response to operation, but only 25% were cured. It is among the latter subgroup of patients with extensive atherosclerosis that this series' only surgical mortality occurred. It is outcome data such as this to which other treatment modalities must be compared in assessing appropriate management of renovascular hypertension.

BIBLIOGRAPHY

1. Dean RH, Krueger TC, Whiteneck JM, et al: Operative management of renovascular hypertension. Results after a follow-up of fifteen to twenty-three years. *J Vasc Surg* 1984; 1:234–242.
2. Moncure AC, Brewster DC, Darling RC, et al: Use of the splenic and hepatic arteries for renal revascularization. *J Vasc Surg* 1986; 3:196–203.
3. Novick AC, Stratton RA, Stewart BH, et al: Diminished operative morbidity and mortality in renal revascularization. *JAMA* 1981; 246:749–753.

4. Stanley JC, Fry WJ: Pediatric renal artery occlusive disease and renovascular hypertension. Etiology, diagnosis and operative treatment. *Arch Surg* 1981; 116:669–676.
5. Stanley JC, Whitehouse WM Jr, Graham LM, et al: Operative therapy of renovascular hypertension. *Br J Surg* 1982; 69 (Suppl): S63–S66.
6. Stanley JC, Ernst CB, Fry WJ: *Renovascular Hypertension.* Philadelphia, WB Saunders, 1984.
7. Stanley JC, Whitehouse JM Jr, Zelenock GB, et al: Reoperation for complications of renal artery reconstructive surgery undertaken for treatment of renovascular hypertension. *J Vasc Surg* 1985; 2:133–144.
8. Stoney RJ, DeLuccia N, Ehrenfeld WK, et al: Aortorenal arterial autografts. Long-term assessment. *Arch Surg* 1981; 116:1416–1422.

31 Poor Risk Patient with Renal Artery Stenosis and Diseased Aorta

A 77-year-old gentleman is referred for severe hypertension and deteriorating renal function. Past history includes several myocardial infarctions, and nonreconstructible severe coronary artery disease has been demonstrated by coronary angiography. BUN and creatinine have slowly increased over the past several years, with current values 55 and 2.9 mg per 100 ml, respectively. Angiography demonstrates total occlusion of the left renal artery without visualization of the left kidney and severe origin stenosis of the right renal artery. The infrarenal aorta is ectatic with extensive atheromatous disease evident.

Consultant: Ashby C. Moncure, M.D.

A variety of alternatives are available to accomplish renal artery revascularization. In most circumstances, aortorenal bypass grafting, utilizing autogenous vein, arterial autografts, or prosthetic conduits, is felt to be the preferred method of renal revascularization because of the predictability of high inflow, relative simplicity of the operation and well-documented durability of result. Thromboendarterectomy is a more complex procedure and patch angioplasty is rarely applicable to adults with atherosclerotic disease. Renal artery reimplantation is a very useful procedure, particularly in combination with replacement of a diseased distal aorta with Dacron graft, but is quite difficult to successfully achieve in the presence of a diseased aorta. Percutaneous transluminal angioplasty has not proven to be a durable procedure in the presence of disease at or near the renal artery ostia, the commonest location of atherosclerotic disease leading to renal artery stenosis or occlusion.

The clinical summary above outlines the features of a clinical category of patient seen with increasing frequency by vascular surgeons, i.e., a medically poor risk patient with uncontrolled hypertension, deteriorating renal function and a severely diseased aorta. Such patients with advanced renovascular occlusive disease will present with widespread atherosclerosis involving not only the renal arteries and adjacent aorta, but also coronary, peripheral vascular and occasionally cerebral territories. Not infrequently, renal artery disease producing hypertension and deterioration of renal function is but one manifestation of severe end stage generalized atherosclerosis and in such a circumstance, a severely diseased aorta may prove difficult to work with if conventional aortorenal bypass grafting is being considered for revascularization of the ischemic kidney. Aortic clamping may also prove a significant deleterious hemodynamic event in those patients with severe cardiac disease. Because of greater risk of combined renal arterial revascularization and grafting of aortoiliac occlusive disease to replace the diseased aorta, an "extraanatomic" approach to renal artery reconstruction is an attractive concept. A "lesser procedure" in terms of incision, operative time, and operative blood loss may be an extremely useful alternative to conventional aortorenal bypass grafting in such circumstances.

The splenic and hepatic arterial circulations can be utilized to revascularize the left and right renal arteries, respectively. In selected circumstances, these procedures have been found to be quite useful, in particular in those patients where it is desirable to avoid using the aorta for inflow because of severity of disease within the aorta itself, or because of the lack of cardiac reserve needed to accommodate to the hemodynamic shifts occurring during clamping and declamping of the aorta.

REVERSAL OF RENAL DYSFUNCTION

Wide experience with preservation or retrieval of functioning renal tissue has documented the potential retrievability of renal function in ischemic kidneys with negligible residual excretory function. Although the renal arteries are essentially end arteries, slowly progressive arterial occlusive disease promotes the enhancement of collateral arterial flow to the renal cortex through capsular, peripelvic, and periureteral branches, frequently maintaining renal viability even in chronic total renal artery occlusion. Variables influencing the choice between renal revascularization and nephrectomy appear to be renal size, histologic characteristics of renal biopsy specimens, split renal function studies, and the arteriographic demonstration of a patent distal renal artery without evidence of severe intrarenal stenoses. Retrieval of function in kidneys measuring less than 8 cm long is thought to be extremely unlikely, reflective of the severity of the ischemic process with loss of parenchymal mass. Although a renal biopsy may not be representative of the state of the entire kidney, obliteration of all glomeruli and tubules with fibrosis would probably be predictive of irreversible loss of renal function. The presence, however, of atrophic glomeruli and tubules may not predict irreversibility of ischemic injury. Split renal function studies have demonstrated no change in excretory function after revascularization in kidneys with preoperative creatinine clearances greater than 30 ml per minute, but statistically significant improvement has been seen in kidneys with less than 20 ml per minute creatinine clearances preoperatively.

The most predictable predictor of success in the management of both renovascular hypertension and retrieval of renal function in patients with renal arterial occlusive disease is the presence of an arteriographically demonstrated patent renal artery distal to the occlusion or stenosis without significant intrarenal arterial disease. Because of the extreme morbidity associated with significant loss of renal function with the attendant need for chronic renal dialysis, operative revascularization has become a more frequently utilized therapeutic option in these patients.

PREOPERATIVE ASSESSMENT

In the case under discussion it seems highly likely that the severe hypertension is related to the bilateral renal artery disease, and the deteriorating renal function documents both the severity of the disease, its progressive nature, and it underlines the urgency of need for revascularization. In view of the poor risk category of the patient, primarily due to his severe cardiac disease and the diseased infrarenal aorta, the possibility of revascularizing the right renal artery from the hepatic circulation should be seriously considered. The preoperative evaluation necessary includes midstream biplane aortography demonstrating the origin of the celiac axis as well as the origin of the superior mesenteric artery. Because the gastroduodenal artery is usually divided in the course of hepatorenal grafting, it is necessary to assure patency of the superior mesenteric artery as it would be unwise to interrupt a major collateral source if ostial disease of the superior mesenteric artery is found to be present. Angiography is also utilized to document anatomic variations involving the celiac axis and superior mesenteric arterial circulations.

Although selective renal vein renin determinations, or split function studies, may be obtained, I do not think they would seriously influence my recommendations for treatment. Therefore, I would probably not obtain them. In this case, the primary operative objective is to preserve, or perhaps even improve, existing renal function. If untreated, the anatomic findings of occlusion of one renal artery and severe stenosis of the solitary remaining renal artery suggests that progression to renal failure and the need for chronic dialysis is likely. Therefore, renal artery reconstruction of the remaining patent renal vessel is indicated despite renin values or lateralization. Relief of possible renovascular hypertension is of secondary importance. Strong lateralization of renins to the left might suggest that concomitant left nephrectomy might be considered at the time of right renal grafting. However, as my procedure of choice in this patient would be a hepatorenal graft, adequate exposure for left nephrectomy would not exist, and I would therefore not consider adding this in this patient.

In addition to good preoperative angiography, other aspects of preoperative preparation should be directed at ensuring a stable cardiac status and as optimal a renal function as is possible to achieve. Cardiac consultation should be obtained, the patient's medication program reviewed, and any abnormalities corrected, as feasible. Adequate hydration is important. Operation should be postponed for a period following diagnostic angiography to make sure that any element of contrast-induced renal failure is not present or that it has cleared.

OPERATIVE MANAGEMENT

The patient is placed supine with the legs externally rotated, and the abdominal wall, groins, and medial thighs prepared and draped as a sterile field. A right subcostal incision extending medially across the midline and laterally to the tip of the right eleventh rib (Fig 31–1A) allows good access to the porta hepatis and the right renal artery. The hepatoduodenal ligament is incised (Fig 31–1B), and the common hepatic artery both proximal and distal to the gastroduodenal artery origin is encircled (Fig 31–1C).

The descending duodenum is mobilized by Kocher's maneuver (Fig 31–2A), and dissection is carried down along the gastroduodenal artery, which serves as a relatively constant and helpful reference point. If the gastroduodenal artery is 3 cm in length prior to its bifurcation and appears to have an internal diameter of 3.5 mm after dilatation, the surgeon may consider use of this vessel for primary end-to-end anastomosis to the right renal artery. In most instances, however, the gastroduodenal artery will not be of sufficient length or adequate caliber after gentle dilatation with a No. 3 Fogarty catheter. The surgeon must then be prepared to harvest the proximal greater saphenous vein in order to lead a graft from the hepatic artery, usually at the gastroduodenal artery origin, down to the right renal artery.

Following the Kocher maneuver, the inferior vena cava and right renal vein are readily located. The right renal artery is identified as it emerges from behind the vena cava, usually just above or below the renal vein (Fig 31–2B). Frequently, the most favorable part of the renal artery with which to work is that part involved with poststenotic dilatation, found immediately distal to the area of stenosis, which is usually at the renal artery ostium. To make this area available for anastomosis as well as to acquire as much length of renal artery as possible, the inferior vena cava may be mobilized and the proximal right renal artery isolated subjacent to it, along the left border of the vena cava. To assure the appropriate axial orientation of the right renal artery as it is rotated up for end-to-end anastomosis to the gastroduodenal artery or saphenous vein graft, an adventitial strip of fine silk suture material may be passed along the cephalad border of the renal artery.

If the gastroduodenal artery is to be utilized primarily, the origin of the gastroduodenal artery is occluded with a find bulldog clamp and the gastroduodenal artery transected at its bifurcation, ligated distally, and thereafter a No. 3 Fogarty embolectomy catheter is passed through the end of the gastroduodenal artery up into the hepatic artery, the balloon inflated with 0.6 ccs of sterile injectable saline, and then brought back through the gastroduodenal artery in the inflated position. The gastroduodenal artery is quite elastic and can usually be safely dilated without inflicting harm on the artery. The occluding bulldog clamp at the origin of the gastroduodenal artery may be released subsequently to assess the adequacy of flow through the artery.

If the gastroduodenal artery is not believed to be adequate to serve as source for inflow, a segment of reversed greater saphenous vein is anastomosed to the hepatic artery after it is occluded proximally and distally, the site of proximal anas-

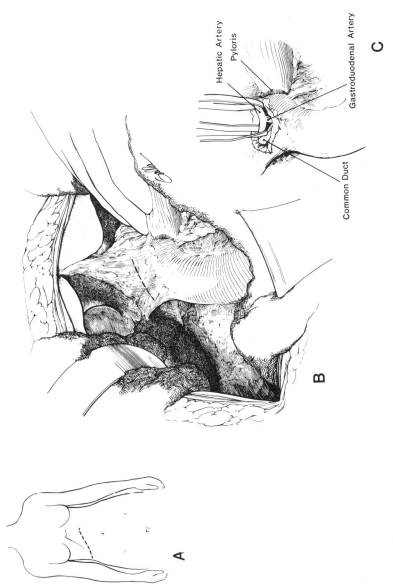

FIG 31–1.
A, A right subcostal incision extending medially across the midline and laterally to the tip of the right eleventh rib allows access to the porta hepatis and the right renal artery. **B,** The hepatoduodenal ligament is incised. **C,** The common hepatic artery is encircled both proximal and distal to the gastroduodenal artery origin. (From Moncure, et al: *J Vasc Surg.* Used by permission.)

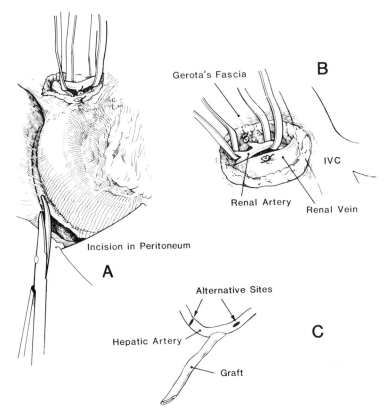

FIG 31–2.
A, The descending duodenum is mobilized by Kocher's maneuver, and dissection is carried down along the gastroduodenal artery, which serves as a relatively constant and helpful reference point. **B,** The inferior vena cava and the right renal vein are identified, and the right renal artery encircled where found, either immediately cephalad, behind, or caudad to the renal vein. **C,** A segment of reversed greater saphenous vein is anastomosed to the hepatic artery after it is occluded proximally and distally, the site of proximal anastomosis usually lying at the origin of the gastroduodenal artery at its takeoff from the hepatic artery. (From Moncure, et al: *J Vasc Surg.* Used by permission.)

tomosis usually lying at the origin of the gastroduodenal artery at its takeoff from the hepatic artery (Fig 31–2C).

The right renal artery is then ligated at its origin, and divided beyond all palpable occlusive disease. The distal renal artery is perfused with chilled heparinized Ringer's lactate solution, and gently dilated with graduated coronary probes (Fig 31–3A). It is not wise to dilate this vessel with a Fogarty catheter because the intima is easily split. When rotated cephalad, the right renal artery is spatulated on its superior surface and anastomosed end-to-end to the spatulated end of the re-

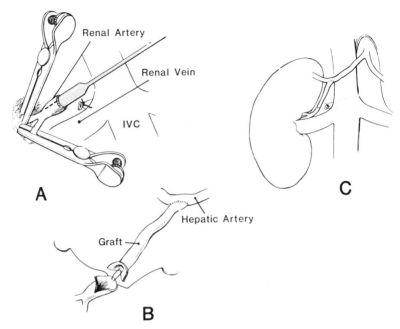

FIG 31–3.
A, The right renal artery is ligated at its origin, divided, perfused with chilled heparinized Ringer's lactate solution, and gently dilated with graduated coronary probes. **B,** The distal right renal artery is spatulated on its superior surface and anastomosed end-to-end with the spatulated end of the reversed greater saphenous vein graft with an oblique anastomosis of 6–0 Prolene. **C,** The completed hepatorenal vein graft is illustrated. (From Moncure, et al: *J Vasc Surg.* Used by permission.)

versed greater saphenous vein graft with an oblique anastomosis of 6–0 Prolene (Fig 31–3B). After release of clamps, the pulse can be assessed within the distal vein graft and the right renal artery (Fig 31–3C).

RESULTS

Blood flow through the hepatic artery has been adequate for revascularization in all but one instance in a Massachusetts General Hospital series of 44 revascularizations of the right renal artery from the hepatic circulation. Occasionally, the hepatic artery may seem small in caliber, but if proximal occlusive lesions in the celiac axis or main hepatic artery have been ruled out by adequate preoperative arteriography, inflow through the hepatic artery has been sufficient for both the revascularized right kidney and liver in all instances. Occasionally, a replaced right hepatic artery will originate from the superior mesenteric artery. Such infrequent occurrences should be identifiable by good preoperative arteriography; despite the smaller caliber of either right or left hepatic arteries in such cases, one or the other will generally prove satisfactory for an inflow site. On no occasion was hepatic dysfunction seen.

At the time of the revascularization of the right renal artery, if the left kidney is felt to be nonsalvageable, contralateral nephrectomy might be considered. To accomplish this, extension of the incision across the midline in a "frown" configuration will be necessary. I might consider this if severe, poorly controlled hypertension were present, particularly if renins had been obtained and lateralized to the left. In general, however, concomitant nephrectomy is not done, as it increases the length and scope of the procedure in an already compromised patient. Most importantly, the primary goal of the procedure in such a patient is stabilization of function by revascularization of the still functioning kidney. In addition, even though the kidney is not visualized on preoperative angiography, collateral flow may preserve some functional capacity in the patient with severe renal dysfunction. In some instances, actual revascularization of such a kidney may be feasible even though no reconstituted distal renal artery or nephrogram is seen on the preoperative arteriogram. If so, the situation might be suitable for a staged bilateral extraanatomic reconstruction, using the splenic artery for left-sided revascularization.

SUMMARY

A wide variety of alternatives are available to accomplish renal artery revascularization. Many operative techniques are not applicable in all clinical situations, and the surgeon must carefully select the method of renal revascularization appropriate to each patient. Although in most circumstances direct aortorenal grafting has become accepted as the preferred method of renal revascularization, selected clinical situations involving poor risk medical patients or the desire to avoid an aortic operation may make use of the hepatic or splenic circulation for inflow for renal revascularization preferable. These procedures have been shown to be effective in revascularizing the renal artery with low mortality and morbidity. Therefore, I believe our patient would be best managed with a hepatorenal bypass graft.

BIBLIOGRAPHY

1. Brewster DC, Moncure AC: Hepatic and splenic artery for renal revascularization, in Bergan JJ, Yao ST (eds): *Arterial Surgery: Diagnostic and Operative Techniques.* New York, Grune & Stratton, Inc, 1987, pp 389–405.
2. Dean RH: *Renovascular Hypertension. Current Problems in Surgery XXII, No. 2.* Chicago, Year Book Medical Publishers, Inc, 1985.
3. Moncure AC, Brewster DC, Darling RC, et al: Use of the splenic and hepatic arteries for renal revascularization. *J Vasc Surg* 1986; 3:196–203.
4. Stanley JC, Whitehouse WM Jr: *Occlusive and Aneurysmal Disease of the Renal Arterial Circulation, Disease-a-Month XXX, No. 7.* Chicago, Year Book Medical Publishers, Inc, 1984.

32 Acute Mesenteric Ischemia

An 80-year-old woman is seen in the emergency room for the sudden onset of severe abdominal pain two hours previously. Other than chronic atrial fibrillation, there have been no outstanding medical problems. Abdominal examination reveals minimal diffuse tenderness without rebound, and no organomegaly or masses. Bowel sounds are diminished. Flat and upright plain X-rays of the abdomen are unremarkable.

Consultant: John J. Bergan, M.D., F.A.C.S., Hon. F.R.C.S. (Eng.)

"Mesenteric arterial occlusion is not difficult to recognize at its immediate onset if the following three criteria are kept in mind: it occurs almost invariably after the age of 50, it occurs in individuals with known or easily recognizable cardiovascular disease, it occurs suddenly with abdominal pain."

—A.A. Klass, 1958

Thirty years following the wise statement by Alan Klass, quoted above, we still find that the diagnosis and treatment of acute mesenteric artery occlusion is in disarray. In reviewing a ten-year experience in 18 hospitals in Ireland, Gorey found that of 65 patients with intestinal gangrene seen, 46 died (70.8%); radiologic investigations were confined to plain abdominal films; preoperative angiography was not carried out; and in the 49 patients with laparotomy, 29 had intestinal resections, revascularization was attempted in only six, and two patients had operations inappropriate to mesenteric vascular disease. In Glasgow, similar results were obtained at the Royal Infirmary, where of 102 patients with acute mesenteric ischemia, the mortality was 92% with half of the patients first diagnosed at postmortem. The depressing conclusions reached by the authors of those two reports echo the words of surgeons writing on this subject 50 years ago. "Improvements in intensive care and nutritional support with the greater use of revascularization procedures . . . have barely influenced mortality." "Death was related to three factors: the mean age of survivors . . . the interval [from onset] to laparotomy . . . and the length of ischemic bowel.''

In this patient, an 80-year-old woman, clearly in the atherosclerotic age group, we learn that a cardiac arrhythmia is present. She is otherwise well and presents herself in an emergency room with an abdominal problem in which physical findings are minimal, yet the patient is quite ill and had ''severe abdominal pain.'' Given the facts above, the surgeon called to see such a patient should think that an acute mesenteric artery occlusion has occurred, probably due to embolization. He will want to ask questions which will reveal the diagnostic triad of mesenteric artery embolization and initiate studies that will confirm the diagnosis, so that a rapid laparotomy, embolectomy, and/or intestinal resection can be carried out.

First, the history. Has the patient experienced bowel emptying by defecation following the abdominal pain? Has she experienced vomiting? The first response of the gastrointestinal tract to ischemia is spasm. This is perceived by the patient as pain and, physiologically, by gut emptying. Next, has the patient experienced previous embolic episodes? Has she had transient ischemic attacks or a frank stroke? Has she experienced acute limb ischemia that did not result in amputation but which may have compromised her physiologically? Ninety percent of patients with mesenteric artery embolization experience an acute onset of abdominal pain, 80% will have manifestations of gut emptying, and one third will experience a previous embolus to extremity or brain. Following the taking of the history, or perhaps simultaneous with it, will be the completion of the physical examination that will add to the findings above. The presence or absence of pulses in the major arteries of the extremities may confirm the presence of a previous embolus or refute that assumption.

Next, diagnostic studies must be initiated, and among these will be the blood count, searching for leukocytosis, the arterial blood gases estimating the degree of acidosis that must be corrected, and the rapid progress of the patient to the radiology suite for an aortogram and perhaps selective visualization of the mesenteric vessels.

PHILOSOPHY

It is unusual to speak about philosophy in discussing treatments of surgical disease. Nevertheless, in acute intestinal infarction, philosophical decisions must be made. The age of the patient, his physical condition, presence of senility or organic brain disease all weigh heavily on surgical decisions. Because patients with mesenteric infarction are seen late in the course of their disease process, resuscitative efforts may be so vigorous that the patient will not survive them. It is appropriate that definite philosophic decisions be made early, perhaps even before the patient proceeds to the X-ray department. Influencing the philosophic decision is the fact that nondefinitive treatment will result in death. Also, surgical resection of the involved intestine without concomitant revascularization will have a disastrously high mortality, in excess of 80%. If therapy is decided on, revascularization must precede the thought of intestinal resection.

DIAGNOSTIC ANGIOGRAPHY

The diagnosis of acute mesenteric artery occlusion can be made clinically, and the patient taken to the surgical suite with the history of acute onset of abdominal pain, bowel emptying, and leukocytosis in excess of 15,000. However, angiography is useful in corroborating the diagnosis and can be done swiftly so that delay in definitive surgery is not experienced. The lateral projection is essential for demonstrating characteristic features of occlusion of the first segment of the superior mesenteric artery, a characteristic of mesenteric thrombosis. Furthermore, in mesenteric artery thrombosis, it would be expected that the celiac axis and/or the inferior mesenteric artery would also be occluded. In mesenteric embolization, which would be expected in the case under discussion, demonstration of the embolus would be obtained 3 cm to 8 cm from the aortic origin of the superior mesenteric artery (Fig 32–1). The characteristic "mercury meniscus" sign would be in the region of the midcolic artery. Proximal jejunal arteries would be demonstrated, but a distal jejunal and ileal arterial branches would not be visualized. Nonorganic arterial occlusion (an oxymoron), a low-flow state without major vascular occlusion, will also be diagnosed by the angiogram. In this situation, the arterial tree is unobstructed, primary and secondary arterial branches are easily seen, and segmental concentric spasm of vessels, particularly origins of vessels, is demonstrated. In such a situation, the arterial catheter is left in place for infusion of appropriate vasodilating drugs. In all other situations the mesenteric artery catheter can be removed and the patient taken to surgery.

DIFFERENTIAL DIAGNOSIS

Although it is acknowledged that acute superior mesenteric artery embolization will account for more than half of the cases of acute intestinal infarction, and the addition of thrombotic occlusion of the mesenteric artery and nonorganic occlusion will encompass more than 90% of all cases of acute mesenteric infarction, the well-educated surgeon must have in his diagnostic armamentarium a variety of other conditions. Nearly all of these are ruled out by the clinical presentation of the patient. However, a mental run-through of the following conditions might be in order. Acute visceral ischemia may be produced by arteritis, such as polyarteritis nodosa, Kawasaki's syndrome, drug abuse arteritis, necrotizing arteritis of Cogan, radiation arteritis, septic embolization, and the spontaneous dissection of fibromuscular dysplasia of mesenteric arteries.

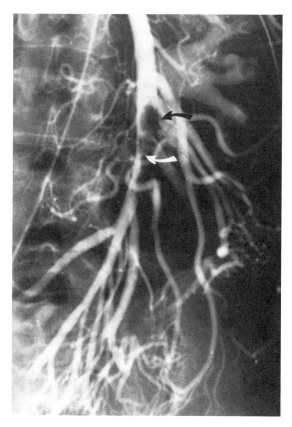

FIG 32–1.
Mesenteric angiogram in a patient with sudden onset of abdominal pain and a cardiac valve prosthesis showing the typical location of a mesenteric embolus distal to jejunal arteries.

Spontaneous mesenteric artery occlusion occurs when there is extrinsic mechanical vessel obstruction, severe intraabdominal inflammation, and hypercoagulable states such as antithrombin III, protein C, and protein S deficiencies. Other coagulopathies include thrombophilia following splenectomy, a nonspecific coagulopathy seen in combination of oral contraceptive agents and heavy smoking in young women, polycythemia rubra vera, and sickle cell anemia. Traditionally, mesenteric venous thrombosis has been included in the differential diagnosis of mesenteric infarction. However, the syndrome of presentation of mesenteric venous thrombosis is markedly different from that seen in intestinal infarction due to arterial occlusion.

FIBRINOLYTIC AGENTS

Although fibrinolytic agents have been available to clinical practice for more than 30 years, their definitive place in the surgeon's therapeutic armamentarium has not been achieved. Promises of efficacy and safety of streptokinase, urokinase, and tissue-specific plasminogen activator have remained tantalizing as carrots before the nose of the surgical donkey. The ideal patient for fibrinolytic therapy can be defined: a younger individual without known blood dyscrasia, not recently postoperative or subjected to multiple vascular punctures, who has encountered reversible ischemia of the bowel, and in whom the arterial catheter used for angiography can be placed proximal to a distal occlusion. Low-dose urokinase infusion followed by serial arteriography to confirm effectiveness or failure of such treatment might be employed. A perfect result would include total lysis, restoring a normal vascular tree to the patient without need for laparotomy. Complications of such therapy are formidable, indeed, and include hemorrhage into necrotic bowel, catheter thrombosis with subsequent embolization, partial thrombolysis with distal embolization, and induction of a systemic lytic state, with central nervous system hemorrhage with or without remote hematoma formation.

EXPLORATORY LAPAROTOMY

One must assume that the prudent surgeon will have exercised the good practices learned in treating desperately ill patients. A large bore intravenous access is as requisite as a bladder catheter. Central venous or pulmonary artery catheter monitoring is mandatory, as is an arterial line. Metabolic acidosis, so characteristic of mesenteric infarction, must be corrected. The low-flow tissue perfusion, hemoconcentration, and absorption via peritoneal surfaces and intestinal lymphatics of the products of bacterial and gut necrosis can be lethal. The elderly patient afflicted with acute mesenteric artery occlusion may bring with him an impaired ventilatory status, contributed to by impaired respiratory movements, increased blood viscosity, intrapulmonary sludging, and obstructive pulmonary disease.

The incision used for laparotomy should be the generous midline incision learned in arterial reconstructive surgery and not the limited incision used in gynecology or general surgical procedures. Inspection of the entire intestine is mandatory. Very early after acute arterial occlusion, the bowel may appear sufficiently normal for the diagnosis to be missed. However, close inspection shows it to be more gray than usual, lacking sheen, and exhibiting pulseless *vasa recta*. Later, the bowel may exhibit a boggy, bluish appearance, and finally hemorrhage into the mesentery may occur with the intestine becoming deeply cyanotic or frankly necrotic. The surgeon, by passing his right hand behind the small bowel mesentery, allows palpation of the superior mesenteric artery between the thumb and index finger. In mesenteric artery thrombosis, the entire vessel is pulseless because occlusion commonly occurs at the origin of the artery. Mesenteric embolization appears distally, as described above in the paragraphs on angiography. Therefore, the proximal mesenteric artery is pulsatile, and the first jejunal branches are vascularized. A confusing picture may be seen when the embolus has shattered in its transit from the heart to the mesenteric arborization (Fig 32–2). In this situation, skip areas of normal intestine will be seen between areas of frankly ischemic or necrotic bowel. Mesenteric venous thrombosis is also characterized by segmental necrosis, but in that situation profound edema of the bowel wall, venous congestion, and mesenteric edema is present.

It is a waste of time to assess bowel viability at this stage or to begin resection of necrotic intestine. Instead, one must give consideration to the elements of revas-

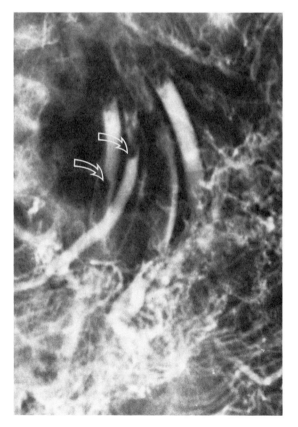

FIG 32–2.
This mesenteric angiogram illustrates embolic fragments in peripheral mesenteric arteries. Such clot fragmentation explains segmental ischemia and skip areas of necrosis sometimes seen in mesenteric infarction.

cularization. For example, where is the inflow to be obtained? What will be the mechanism of revascularization? In the situation of mesenteric embolus, the inflow will be the normal origin of the mesenteric artery from the aorta. In mesenteric artery thrombosis, the inflow should be from the aorta itself.

In the case under discussion, the procedure will undoubtedly be embolectomy. The proximal superior mesenteric artery is exposed by incising the ligament of Treitz, mobilizing the fourth portion of the duodenum and upper jejunum after retracting the transverse colon upward and drawing the small bowel mesentery downward. The patient is systemically heparinized, and the superior mesenteric artery skeletonized. It is entered through a transverse incision which allows balloon catheter embolectomy and irrigation of the arterial tree with heparinized saline solution.

When organic occlusion of the superior mesenteric artery is caused by thrombosis, a formal, full-scale vascular reconstruction is required. Extensive thromboendarterectomy of the aorta and mesenteric vessels has been advocated by some for this condition. However, the desperate metabolic state of the patient with intestinal infarction must be considered when one contemplates the magnitude of an aortomesenteric endarterectomy.

Bypass grafting for thrombosis is usually the procedure of choice. In advanced bowel ischemia, with or without bowel infarction, an autogenous saphenous vein is preferred. The infrarenal aorta may serve as the origin of the graft if it is relatively free of atherosclerotic degenerative disease. Alternatively, grafts to the superior mesenteric artery and/or the celiac axis can take their origin from the supraceliac aorta. This portion of the aorta is mercifully spared from atherosclerotic degenerative change and can be exposed with minimum time and trauma. The most direct route is through the gastrohepatic omentum, which is divided vertically, with incision of the triangular ligament of the left lobe of the liver, retraction of the esophagus and upper portion of the stomach to the left, incision of the thickened solar plexus surrounding the celiac axis, and division of the arcuate ligament and muscular fibers of the left crus of the diaphragm. This exposes the anterior aspect of the lower thoracic aorta just above the celiac axis.

A word of caution about the inferior phrenic arteries is in order. These are variable in origin and must be identified if they are encountered during exposure of the supraceliac aorta. They may originate from the aorta itself, rather than from the celiac trunk or its branches. Also, intercostal arteries arising from the posterior part of the aorta should be identified and preserved so that they can continue to supply blood flow to the terminal spinal cord and conus medullaris. An inch or two of exposed lower thoracic aorta can be isolated between atraumatic vascular clamps, and a disk of anterior aortic wall punched out to receive the origin of the saphenous vein graft, which can then be passed distally to the superior mesenteric artery. The tunneling maneuver which allows passage of the graft is along the anterior aspect of the aorta, just to the right of the celiac axis, coursing behind the pancreas. The anastomosis may be end-to-end, using 6–0 or 7–0 monofilament suture. Such revascularization allows reconstruction of the celiac axis simultaneous with superior mesenteric artery revascularization.

Alternative revascularization maneuvers include anastomosis of the ileocolic artery to the right common iliac artery, implantation of the superior mesenteric artery on the aorta, and/or implantation of the inferior mesenteric artery.

BOWEL VIABILITY, SECOND LOOK

Once revascularization has been accomplished and the bowel returned to the abdominal cavity for 20 to 30 minutes, the viscera can be inspected. In a fortunate and early case such as the one under discussion, the bowel will be expected to be clearly viable, and the abdomen can be closed with the decision made not to perform a second-look procedure. In other situations, the need for resection may be obvious, and the surgeon's clinical judgment employed regarding extent of resection.

A number of tests of bowel viability have become available because of surgical research interest on this subject. Clinically, return of arterial pulsation in the mesenteric vessels is a good indicator of viability, as is peristalsis. Methods in use to assess intestinal viability following revascularization include Doppler tests, dye infusions, electromyography, pH recordings, temperature, oxygen electrodes, chemical tests and radionuclides. Experience has shown that there is a good correlation between loss of Doppler signals at the antimesenteric border and subsequent bowel necrosis. Doppler-predicted intestinal viability is reliable except in mesenteric venous thrombosis. The Doppler probe has a high specificity in arterial occlusions, and if the surgical team favors the fluorescence technique, the Doppler probe can be used to selectively study a suspected underperfused area. In using the fluorescence technique, it is necessary to illuminate the intestine with an ultraviolet light after systemic intravenous injection of fluorescein. The fluorescein is taken up by living cells, which indicate cell viability as well as reperfusion. The entire small bowel must be exposed before the injection of fluorescein, as peritoneal fluid stained with fluorescein can cloud the accuracy of the test.

If segmental resection of the intestine is done, and even if the bowel is returned to the abdominal cavity without resection, a decision must be made at this time whether or not to do a second-look procedure. The second look must be planned at the time of the first operation, as no element of the patient's postoperative course will allow such a determination to be made. The physical findings and laboratory studies will be of no help whatsoever in determining the need for a second laparotomy. The second-look procedure is not an absolute necessity and should be applied selectively in the critically ill, elderly patient with intestinal infarction.

ANCILLARY CARE

Anticoagulant use is debated in discussions of treatment of intestinal infarction. Guidelines can include the following elements:

The patient should be systemically heparinized whenever a major artery is occluded. Therefore, all patients are heparinized during arterial reconstruction.

Patients with embolic occlusion of major vessels should be considered for long-term anticoagulation, and therefore the heparin is given from the time of diagnosis through the postoperative period, when the patient is converted to prothrombin depressant medications in consideration for long-term use.

Thrombotic occlusion of mesenteric vessels does not require long-term anticoagulation, and therefore the operative heparinization will be sufficient.

Unfortunately, ischemic bowel undergoing revascularization will be the subject of mucosal slough with intraluminal hemorrhage. Therefore anticoagulation may be dangerous in the patients who need such therapy the most.

With regard to antibiotics, surgical exploration for mesenteric infarction should be classified as contaminated surgery, and antibiotic use is regarded as therapeutic rather than prophylactic. Aerobic and anaerobic gastrointestinal organisms such as *E coli, B fragillis,* along with *S aureus,* are important causes of the infectious complications. Therefore, the first bottle of resuscitative fluid should contain cefazolin, 2 gr, followed by 3 gr to 4 gr per day, or cefoxitin, 2 gr, followed by 4 gr to 6 gr per day, or clindamycin, 600 mg, followed by similar amounts every six hours and tobramycin, 1.5 mg per kg of body weight every eight hours, intramuscularly or intravenously.

CONCLUSIONS

Mesenteric infarction is a generic term now used to describe intestinal necrosis caused by vascular occlusion. It does not connote etiology and therefore cannot suggest therapy. Therefore, a syndrome of mesenteric infarction due to embolization to the superior mesenteric artery, as described in the case discussed above, must be differentiated from thrombosis of the mesenteric vessels. These in turn must be differentiated from mesenteric venous thrombosis and nonorganic arterial occlusion.

Radiologic imaging techniques corroborate the diagnosis and suggest surgical therapy. Vigorous resuscitation, correction of metabolic disturbance including acidosis, optimization of cardiac function, precise surgical intervention, accurate estimation of bowel viability, and judicious use of a second-look procedure characterize management of cases of acute mesenteric artery occlusion in this modern era.

Despite changes in surgical philosophy, techniques, and ancillary support such as intensive care, the wisdom of A.A. Klass expressed 30 years ago still guides us in care of patients with mesenteric embolization.

BIBLIOGRAPHY

1. Bailey RW, Bulkley GB, Hamilton SR, et al: Protection of the small intestine from nonocclusive mesenteric ischemic injury due to cardiogenic shock. *Am J Surg* 1987; 153:108–116.
2. Baur GM, Millay DJ, Taylor LM, et al: Treatment of chronic visceral ischemia. *Am J Surg* 1984; 148:138–144.
3. Bergan JJ, Yao JST: Acute intestinal ischemia, in Rutherford RB (ed): *Vascular Surgery*, ed 2. Philadelphia, WB Saunders, 1984, pp 948–963.
4. Gorey TF, O'Sullivan M: Prognostic factors in mesenteric vascular disease. *Br J Surg* 1988; in press.
5. Hollier LH: Revascularization of the visceral artery using the pantaloon vein graft. *Surg Gynecol Obstet* 1982; 155:415–416.
6. Jaxheimer EC, Jewell ER, Persson AV: Chronic intestinal ischemia: The Lahey Clinic approach to management. *Surg Clin North Am* 1985; 64:123–130.
7. Klass AA: Embolectomy for acute mesenteric vascular occlusion. *Can J Surg* 1958; 1:358–361.
8. Kwaan JHM, Connolly JE: Prevention of intestinal infarction resulting from mesenteric arterial occlusive disease. *Surg Gynecol Obstet* 1983; 157:321–324.
9. Poole JW, Sammartano RJ, Boley SJ: Hemodynamic basis of the pain of chronic mesenteric ischemia. *Am J Surg* 1987; 153:171–176.
10. Ricotta JJ, Williams GM: Endarterectomy of the upper abdominal aorta and visceral arteries through an extraperitoneal approach. *Ann Surg* 1980; 192:633–638.
11. Wilson C, Gupta R, Gilmour DG, et al: Acute superior mesenteric ischaemia. *Br J Surg* 1987; 74:279–281.

33 Chronic Mesenteric Ischemia

A 61-year-old woman has been admitted for a six-month history of postprandial abdominal pain. She has lost 40 lbs. in weight over this interval. Numerous previous gastrointestinal X-rays, studies, and endoscopic procedures have been unremarkable. Aortography demonstrates high-grade stenoses of both the celiac axis and superior mesenteric arteries, and total occlusion of the inferior mesenteric artery.

Consultants: Kimberley J. Hansen, M.D.
and William K. Ehrenfeld, M.D.

This patient demonstrates the key clinical and etiological features of chronic mesenteric ischemia. Recognition of these key features is essential for successful surgical management. The goals of surgical management are: (1) to relieve postprandial abdominal pain, (2) to halt and reverse weight loss and, (3) to prevent intestinal infarction.

To meet these goals, a number of surgical procedures have been proposed. These procedures include: (1) transarterial and transaortic endarterectomy, (2) visceral vessel reimplantation, (3) antegrade or retrograde aortovisceral bypass and, (4) percutaneous transluminal angioplasty. Based on our experience with these procedures in treatment of over 100 patients with chronic visceral ischemia, we believe that patients are best managed with either transaortic endarterectomy or antegrade aortovisceral bypass. This discussion will emphasize our preoperative and operative management and our results of operative treatment.

ANATOMY AND PATHOLOGY

The visceral arteries (celiac, superior, and inferior mesenteric) that supply the splanchnic circulation are arranged in parallel fashion (Fig 33–1). Despite this parallel arrangement, three major collateral pathways may develop to bypass proximal obstruction in the visceral arteries. First, the celiac and superior mesenteric arteries may communicate through the pancreaticoduodenal arteries. Similarly, the superior

214

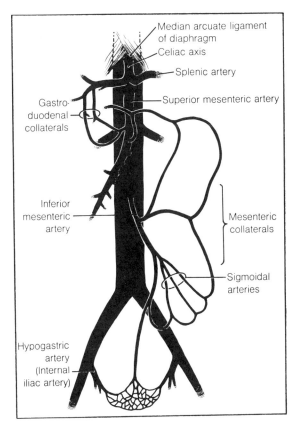

FIG 33–1.
Diagramatic representation of the splanchnic circulation and major collateral pathways.

and inferior mesenteric arteries may communicate through the "meandering mesenteric artery." Finally, the inferior mesenteric and internal iliac arteries may communicate through sigmoidal and hemorrhoidal arteries. The clinical importance of the latter collateral pathway may be confirmed in aortoiliac reconstruction, when critical collateral flow through the internal iliac artery is sacrificed causing infarction of the rectosigmoid.

Of these three collateral pathways, the arteriographic demonstration of the "meandering mesenteric artery" is pathognomonic for significant obstruction in the visceral arteries (Fig 33–2). The "meandering" mesenteric artery is located deep within the colonic mesentery. It is different from the marginal artery of Drummond which is located close to the colonic wall. The demonstration of the meandering mesenteric artery alerts the surgeon to significant underlying visceral vessel disease regardless of the patient's presenting symptoms.

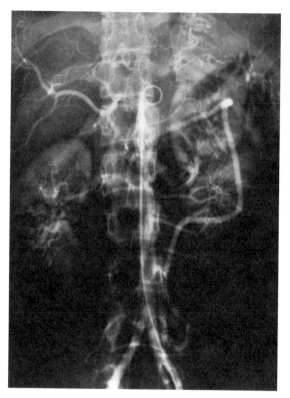

FIG 33–2.
Late phase of an A-P aortogram demonstrates the meandering mesenteric artery.

The pathologic lesion responsible for visceral artery occlusion is atherosclerosis in over 90% of patients. They are usually "ostial" lesions that represent atherosclerosis of the aortic wall that encroaches on the lumen of the visceral vessel at its origin. The atheroma characteristically extends 1 cm to 2 cm into the vessel and in that position it can be removed by thromboendarterectomy. However, atherosclerosis in the superior mesenteric artery may extend 4 cm to 5 cm distal to its origin. Extensive atherosclerosis of this type is usually treated by aortovisceral bypass.

CLINICAL PRESENTATION AND DIAGNOSIS

The patient presented is representative of our clinical experience with chronic visceral ischemia. Our patients are typically women (76%) in their fifth decade (mean, 59 years). Although the pathophysiology of the accompanying abdominal pain is poorly understood, pain is present in nearly all of the patients (98%). The pain has its onset from 15 to 30 minutes after meals and may persist from one to four hours. The pain, which is described as gnawing and dull in quality, is periumbilical or epigastric in location. As the obstruction of the visceral arteries progresses, smaller amounts of food result in more severe and persistent abdominal pain. Finally, the patient demonstrates food avoidance or "food fear," which eventually leads to significant weight loss (15% loss of body weight in 80% of the patients).

On physical examination these patients demonstrate signs of significant weight loss and they typically have an audible epigastric bruit (86%). In addition to their visceral artery disease, they frequently demonstrate signs of additional peripheral vascular disease (34%).

Diagnosis of this condition depends on a high index of suspicion. It is considered in any patient who presents with postprandial pain and food avoidance with weight loss. Definitive diagnosis of chronic visceral ischemia requires aortography in both lateral and A-P projections. The lateral projection best demonstrates the proximal visceral artery stenosis or occlusion, while the A-P view best demonstrates the collateral pathways and additional peripheral vascular disease. We have not been satisfied with intravenous digital subtraction angiography as an alternative to conventional aortography or digital subtraction studies obtained by an intraarterial approach. Intraarterial digital subtraction angiography provides satisfactory arterial imaging while minimizing the contrast load in patients with renal dysfunction.

Diagnostic aortography in our patients usually reveals combined patterns of stenosis or occlusion of both the celiac axis and superior mesenteric artery (94%). In addition, half of these patients (49%) have significant occlusive disease involving the inferior mesenteric artery. Our patients often have atherosclerotic stenosis or occlusion of one or both renal arteries (34%); one fourth (26%) will have significant aneurysmal or occlusive disease of the infrarenal aorta.

Similar to the patient described in the case presentation, most of our patients are referred to us following an extensive evaluation for abdominal pain and weight loss. Ideally, the extravascular evaluation of these patients should be guided by their history and physical findings. In patients with classical intestinal angina and a positive aortogram, we have not encountered unexpected extravascular pathology at laparotomy.

OPTIONS OF SURGICAL RECONSTRUCTION

Surgical revascularization is indicated in all patients with symptomatic chronic visceral ischemia. As noted, the goals of surgical reconstruction are: (1) to relieve postprandial abdominal pain, (2) to halt and reverse weight loss and, (3) to prevent intestinal infarction.

As previously stated, we believe transaortic thromboendarterectomy and antegrade aortovisceral bypass are the preferred methods of surgical repair. These techniques are preferred because: (1) they originate from undiseased or endarterectomized aorta, (2) they provide optimal nonturbulent flow and, (3) they avoid problems of alignment and compression inherent to retrograde grafting.

Other modes of revascularization have a number of deficiencies. Transarterial endarterectomy fails to directly visualize the aortic atherosclerosis which constitutes the ''ostial lesion.'' Visceral vessel reimplantation into adjacent undiseased aorta without tension or narrowing is rarely possible. Retrograde aortovisceral bypass frequently originates from diseased infrarenal aorta; in addition, such retrograde grafts are without distal kinking or compression. Percutaneous transluminal dilatation should be considered only as a temporizing procedure that may help to correct severe nutritional deficits in cachectic patients prior to definitive surgical repair. Collectively, these methods have resulted in late failure rates of 14% to 50%. In contrast, transaortic thromboendarterectomy and antegrade aortovisceral bypass have resulted in long-term relief of abdominal pain and have prevented intestinal infarction in 93% of our patients.

SURGICAL TECHNIQUE

We believe the optimal operation for chronic visceral ischemia is one that restores normal blood flow to both the celiac axis and superior mesenteric artery. If revascularization of both of these vessels is not feasible, our priority for revascularization in order of importance is, the celiac followed by the superior mesenteric and, lastly, the inferior mesenteric arteries. No patient in our series has had recurrent symptoms or intestinal infarction with a patent celiac artery repair.

Transaortic thromboendarterectomy performed through a thoracoretroperitoneal exposure is particularly applicable to the correction of simultaneous visceral, renal, and infrarenal aortic disease. However, if the visceral occlusive disease is not ostial in character, or if the patient is older, with significant cardiopulmonary disease, we select antegrade aortovisceral bypass. In these patients, antegrade bypass avoids the risk of morbidity, associated with combined abdominal and thoracic exposure.

Both thromboendarterectomy and antegrade bypass require temporary supraceliac aortic occlusion. During this period of increased cardiac afterload, we feel transesophageal two-dimensional echocardiography is the best technique for cardiac monitoring. This technique images the heart in real time. From this image the anesthesiologist can assess cardiac chamber volumes and abnormalities in segmental wall motion.

Transaortic thromboendarterectomy of the mesenteric vessel is performed through a thoracoretroperitoneal approach. The incision extends in oblique fashion from the midline, 2 cm to 4 cm below the umbilicus to the posterior axillary line in the eighth intercostal space. After excising 1 cm to 2 cm of the costal margin, the chest is entered and the diaphragm is incised circumferentially 1 inch from the chest wall. Further dissection proceeds in an extraperitoneal plane reflecting the peritoneal envelope medially. The most difficult aspect of this dissection is developing a plane anterior to the kidney and adrenal gland, but remaining posterior to the peritoneum. Early identification of the left renal vein as a surgical landmark will prevent entry into the peritoneal cavity.

The left crus of the diaphragm is detached posteriorly to expose the dense neuroplexus over the upper abdominal aorta. This plexus is resected and the aorta, celiac and superior mesenteric arteries are circumferentially dissected. At this point, the surgeon must carefully assess the extent of disease within the visceral vessels. If the disease extends well beyond the ostia (most often seen in the superior mesenteric artery) antegrade bypass is performed. If careful assessment confirms ostial disease ending within 1 cm to 2 cm of the vessel's origin, a thromboendarterectomy is performed.

After heparinization (2,000–4,000 units heparin), clamps are placed on the supraceliac and infrarenal aorta. The visceral vessels are individually controlled, and the lumbar arteries are controlled with bulldog clamps. If only visceral thromboendarterectomy is being performed, a trap-door incision surrounding the two arterial orifices is made. Since the atheromatous disease usually involves the full circumference of the aorta, the visceral endarterectomy is accomplished with a sleeve of aortic intima. The remaining distal ledge of transected aortic intima has never caused obstruction or intramural dissection (Fig 33–3).

After the aortotomy is closed and flow is reestablished, the repair is evaluated with intraoperative duplex scanning. We feel this technique, which combines real

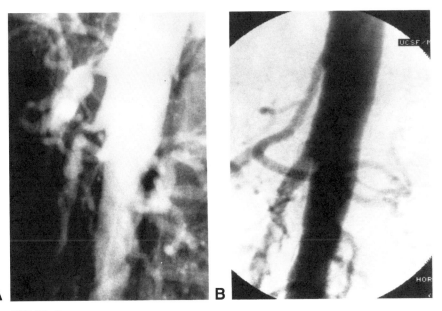

A   B

FIG 33–3.
Lateral aortograms demonstrate preoperative **(A)** and postoperative **(B)** celiac and SMA anatomy after thromboendarterectomy.

time B-mode ultrasound with Doppler flow detectors provides the best method to ensure technical perfection of the endarterectomy. Duplex scanning can be performed rapidly and is very sensitive to the technical defects which could jeopardize the immediate or long-range patency of the reconstruction.

In older patients with significant cardiopulmonary disease or in those patients with occlusive disease extending well beyond the vessel origin, an antegrade aortovisceral bypass graft is performed. The incision extends from the xyphoid to just below the umbilicus. After thorough exploration of the abdominal cavity, the left lobe of the liver is retracted to the right and the esophagus is retracted to the left. The lesser omentum is opened in an avascular space to expose the posterior diaphragm. After division and separation of the preaortic fibers of the diaphragm, the dense neuroplexus surrounding the celiac artery and overlying aorta is resected. This exposes the origin of both celiac and mesenteric arteries. When the body of the pancreas is freed from its posterior attachments and retracted caudally the first 4 cm to 5 cm of the superior mesenteric artery is easily exposed (Fig 33–4).

A 12 × 6 mm or 10 × 5 mm bifurcated prosthetic graft is used to accomplish simultaneous celiac and superior mesenteric artery revascularization. The supraceliac aorta is segmentally controlled proximally and distally and an elliptical antero-

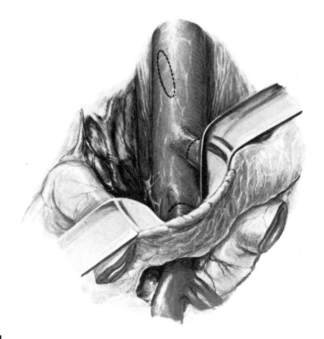

FIG 33–4.
Division of the preaortic fibers of the diaphragm and the neuroplexus exposes the descending thoracic aorta and both major visceral arteries. (From Wylie EJ, Stoney RJ, Ehrenfeld WK: *Manual of Vascular Surgery.* New York: Springer-Verlag, 1981. Used by permission.)

lateral aortotomy is made for the proximal anastomosis. The graft is positioned so the left limb extends along the left anterior aspect of the aorta for end-to-end anastomosis with the celiac artery. The right limb extends along the right anterior lateral aspect of the aorta in a retropancreatic position for end-to-end anastomosis with the superior mesenteric artery. Both anastomoses are accomplished with fine interrupted Dacron sutures (Fig 33–5). As with mesenteric thromboendarterectomy, the technical perfection of the arterial repair is assessed with intraoperative duplex scanning (Fig 33–6).

RESULTS

Since 1959, we have treated over 100 patients with chronic visceral ischemia. Of these, 76 patients were treated with transaortic thromboendarterectomy or antegrade aortovisceral bypass; 52 had endarterectomy and 24 had antegrade bypass. During

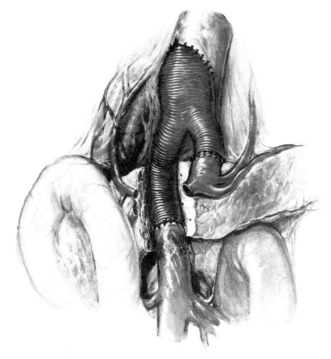

FIG 33–5.
Bifurcated antegrade aortovisceral graft. Contrary to the artists' depiction, the proximal anastomosis is performed with continuous suture technique. (From Wylie EJ, Stoney RJ, Ehrenfeld WK: *Manual of Vascular Surgery*. New York: Springer-Verlag, 1981. Used by permission.)

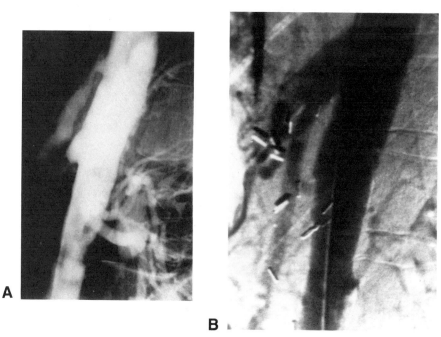

FIG 33–6.
Lateral aortograms demonstrate preoperative **(A)** and postoperative **(B)** visceral artery anatomy after antegrade aortovisceral bypass.

late follow-up (mean 53 months), one patient from each group had recurrent symptoms of mesenteric ischemia and both patients underwent successful reoperation. Three patients died in the perioperative period; two patients treated with endarterectomy and one patient treated with antegrade bypass. Nineteen percent of patients had perioperative cardiopulmonary complications which were primarily postoperative atelectasis and cardiac dysrhythmia. All other surviving patients have remained asymptomatic. We are not aware of a single case of enteric paraprosthetic fistula complicating an antegrade graft.

SUMMARY

The successful surgical management of chronic visceral ischemia requires prompt recognition of the clinical syndrome and a thorough understanding of the anatomy of the visceral vessels. Patients present with postprandial abdominal pain which becomes progressively more severe and may culminate in "food fear" with significant weight loss.

Although a number of surgical procedures for revascularization have been proposed, we feel these patients are best managed with either transaortic endarterectomy or antegrade aortovisceral bypass. Revascularization by both of these techniques has relieved postprandial pain and prevented intestinal infarction in 93% of our patients.

BIBLIOGRAPHY

1. Okuhn SP, Reilly LM, Ehrenfeld WK, et al: Intraoperative assessment of renal and visceral artery reconstruction: The role of duplex scanning and spectral analysis. *J Vasc Surg* 1987; 5:137–144.
2. Roizen MF, Beaupre PN, Ehrenfeld WK, et al: Monitoring with two dimensional transesophageal echocardiography: Comparison of myocardial function in patients undergoing supraceliac, suprarenal-infraceliac or infrarenal aortic occlusion. *J Vasc Surg* 1984; 1:300–305.
3. Stoney RJ, Ehrenfeld WK, Wylie EJ: Revascularization methods in chronic visceral ischemia caused by atherosclerosis. *Ann Surg* 1977; 186:468–476.
4. Wylie EJ, Stoney RJ, Ehrenfeld WK: *Manual of Vascular Surgery*, vol I. New York, Springer-Verlag, 1980.

34 Acute Lower Extremity Ischemia

A 64-year-old physician's wife is seen in consultation for a 12-hour history of right leg ischemia. Two months previously she underwent mitral valve replacement and double coronary artery bypass surgery for angina and dyspnea on exertion, with a satisfactory recovery. She has a history of intermittent atrial arrhythmias. She denies prior claudication, but has been relatively inactive. Examination shows an intact right femoral pulse and absent distal pulses. The right foot is cool but viable. Left leg pulses are normal.

Consultant: Richard P. Cambria, M.D.

OVERVIEW

Few clinicians would have difficulty in recognizing this case scenario as typical of acute ischemia secondary to peripheral arterial embolism. The case is illustrative of certain clinical and demographic characteristics that are associated with arterial embolism, namely, the abrupt onset of symptoms, female sex, and the presence of heart disease with arrhythmias. Cardiac pathology accounts for all but a few arterial emboli, although the primary nature of that pathology has gradually shifted from rheumatic valvular heart disease to the sequellae of atherosclerotic coronary occlusive disease. Coincident with that evolution over the past 50 years has been an increase in the average age (mean age, 70 years) in patients seen with peripheral arterial embolism. Thus, the patient population at risk for arterial embolism is likely to have a high incidence of concomitant peripheral occlusive disease. This is important in so far as it affects one of the more important clinical distinctions to be made when seeing such a patient, namely, the differentiation between acute embolism and *in situ* thrombosis on preexistent occlusive disease. The ability of the clinician to predict the level of obstruction and the responsible pathology will have major import in the wisdom of obtaining pretreatment angiography, the timing of operative intervention, and in the nature of the definitive treatment itself.

INITIAL PATIENT EVALUATION

The important historical points in a patient who presents with acute lower extremity ischemia are referable to antecedent cardiac and/or peripheral vascular disease. While a history of claudication in the appropriate leg would make the clinician suspect that the acute problem was *in situ* arterial thrombosis, only 40% of patients we reviewed with acute arterial thrombosis gave such a history. This seems consistent with the relatively sedentary lifestyle that this patient population may manifest. Alternatively, fully 75% of our patients seen with peripheral arterial embolism were in atrial fibrillation at the time of presentation. Consequently, a history of any cardiac disease, and particularly arrhythmias, should alert the clinician to suspect arterial embolism. Of course, a recent history of myocardial infarction is strongly correlated with peripheral embolism, and the highest risk is between seven and ten days postinfarction. Yet it must also be recognized that acute cardiac decompensation can precipitate thrombosis on preexistent atherosclerotic disease due to a reduction in cardiac output.

On physical examination, the presence of normal pulses in the unaffected limb suggests the problem is acute embolization to a previously undiseased vascular tree. Similarly, the presence of chronic changes of peripheral vascular insufficiency suggests the problem is acute occlusion on antecedent occlusive disease. Several other findings on pulse examination can be quite helpful in arriving at the correct diagnosis. Since the femoral bifurcation is the most common site (nearly 50%) for an arterial embolism to lodge, the femoral pulse in the affected limb is usually present and, in fact, is often accentuated due to a water-hammer type affect. However, if the femoral bifurcation is high, or if presentation is delayed so that proximal propagation of clot in the common femoral artery has occurred, the groin pulse may be absent. If such is the case, the examiner should make an attempt to insinuate the hand superiorly over the inguinal ligament and attempt to palpate the external iliac pulse as it arises from the depths of the pelvis. The presence of such a pulse implies that the obstruction is at the femoral bifurcation, and likely secondary to arterial embolism. Iliac occlusions which occur on the basis of antecedent occlusive disease generally occur in the common iliac artery and its bifurcation, thereby obliterating both the external iliac and common femoral artery pulse. Similarly, if the femoral pulse is present, an attempt should be made to trace it medially in the leg and palpate the superficial femoral artery pulse. If such is present, the block is distal to the femoral bifurcation, implying an occlusion at the level of Hunter's canal. Since this is the typical location for occlusive disease in the superficial femoral artery, this finding would imply that the problem was thrombosis of the superficial femoral artery at this location. Furthermore, embolism to the popliteal artery generally lodges at its division into the anterior tibial artery and tibioperoneal trunk, thereby preserving a prominent popliteal pulse. This finding has important clinical implications for initial surgical management as discussed below. A thrombosed popliteal aneurysm may give a similar clinical picture, although, more commonly, the popliteal pulse will be absent. A history of aneurysmal disease and the status of the contralateral popliteal artery (50% popliteal aneurysms are bilateral) are further diagnostic clues.

Other important elements of the physical exam relate to the status of the skeletal muscle in an ischemic extremity. The decision to proceed with revascularization as opposed to primary amputation is an important point of surgical judgment, because the consequences of inappropriate revascularization may not be limited to limb loss. Specifically, the revascularization of a limb with advanced ischemia may precipitate the "myonephropathic syndrome," describing the clinical problem of gross limb swelling, hyperkalemia, and myoglobinuric renal failure, which is associated with a high mortality. The presence of calf tenderness is an ominous sign, and the presence of calf rigidity should indicate that primary amputation is the best alternative.

The decision to obtain an angiogram is a function of the initial clinical assessment. Patients diagnosed with arterial embolism are treated with prompt surgical embolectomy, and the angiogram will only add redundant information at the expense of fluid shifts and a dye load in patients with compromised cardiac function. Alternatively, angiography is necessary to plan the potential method of revascularization in patients with *in situ* thrombosis. Of course, the clinician must weigh the potential benefit of angiography in view of the overall clinical picture of the patient. In the absolute best scenario, complete angiography will delay definitive surgery a minimum of two and more probably four or more hours. Should the patient have an imminently threatened limb, we would proceed directly to the operating room, relying on intraoperative angiography to plan potential reconstructions.

PATIENT MANAGEMENT

The initial management of a patient with acute arterial ischemia is directed not so much at the obstruction itself, but rather at protecting the distal vascular tree from thrombosis in the microcirculation. Indeed, this is the crucial anatomic level that will ultimately determine limb prognosis, and most surgeons are familiar with the unfortunate circumstance of reestablishing circulation in the named vasculature, yet losing the limb because of thrombosis in the microcirculation. Thus patients with all forms of acute extremity ischemia should be treated with intravenous heparin *while the initial evaluation is proceeding*. The initial response of the vascular tree downstream from an acute obstruction is intense vasoconstriction. This is usually accompanied by a profound symptom complex, consisting of intensive pain, numbness, and a feeling of paralysis in the leg. Hours later, as the products of anaerobic metabolism build up in the skeletal muscle, the microcirculation will experience vasodilatation mediated by local tissue acidosis. It is this subsequent stage of vasodilatation with stagnant circulation where thrombosis in the smaller blood vessels may occur, and it is toward this event that early and aggressive heparin therapy is directed. Paradoxically, the patient will ordinarily have less pain at this juncture and the inexperienced examiner may erroneously interpret this as adequate recruitment of collateral circulation.

Two additional considerations must be addressed when dealing with the topic of anticoagulation. First, is high dose heparin therapy alone in lieu of catheter embolectomy an acceptable treatment alternative? Second, what is the role of thrombolytic therapy? Use of high dose heparin therapy alone as the primary treatment, as advocated by Blaisdell, has not gained wide acceptance. This treatment plan was originally predicated on the assumption that revascularization of a markedly ischemic limb contributed significantly to the high mortality associated with peripheral arterial embolism. Indeed, our own experience (20% in-hospital mortality for arterial embolism patients) mirrors that which is reflected in the literature. However, it is clear that the excessive mortality in these patients is a function of their underlying cardiac disease and not related to the limb ischemia *per se*. The most commonly performed surgical approach in these patients is a femoral embolectomy which we usually perform with local anesthesia and which constitutes a minimal surgical insult to the patient. Furthermore, it is our belief that mortality in these patients is similar, irrespective of whether primary amputation or attempts at revascularization are carried out. In our practice, the treatment of peripheral arterial embolism is prompt catheter embolectomy and *permanent* anticoagulation thereafter.

Does thrombolytic therapy play any role in the treatment of the patient with acute lower extremity ischemia? This issue must be considered unanswerable at the moment as more selective thrombolytic agents such as tissue plasminogen activator are becoming available. Yet the experience to date allows some comments on the efficacy of thrombolytic therapy. Certain considerations would seem to preclude its use in the patient with arterial embolism. The chronicity of cardiac clot may prevent lysis by the fibrinolytic system; the theoretic possibility of cleaving fragments of large mural thrombi is present, and the potential for concomitant or subsequent cerebral embolization and superimposed hemorrhage are all reasons to avoid its use in the patient with arterial embolism. Certainly, the same arguments do not pertain to the patients with arterial thrombosis, and lytic therapy may occasionally be considered initially in such patients, hoping to reveal a limited area of disease perhaps suitable to balloon angioplasty. The guiding principle, however, in the use of thrombolytic therapy in any form of acute arterial ischemia must remain the clinical status of the limb. The luxury of time must be available in order to utilize thrombolytic therapy in this setting. Selective intraarterial thrombolytic therapy usually requires multiple trips to the angiography suite, monitoring in an intensive care type setting, repeated dye loads, and time. Thus, an immediately threatened limb is not an appropriate circumstance in which to use thrombolytic therapy.

OPERATIVE MANAGEMENT

As noted above, my approach to definitive surgical management depends on the clinical diagnosis. In patients with acute arterial embolism, I favor proceeding with prompt surgical embolectomy. In patients with aortic saddle embolism, or iliac/femoral bifurcation emboli, the approach is via the femoral artery in the groin, and the operation is usually conducted under local anesthesia. If, however, on the basis of a palpable popliteal pulse, the clinical diagnosis is popliteal embolism, I recommend a direct approach to the popliteal artery; this facilitates complete, selective embolectomy of the runoff vessels. An embolectomy catheter placed from the groin will generally proceed to either the posterior tibial or peroneal artery, seldom both, and quite rarely will embolectomy of the anterior tibial artery be feasible from the groin. This strategy does have the potential disadvantage of increasing the operative insult to the patient, as it will ordinarily not be possible to explore the popliteal artery under local anesthesia alone. Furthermore, since these patients should, by the time they arrive in the operating room, be fully anticoagulated, a spinal type anesthetic may be unsafe, thereby committing the patient who requires a popliteal artery exploration to general anesthetic.

In an undiseased common femoral artery, I prefer a 180° transverse arteriotomy placed just proximal to the femoral bifurcation. All femoral artery branches are selectively catheterized and following extraction of embolic material, regional heparin is instilled into these vessels. If there is significant atherosclerotic disease in the common femoral artery, I do not hesitate to use a longitudinal arteriotomy and closure with a vein patch. In the popliteal artery, the arteriotomy is routinely made in longitudinal fashion, placed in such a location as to directly visualize the orifice of the anterior tibial artery. Furthermore, the tibioperoneal trunk is sufficiently dissected to permit selective catheterization of both the peroneal and posterior tibial arteries. Closure of the longitudinal popliteal arteriotomy is carried out with a vein patch.

It is imperative that the surgeon verify the completeness of embolectomy. In our practice we make frequent use of intraoperative monitoring with the pulse volume recorder, and this has alleviated the need for routine intraoperative angiography. However, we have a low threshold for proceeding with the latter in circumstances where the PVR tracing may be unsatisfactory. Furthermore, intraoperative angiography becomes a necessity if the preoperative diagnosis of acute embolism should prove to be in error, and *in situ* arterial thrombosis is found. In fact, this occurred at a rate of 20% in a series of patients we reviewed with acute arterial thrombosis.

While there are few absolutes in surgery, one which I strictly adhere to is that catheter thrombectomy alone never suffices for acute atherosclerotic thrombosis. The mechanical obstruction must be dealt with definitively, usually by some form of bypass graft.

The earlier literature on this topic suggested that, in the circumstance of acute ischemia on the basis of atherosclerotic thrombosis, the prognosis for limb salvage was poor and reconstruction conducted in such a setting was seldom successful. This engendered a teaching wherein acute thrombosis was treated with anticoagulant therapy until such time that the patient could be prepared for elective surgical correction. Indeed, this is frequently possible but as emphasized in our review, definitive surgical correction on an urgent or emergent basis will sometimes be required in these patients. Such a determination is made on the basis of the degree of ischemia seen on initial evaluation. We reviewed 52 patients with acute ischemia (hospitalization within seven days of the sudden onset of ischemic symptoms) secondary to arterial thrombosis and determined that two thirds of these required surgery during their initial hospitalization. Urgent or emergent (within 48 hours of admission to the hospital) femoropopliteal reconstruction was accompanied by favorable (86%) early patency rates and good clinical results. We recommended, on the basis of this experience, that there should be no reluctance to proceed with indicated vascular reconstruction in the setting of acute limb ischemia secondary to arterial thrombosis.

TREATMENT RESULTS

Patient outcome in acute arterial ischemia is stratified along the spectrum of the various anatomic conditions which may produce limb ischemia. Clearly, in the patient with acute arterial embolism, one should anticipate functional restoration of the limb in the majority of cases. In our own collective review, limb salvage with surgical embolectomy was achieved in 86% of cases, and this is consistent with a range of 75% to 95% salvage rate as determined from a review of the recent literature. However, mortality rates in patients hospitalized for acute peripheral arterial embolism continue to range from 11% to 30%. While limb salvage was statistically inferior in our acute thrombosis patients (64%), the coincident mortality (8%) was also much lower. Dale has reported similar figures when patients with embolism are compared to those with acute thrombosis. Excessive mortality, in the range of 50%, has been reported for patients sustaining acute aortic occlusion, irrespective of the underlying pathology. Clearly, treatment delay in this circumstance is strongly correlated with an unfavorable outcome due to the large bulk of muscle at risk for ischemia and reperfusion injury.

SUMMARY

Successful management of the patient with acute lower extremity ischemia is predicated on the principles of prompt anticoagulation and the establishment of an anatomic and pathologic diagnosis based on clinical findings. Such evaluation determines the need for angiography which is unnecessary in embolic disease, yet desirable in patients with arterial thrombosis. Definitive therapy involves catheter thrombectomy for embolic disease and correction of the precipitant obstruction in patients with arterial thrombosis.

BIBLIOGRAPHY

1. Abbott WM, Maloney RD, McCabe C, et al: Arterial embolism: A 44 year perspective. *Am J Surg* 1982; 143:460–464.

2. Abbott WM, McCabe C, Maloney RD, et al: Embolism of the popliteal artery. *Surg Gynecol Obstet* 1984; 159:533–536.

3. Blaisdell FW, Steele M, Allen RE: Management of acute lower extremity arterial ischemia due to embolism and thrombosis. *Surgery* 1978; 84:822–824.

4. Cambria RP, Abbott WM: Arterial thrombosis of the lower extremities: Its natural history contrasted with embolic occlusion. *Arch Surg* 1984; 119:784–787.

5. Dale WA: Differential management of acute peripheral arterial ischemia. *J Vasc Surg* 1984; 1:269–278.

35 The Patient with Claudication Alone

A 55-year-old management consultant is seen for right calf claudication occurring after walking one or two blocks. He smokes one pack of cigarettes daily, but denies significant medical problems. He has no pain at rest. The symptoms are very troublesome to him during the extensive travel and walking that he must do for his occupation and interferes significantly with his active lifestyle.

Consultant: John A. Mannick, M.D.

The above patient is typical of those seeking relief from intermittent claudication caused by femoropopliteal occlusive disease. In my opinion, the fact that this patient has no symptoms suggestive of ischemia at rest does not necessarily make him ineligible for surgical treatment. Between 20% and 30% of patients operated on our Vascular Service for infrainguinal arterial occlusive disease undergo femoropopliteal bypass grafting for symptoms of disabling intermittent claudication. However, most individuals with claudication on the basis of superficial femoral artery occlusion do not require arterial reconstructive surgery and do not have symptoms of sufficient severity to interfere significantly with their daily lives.

If surgical therapy is to be offered for disabling intermittent claudication, then the early and late results of surgery should be superior to the outcome anticipated from the natural history of the disease itself. It is apparent from several large studies reported in the medical literature that the natural history of intermittent claudication is, in general, benign, with 80% of patients remaining stable symptomatically or showing improvement over a period of five years from the onset of symptoms. Certainly less than 10%, perhaps about 5%, of such individuals will have sufficient progression of atherosclerotic disease to require amputation over the same five-year period.

INITIAL EVALUATION AND MANAGEMENT

The patient presenting with symptoms of intermittent claudication deserves a careful history and physical examination, with particular attention paid to the state of the peripheral circulation and to possible risk factors for atherosclerosis. The patient in question is a smoker and should clearly be advised to cease cigarette smoking. He should be checked for hypertension and should be placed under treatment for this condition if it is present. Similarly, detection of elevated blood lipids is important, and should be treated with dietary modification or drug therapy, as necessary.

On physical examination one would anticipate finding that the patient had normal femoral pulses bilaterally with no pulses palpable below the femoral level in the right limb. Calf claudication is usually a sign of femoropopliteal occlusive disease; however, in our experience 25% of patients with principally aortoiliac occlusive disease have only calf claudication as a symptom of this disorder. This fact should be born in mind when evaluating any individual with calf claudication.

Careful inspection of the patient's foot is also mandatory to detect evidence of ischemia at rest including rubor on dependency, coolness, trophic changes of the skin, ischemic ulceration or even incipient gangrene. It is, of course, highly unlikely that the patient under discussion will have such changes.

Laboratory examination of the patient with claudication is often helpful in determining his or her management. It is our belief that segmental lower extremity pressures measured with the Doppler at rest and a pulse volume recording are adequate evaluation in most instances. A patient with an ankle/brachial blood pressure index of 0.4 or less, or an absolute ankle blood pressure of 60 mm of mercury or less, might well be considered a candidate for surgery on the basis of hemodynamic evidence for resting ischemia even though he or she denied resting symptoms. We have not found segmental limb pressures to be particularly useful in predicting the level of occlusive disease in patients with claudication.

Measurement of Doppler ankle pressures, before and after a period of standard exercise on a treadmill, may be useful in making the diagnosis of intermittent claudication in an individual in whom this diagnosis, based on history and physical examination, is in doubt. However, we have not felt that exercise testing was mandatory in evaluating all patients with intermittent claudication.

We have recently begun to study patients who present with calf claudication by Doppler imaging of the superficial femoral artery. The duplex scanner is used for this purpose at our hospital. If the patient is found to have a localized stenotic lesion of the superficial femoral artery, balloon angioplasty might be offered. In the hands of an experienced radiologist, percutaneous balloon angioplasty of short stenotic superficial femoral lesions is associated with low morbidity, few complications, and an acceptable success rate. Thus angioplasty might be considered for a subgroup of patients with localized and therefore favorable superficial femoral lesions whose symptoms were not sufficiently severe to warrant arterial reconstructive surgery. (Fig 35–1A and B).

TREATMENT

In managing the patient with intermittent claudication caused by infrainguinal occlusive disease, there is fortunately no urgency about proceeding to surgical therapy

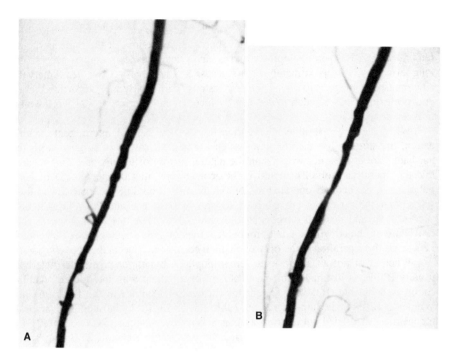

FIG 35–1.
A. Angiogram of patient with intermittent claudication on the basis of a high grade mid-superficial femoral artery stenosis. **B.** Completion angiogram on the same patient after therapy with percutaneous transluminal balloon angioplasty.

or angioplasty. In my practice, arterial reconstruction is seldom offered to a patient with only claudication at the time of the first office visit. This is particularly true of the patient with calf claudication of recent onset. In such individuals cessation of smoking, if the patient can be persuaded to do so, and regular exercise of the affected leg, usually a program of walking gradually increasing distances, will not infrequently produce symptomatic improvement so that surgery is unnecessary. If at the end of three months of such a regimen the patient is still having disabling claudication, then surgical therapy or possibly balloon angioplasty is appropriate.

On our service we have been disappointed with the results of Pentoxifylline therapy for patients with intermittent claudication. Even in the controlled studies which led to the introduction of this drug into the US market, the percentage increase in walking distance associated with Pentoxifylline therapy, while statistically significant, was probably not of great clinical significance. Certainly this has been our experience.

If the patient's claudication is of long duration, increasing in severity and seriously interfering with his or her ability to work, then clearly less time can be spent in conservative therapy and surgery or angioplasty should be offered sooner. As noted above, balloon angioplasty for superficial femoral occlusive disease has been most successful in individuals with short stenotic lesions of the midsuperficial femoral artery. Balloon angioplasty under such circumstances produces acceptable long-term results, approximately 50% success at the three- to five-year interval. Angioplasty of longer superficial femoral lesions, particularly long superficial femoral occlusions, has a much lower rate of success and is probably not worthwhile in most instances.

When offering operative intervention for the treatment of intermittent claudication, the surgeon has the obligation to ensure that the results of surgery in his or her hands are at least not worse than the natural history of the disease. This means that the operative mortality should be at or near zero, that the percentage of amputations in the patients operated on for claudication should be less than 5% in five years, that the operative procedure itself should have an acceptably high initial success rate, and that this success should be durable. Thus, for most surgeons the procedure of choice will be a femoropopliteal bypass graft of autogenous saphenous vein since this operation is the only one which consistently meets the above criteria.

Whether or not an above knee femoropopliteal bypass of prosthetic material, usually PTFE, is justifiable for the treatment of a patient with intermittent claudication is debatable. Relevant experience on our own service at the Brigham and Women's Hospital is summarized in Table 35–1. Of 1,173 infrainguinal arterial reconstructions carried out on the Vascular Service over the past decade, 249 (21%) were femoropopliteal bypass grafts performed for disabling claudication in 208 patients. There were 167 autogenous vein grafts and 82 PTFE grafts. There were two deaths occuring within 30 days of operation, for an operative mortality rate of 0.8%. As can be seen from the table, neither vein grafts nor PTFE grafts led to an unacceptably high five-year amputation rate. In fact, the percentage of amputations (2.4%) was the same for both types of reconstruction. However, the late patency was clearly and statistically significantly superior for vein grafts.

It is my opinion from this experience that PTFE grafts should not be done for intermittent claudication because of the rather low (approximately 50%) late pa-

TABLE 35–1.
Femoropopliteal Bypass for Claudication (1977–1987)

RECONSTRUCTION	NUMBER LIMBS	5-YEAR AMPUTATION RATE	5-YR. CUMULATIVE PRIMARY GRAFT PATENCY (%)
Autogenous	AK 87	2	72
Vein	BK <u>80</u>	<u>2</u>	<u>84</u>
	Total 167	4 (2.4%)	78*
PTFE	AK 63	1	55
	BK <u>19</u>	<u>1</u>	<u>42</u>
	Total 82	2 (2.4%)	52*

*p<0.05

tency of such reconstructions. However, the opposite conclusion might legitimately be drawn by others reviewing the same data. My present view is that the only acceptable operative alternative to autogenous vein bypass grafting for the patient with intermittent claudication is localized endarterectomy of the superficial femoral artery with autogenous venous patch graft angioplasty. This procedure has also produced acceptable and durable long-term patency (approximately 70% at five years) and, like vein grafting, has little tendency to produce occlusion of previously patent distal vessels if the reconstruction itself occludes.

The presence of a saphenous vein is, therefore, a factor in deciding whether or not to recommend surgery to a patient with intermittent claudication alone. If the saphenous vein in the affected leg has been surgically removed or is unacceptably diseased, this does not necessarily preclude venous bypass grafting since the lesser saphenous vein and cephalic vein from the arm have been used for this procedure, with success equal to that of reversed greater saphenous vein. However, with our current preference for *in situ* saphenous vein grafting in the infrainguinal position, we are reluctant to sacrifice the greater saphenous vein in the opposite leg for a femoropopliteal bypass for claudication. Therefore, it is our belief that some knowledge of the quality, size, and patency of the greater saphenous vein in the affected limb is important in planning femoropopliteal reconstruction. We currently find the most acceptable method of evaluating the saphenous vein preoperatively is duplex imaging. The exact course of the vein can be drawn with ink on the skin at the time to facilitate operative exposure.

It goes without saying that, in preparing the patient with intermittent claudication for arterial surgery, careful attention to the possible coexistence of coronary artery disease is essential. While femoropopliteal reconstruction in the patient population with claudication is a very low risk procedure, failure to identify an individual who might be in danger of a perioperative myocardial infarction is a tragedy. The patient with EKG or clinical evidence of coronary artery disease should be evaluated preoperatively by a cardiologist for determination of whether or not further detailed investigation of myocardial function and coronary anatomy is necessary.

Adequate arteriography is also clearly necessary in planning arterial surgery for claudication, as for any other indication. This, in our opinion, includes aortography with biplane views of the iliac arteries to rule out hemodynamically significant lesions in the proximal arterial tree, as well as complete views of the femoral, popliteal and tibial vessels.

As noted above, the method of femoropopliteal reconstruction currently preferred on our service is the *in situ* autogenous venous bypass graft. This applies to patients with claudication, as well as those with ischemia at rest.

I prefer to expose the entire length of saphenous vein to be used for the femoropopliteal bypass. The proximal anastomosis is performed first and the vein graft is allowed to fill with autogenous blood under arterial pressure. Valves are incised with a Leather valvulotome inserted through side branches or the distal end of the graft. The distal end of the vein is gently dilated with autologous blood containing papavarine prior to introduction of the valvulotome to avoid injury to the intima.

After pulsatile flow through the end of the graft is achieved, the distal anastomosis is performed. All visible branches of the vein are then ligated. Completion angiography with views of the entire vein graft is mandatory. *In situ* vein grafts performed with this technique have resulted in superior patency when compared with reversed autogenous vein grafts on our Service, although differences did not achieve statistical significance. It appears that this trend toward superior patency is directly related to a lesser incidence of myointimal hyperplasia in *in situ* grafts near the proximal anastomosis to the common femoral artery.

Intermittent claudication is not considered an appropriate indication for femorotibial bypass grafting, in my opinion. However, this conservative policy may need reevaluation in the future in view of the cumulative results of *in situ* vein grafting at our institution. The patency rates at four years for femoropopliteal and for femorotibial *in situ* grafts are identical at 84%. We have previously felt that the chance of long-term success for femorotibial grafts was too low to warrant the use of such procedures for the treatment of even the most disabled claudicators.

To summarize, it is clear that most patients with intermittent claudication alone, on the basis of superficial femoral artery occlusion, do not require arterial reconstructive surgery in order to lead productive and profitable lives. However, for the individual with disabling claudication, femoropopliteal bypass grafting may be carried out with an acceptably low operative mortality and an anticipated amputation rate at least no worse than that associated with the natural history of the disease. While the five-year patency rate, and therefore the symptomatic success rate, is significantly higher for reconstructions utilizing autogenous vein, long-term symptomatic relief may be expected in approximately half the patients treated with above-knee PTFE femoropopliteal bypass grafts.

BIBLIOGRAPHY

1. Boyd AM: The natural course of arteriosclerosis of the lower extremities. *Angiology* 1960; 11:10–14.
2. Cronenwett JL, Warner KG, Zelenock GB, et al: Intermittent claudication: Current results of nonoperative management. *Arch Surg* 1984; 119:430–436.
3. Donaldson MC, Mannick JA: Femoropopliteal bypass grafting for intermittent claudication: Is pessimism warranted? *Arch Surg* 1980; 115:724–727.
4. Imparato AM, Kim GE, Davidson T, et al: Intermittent claudication: Its natural course. *Surgery* 1975; 78:795–799.
5. Kent CK, Donaldson MC, Attinger CE, et al: Femoropopliteal reconstruction for claudication: The risk to life and limb. *Arch Surg* 1987, in press.
6. McAllister FF: The fate of patients with intermittent claudication managed nonoperatively. *Am J Surg* 1976; 132:593–595.
7. Naji A, Barker CF, Berkowitz HD: Femoropopliteal vein grafts for claudication: Analysis of 100 consecutive cases. *Ann Surg* 1978; 188:79–82.
8. Singer A, Rob C: The fate of the claudicator. *Br Med J* 1960; 2:633–636.

36 Femoropopliteal Bypass— Reversed vs *In Situ* Vein Graft

A 64-year-old electrician is admitted with progressive left leg ischemia. He has a history of prior severe claudication and has complained of rest pain in the left foot for the past two months. In the past week, the left fifth toe has been blue and increasingly painful. Examination reveals a satisfactory femoral pulse, absent distal pulses, and dry gangrene of the entire fifth toe. Arteriography reveals scattered atheromatous changes in the aortoiliac segment, and occlusion of the entire left superficial femoral artery. The left popliteal artery reconstitutes 2 cm distal to the adductor canal with a two-vessel runoff.

Consultants: R. Clement Darling, Jr., M.D. and R. Clement Darling, III, M.D.

CLINICAL-ANATOMICAL BACKGROUND

The above scenario is a common problem presenting to the general vascular surgeon. One needs to understand the anatomical pathology that occurs in the superficial femoral artery (SFA). SFA occlusions of a chronic nature may be reasonably well tolerated within the varying limitations of intermittent claudication. Acute atherosclerotic occlusions in the midportion of the SFA (Hunter's canal) may often remain silent until thrombosis progresses centripetally, often to the level of the profunda femoris artery. This vessel provides the major collateral network to the popliteal artery both above and below the knee. The distal outflow pattern may frequently have been established before the SFA occlusion occurs; that is, of the three named outflow vessels (anterior tibial, posterior tibial, and peroneal) some or all may be diseased. The pattern of femoropopliteal occlusive disease may also extend distally from the mid SFA allowing the popliteal artery segment below the knee to remain uninvolved. The severity of clinical symptoms, however, may not relate to the anatomical extent of the disease as much as to the rate of progression to occlusion which may be even more important. The temporal aspects of occlusive disease are related, in order of importance, to (1) active cigarette smoking, (2) age of the patient (the younger, the more virulent), and (3) the presence as well of other risk factors such as diabetes, hypertension, and dyslipidemia.

The case under study is of a relatively young working male with claudication progressing within a few months to ischemic foot pain and then to digital gangrene. This rapid progression is not unlike that seen in many middle-aged male cigarette smokers. The tibial artery occlusion may well have existed along with a chronic SFA occlusion in the mid-thigh but then worsened acutely with more proximal extension of the disease. This might be due to (1) proximal SFA thrombosis, or (2) progressive stenosis of the profunda femoris origin, or (3) development of aortoiliac occlusive disease. In our diagnostic workup it will be important to obtain some measure of inflow and outflow disease either noninvasively or invasively.

NONINVASIVE STUDY

In our experience, wave forms and amplitudes obtained with the PVR, [R] along with pressures obtained with the Doppler probe, are most important. Blood pressure cuffs of appropriate size at the thigh, calf and ankle outline the differences in the pressures at these three areas on the lower extremity. Diminished amplitude and attenuation of pulse volume recordings, as well as Doppler pressures of 50 mm Hg or less at the ankle, are highly suggestive of anatomically severe foot ischemia. However, artificially high pressures may be present in the diabetic who commonly has calcification of arteries below the inguinal ligament. A significant difference of pressure between the calf and the ankle simply attests to the presence of outflow disease in the tibial vessels, this difference usually exceeding 20 mm Hg.

A thigh pressure equal to the systemic pressure suggests in the nondiabetic that the inflow, at least at rest, is adequate. A low thigh Doppler pressure, however, does not necessarily document the presence of a poor inflow since the thigh cuff is often placed distal to the origin of a high SFA occlusion and the profunda femoris may be relatively underdeveloped. The difference in thigh pressure from calf pressure simply documents the degree of the occlusive process and the adequacy of collateral circulation between the two levels. Treadmill exercise testing will emphasize some of these changes. In our experience, and contrary to the extensive literature, there is very little correlation between outcome of bypass procedures and these pressure recordings.

Because of the misleading pressure determinations obtained in the patient with calcified vessels, it is important that the pulse volume recordings be used. Amplitude and wave form characteristics are critical in determining the degree of limb ischemia as well as the extent of collateral artery blood flow. Digital readings by using a small cuff may also help assess the ability of a digital or transmetatarsal amputation to heal. Transcutaneous oxygen tension (TcpO$_2$) on the anterior skin surface of the digit or forefoot, with findings of 50 mm Hg or greater have corre-

[R]Life Sciences, Incorporated, Greenwich, CT

lated with successful healing of amputations either before or after femoropopliteal grafting.

INVASIVE STUDY

Angiography in this case should include the following:

1. Transfemoral puncture of the involved extremity, done primarily to obtain *peak* systolic pressures in the distal aorta as well as in the distal iliac system. A gradient, or what might be more properly called a pressure difference, of 15 mm Hg or more should be considered evidence of an inflow problem.

Experimental work has shown that at higher flow rates, lesions of less than the usual recognized "critical" stenosis will produce increased systolic pressure differences. This is best demonstrated by the intraarterial injection of tolazaline (12.5 mg to 15 mg) which gives a functional reactive hyperemia. Another method is to use aqueous nitroglycerine (100 μg to 200 μg [micrograms]), or 30 mg papaverine intraarterially. Systemic pressures must be monitored in order to provide an adequate relationship with the distal fall in peak systolic pressure. Most of us believe that a 15% fall suggests a hemodynamically significant aortoiliac occlusive process.

2. Good oblique films of the iliac vessels, as well as of the profunda femoris arteries, to assess both the inflow disease as well as the profunda femoris collateral integrity are essential. Again, this relates to the pathology of the atherosclerotic plaque in the aortoiliac segment, particularly the common iliac arteries where crescentic plaquing occurs posteriorly. With obstruction of as much as 60% of the cross-sectional lumen diameter, a standard anterior-posterior aortogram may reveal only "scattered atheromatous changes." These may, in fact, represent hemodynamically important lesions. The same holds true with the physical examination; a good femoral pulse does not necessarily mean an unobstructed inflow. Lateral views of the profunda takeoff are important since worsening of limb ischemia may be related to the inadequacy of the profunda femoris collateral, secondary to occlusive disease at its origin. This, of course, would require profundaplasty at the time of a femoropopliteal bypass.

3. Puncturing the involved side—a consideration for the poor risk patient with distal disease who might not tolerate a concomitant aortofemoral reconstruction. The possibility of balloon angioplasty as a staged procedure prior to femoropopliteal bypass should also be considered.

GENERAL TREATMENT—CHOICES AND OPTIONS

This case demonstrates progressive atherosclerotic peripheral vascular disease with a limb in jeopardy. Treatment should consist of immediate hospitalization with bed rest and control of lower extremity vaso-motor tone. This must be accompanied by complete cessation of cigarette smoking as well as administration of intravenous antibiotics to control regional sepsis. Noninvasive studies can be carried out at rest; usually within a 72-hour period a transfemoral aortogram should be obtained. If coronary artery disease is suggested by history or EKG abnormalities, a Persantine-Thallium stress test should be performed in order to assess the degree of cardiac risk, as well as to predict whether coronary bypass with autogenous vein will eventually be considered.

Bypass should be carried out optimally using autogenous tissue, preferably the long saphenous vein. Whether the vein is used *in situ* or is reversed depends largely on the past experience of the surgeon. With the advent of fine polypropylene sutures, optical magnification, and coaxial fiber optic illumination, patency rates and limb salvage appear comparable, both in prospective and retrospective studies.

We think in this particular instance, we would prefer the use of a reversed saphenous vein graft to the below-knee segment if the vein is of adequate caliber, that is at least 4 mm internal diameter. For over 20 years we have noted the long-term results in both *in situ* and reversed vein grafts. Although the number of reversed grafts is substantially larger, there seems to be little difference when the anastomosis is made to the distal popliteal artery itself. If the vein graft is placed in the below-knee position, the chances of long-term patency in followup of the Linton series are significantly greater than if the anastomosis is to the proximal popliteal artery. We would anticipate an 85% patency rate at five years in the former, while in the latter, grafting to an above-knee segment carries with it about 55% patency rate at five years because of disease progression in the above-knee segment.

An additional problem with an *in situ* vein grafting to an above-knee segment is that it is an unnecessarily tedious procedure. One must free up the proximal vein so that it will reach the common femoral artery since the saphenous vein origin and the profunda femoris takeoff are at the same anatomical level. In addition, in order to avoid angulation as the *in situ* vein dips around the adductor tendon, one has to free the vein up and consequently one ends up taking the majority of branches. Then, instead of reversing the vein which is quite simple, the extra chore of removing the valves simply adds time and unnecessary complexity.

We reject the notion that the vein cannot be compromised by entrapment if one does not pass the vein's distal portion underneath the medial head of the gastrocnemius and its four accompanying tendons. So again one is left with the same setup: extensive freeing up of the vein proximally and distally which might have been avoided by reversing the vein with no need for diddling around with the valves. One would be foolish indeed to think that no endothelial damage occurs when one passes a selected series of strippers, scissors, knives, wires, nuts, or bolts down the lumen of the nonreversed vein to obliterate the bicuspid valves.

Proponents of the *in situ* bypass graft have stated that leaving the vein *in situ* preserves the intact vasa vasorum, which results in improved endothelial preservation and increased vein wall production of prostacyclins. However, the normal vein wall is nourished, for the most part, by the intimal blood flow, in contrast to arteries where two thirds of the wall are nourished by an extensive vasa vasorum. Minimizing the warm ischemia time and temporarily storing the vein distended with heparinized arterial blood has proven clinically to be effective in the reversed vein graft.

Many of us fail to remember that the *weakest point* of a reversed saphenous vein femoropopliteal bypass graft is the proximal anastomosis where the *narrowest* portion of the vein is anastomosed to the *thickest* portion of the proximal artery. It is here that most anastomotic strictures occur—not distally where the *in situ* proponents have laid their money.

Our experience suggests only two potential virtues in an *in situ* vein graft from the femoral to the distal popliteal region. The first would be if the distal vein is of inadequate caliber, i.e., 4 mm or less, to anastomose to the common femoral artery in reversed fashion. In such instances, one might use a nonreversed technique to remove valve function and simply advance or translocate the proximal vein cephalad along with the anterior portion of the femoral vein and suture it to the common femoral artery. A second possible advantage arises from our observation that the late segmental stenoses occurring after two years in reversed vein grafts often relate to the sites of valve seating. It has been adequately demonstrated that in the reversed vein grafts, the valves do not completely allow undisturbed flow of blood. Angioscopy reveals the valves sometimes may continue to flutter in the reversed position. The valve seats are also sites of rings of fibrous tissue deposits in some patients. Possibly the removal of the valve or the valve seat would be advantageous. These considerations are perhaps more of a theoretical proposition since the intraoperative flow rates and postoperative patency rates with both *in situ* vein grafts and reversed vein grafts are similar.

USE OF PROSTHETIC MATERIAL

In the patient with an above-knee segment and with a positive Persantine-Thallium test showing redistribution and suggesting severe coronary artery disease, an option exists for the use of a prosthetic above-knee bypass. At the moment, the use of 6 mm polytetrafluoroethylene (PTFE) with or without a spiral polypropylene strut seems to be a reasonable choice. Patency rates at three years approximate 65% to 80% and suggest that this is a viable alternative. However, the fact remains that though the above-knee segment seems patent by angiography, it is rarely uninvolved with atherosclerosis. It cannot be overemphasized that it is the best judgment in the case of a patient at good risk to spend the extra time to perform an autogenous vein bypass to the below-knee segment when at all possible.

MANAGEMENT OF THE GANGRENOUS TOE

With regard to local amputation of the gangrenous toe, two factors must be considered. First, the extent of the amputation and, second, its timing. In this patient, the involvement of the entire fifth toe precludes button-toe amputation. Transmetatarsal amputation (TMA) of the fifth toe or the entire forefoot will probably be necessary for healing.

The timing of the TMA may be variable depending on (1) excellence of arterial reconstruction, (2) perfusion of the forefoot, (3) character of the outflow vessels, and (4) the extent of demarcation. Some surgeons would wait as long as three weeks; however, there is risk of relighting a latent infection by delaying too long, in addition to the risks of antibiotic resistance or superinfection. A middle of the road approach would be to wait three to five days to allow demonstration of patency of the reconstruction and demarcation of the forefoot.

If one feels comfortable, as we do, with intraoperative monitoring using pulse volume recordings and Doppler pressures or intraoperative angiography, and is convinced that the operative procedure will revascularize the forefoot, one should proceed with amputation at the time of bypass surgery. In this case, it would be a transmetatarsal amputation of the fifth toe with the closure of the skin in loose fashion; and this would be considered an operation for drainage. Often this will be successful. Certainly not much is lost by doing so since, if necessary, this can be converted to a full transmetatarsal amputation at a later time.

BIBLIOGRAPHY

1. Boucher CA, Brewster DC, Darling RC, et al: Determination of cardiac risk by dipyridamole-thallium imaging before peripheral vascular surgery. *N Engl J Med* 1985; 312:389–394.
2. Brener BJ, Raines JK, Darling RC, et al: Measurement of systolic femoral arterial pressures during reactive hyperemia: An estimate of aorto-iliac disease. *Circulation (Suppl II)* 1974; 49 & 50: 259–267.
3. Brewster DC, LaSalle AJ, Darling RC: Comparison of above-knee and below-knee anastomosis of femoropopliteal grafts. *Arch Surg* 1981; 116:1013–1018.
4. Cambria RP, Megerman J, Abbott WM: Endothelial preservation in reversed and in-situ autogenous veins grafts. *Ann Surg* 1985; 202:50–55.
5. Charlesworth PM, Brewster DC, Darling RC: The fate of polytetrafluoroethylene grafts in lower limb bypass surgery—a six year follow-up. *Br J Surg* 1985; 72:896–899.
6. Darling RC, Linton RR: Durability of femoro-popliteal reconstructions: Endarterectomy versus vein bypass grafts. *Am J Surg* 1972; 123:472–479.
7. Darling RC, Raines JK, Brener BJ, et al: Quantitative segmental pulse volume recorder: A clinical tool. *Surgery* 1972; 72:873–887.
8. Hallett JW Jr., Brewster DC, Darling RC: The limitations of polytetrafluoroethylene in femoropopliteal and tibial artery reconstructions. *Surg Gynecol Obstet* 1981; 152:819–821.
9. Harris PL, How TV, Jones DR: Prospectively randomized clinical trial to compare in-situ and reversed saphenous vein grafts for femoropopliteal bypass. *Br J Surg* 1987; 74:252–255.
10. Katsamouris A, Brewster DC, Megerman J, et al: Transcutaneous oxygen tension in selection of amputation level. *Am J Surg* 1984; 147:510–517.

11. Leather RP, Karmody AM: In situ saphenous vein arterial bypass for the treatment of limb ischemia. *Advances in Surgery* 1986; 19:175–219.
12. McNamara JJ, Darling RC, Linton RR: Segmental stenosis of saphenous vein autografts: Preventable cause of late occlusion in arterial reconstruction. *N Engl J Med* 1967; 227:290–292.
13. Raines JK, Darling RC, Buth J, et al: Vascular laboratory criteria for the management of peripheral vascular disease of the lower extremities. *Surgery* 1976; 79:21–29.
14. Taylor LM Jr., Edwards JM, Phinney ES: Reversed vein bypass to infrapopliteal arteries; modern results are superior to or equivalent to in-situ bypass for patency and for vein utilization. *Ann Surg* 1987; 205:90–97.

37 Femorotibial Bypass— Preferred Techniques and Site of Distal Anastomosis

A 70-year-old diabetic has been admitted for a painful nonhealing ulceration of the right heel of three months' duration. Arteriography shows occlusion of the entire popliteal artery. The superficial femoral artery is relatively free of disease. Distally, there is reconstitution of the peroneal artery in the proximal calf and the distal anterior tibial artery 3 cm above the ankle, with runoff into the foot.

Consultants: Robert P. Leather, M.D. and Benjamin B. Chang, M.D.

This patient presents with a fairly typical clinical picture of diabetic patients requiring distal arterial bypass for limb salvage. Distal bypasses for the terminal stages of atherosclerotic occlusive disease manifest by chronic limb threatening ischemia are the most challenging arterial reconstructive procedures for the vascular surgeon today. Their length and low flow rates often exceed the functional limits of synthetic and even free vein grafts. However, the saphenous vein when used *in situ* provides a unique, viable, physiologically active and hence antithrombogenic endothelial flow surface which is ideally suited for such bypasses. In this patient, I believe the revascularization procedure which offers the best chance of successful limb salvage would be an *in situ* saphenous vein graft.

Clearly, use of autogenous vein for the bypass conduit is of crucial importance in patients with advanced ischemia and compromised runoff, as described in our patient. Because the graft must be carried to an infrapopliteal vessel, the size-match characteristics and gradual distal taper of an *in situ* graft results in more optimal flow characteristics and is particularly appealing. With the *in situ* technique, vein utilization is maximal and preservation of the vein endothelium best accomplished. Using the *in situ* method, our results of infrapopliteal grafting have been excellent, and equal or superior to those reported for alternate techniques.

This technique has been tested in over 1,000 consecutive patients requiring distal arterial reconstruction. An *in situ* bypass was attempted in over 95% of those unselected limbs requiring it for limb preservation, and 94% were completed *in*

244

situ, overall. A total of 603 of these were carried out to the infrapopliteal level, and at the distal level of transection the saphenous veins had diameters of less than 3.5 mm outer diameter in over 50% of limbs, suggesting that conventional reversed grafting techniques might have proven difficult. The immediate failure (30 day) rate was less than 5%. Cumulative patency by life table analysis at one, two, three, four, and five years was 89%, 85%, 83%, 79%, 78%, and 75%, respectively. Neither the distal vein diameter nor location of the distal anastomosis had a significant effect on these patency rates. The use of the saphenous vein *in situ*, prepared by the valve incision method, resulted in these improved patency rates in spite of exercising no selective preoperative angiographic criteria, while allowing the successful use of veins as small as 2.5 mm. Hence, I regard this method of revascularization the best for our patient.

PREOPERATIVE EVALUATION

Pulse volume recordings and segmental pressures are obtained both to confirm the need for distal reconstruction and to provide a baseline for comparison with postoperative studies. If the inflow appears adequate, then distal reconstruction is contemplated. If an inflow lesion is suggested by PVRs and physical examination, these are further evaluated by arteriography. The adequacy of inflow may be confirmed by the use of catheter pullout pressures at time of arteriography. Although an unobstructed inflow is ideal, in certain patients with multilevel disease, an *in situ* bypass may be placed below a partial inflow lesion with successful limb salvage.

The arteriograms are reviewed after a decision to operate is made. The femoral vessels are evaluated for use as an inflow source for distal bypass. The profunda femoris artery is known to be relatively spared from the ravages of atherosclerotic disease and thus provides a potentially more satisfactory anastomotic site, as well as a more distal inflow source. This allows for excision of the surgically manipulated proximal vein segment while constructing a tension-free anastomosis. The common femoral artery is the traditional inflow source but requires a greater length of mobilized and manipulated vein for anastomosis. The superficial femoral artery is generally the least suitable inflow source as this vessel is more likely to be thick-walled and involved with significant atherosclerosis. However, if necessary, this artery may be used if vein length is a limitation in the choice of inflow vessel. By description of the artery in our patient, it could be used, if necessary.

The distal arterial tree is then inspected on the angiograms. Frequently, angiograms from outside hospitals do not show below-knee arterial segments in sufficient detail. Repeat studies using digital subtraction techniques with biplane views of the tibial and pedal vessels may be required. In this case, the arteriogram apparently reveals a patent peroneal artery at the mid-calf and a patent anterior tibial artery in the distal leg. In general, the ideal outflow vessel provides direct perfusion of the foot, although the peroneal artery has yielded equally satisfactory limb salvage results. Patency of the pedal arch is not necessary for successful bypass patency and limb salvage. Given more than one vessel patent into the foot, the most proximally patent vessel is selected. If there are two or more vessels reconstituted at the same level, the posterior tibial vessel is the most easily exposed and requires the shortest distal mobilized vein segment. The peroneal artery is, in general, the second artery of choice and would be the appropriate one in this patient. Furthermore, the peroneal artery is statistically most likely to remain patent and disease-free in a manner analogous to the profunda femoris artery. Forty-one percent of tibial bypasses performed at our institution have utilized this outflow vessel (Fig 37–1). The anterior tibial artery requires the use of a relatively long mobilized segment of vein passed over the tibial or through the interosseous membrane and is therefore regarded as the least ideal artery for distal anastomosis unless direct perfusion of a gangrenous forefoot is necessary, and the posterior tibial artery is occluded. *In situ* bypass patency, ultimately, is equally good regardless of the site of distal anastomosis.

After arteriography is completed, preoperative evaluation of the saphenous vein is mandatory. Although venography provides an accurate picture of venous anatomy, this invasive study carries a small but finite complication rate. Currently we have used B-mode ultrasound in the last 345 limbs as a noninvasive means of vein imaging. In the overwhelming majority of the cases ultrasonography is sufficient to adequately define venous anatomy. A map of the vein anatomy is traced on the patient's skin with indelible ink. Vein diameter, however, is best determined at operation, as neither sonographic nor phlebographic measurements of internal vein diameter at venous pressures correlate closely with or should be confused with data where the external diameter of the vein is measured under arterial pressure. In

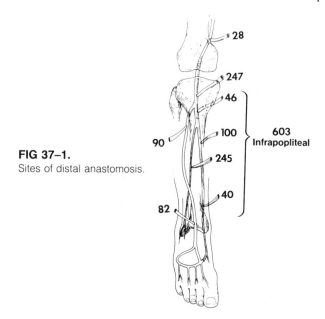

FIG 37–1.
Sites of distal anastomosis.

fact, the question of adequate vein size has been obscured in the literature because of these differences of measuring vein size. Patients are never denied operation on the basis of a "small vein" seen on preoperative studies, be it venography or ultrasound. Of those patients with an intact ipsilateral saphenous vein on preoperative evaluation, fully 94% can be expected to undergo a successful *in situ* bypass; an additional 3% to 4% may require the use of segments of ectopic vein for completion of a "partial" *in situ* bypass.

If a long femorotibial bypass is needed in a patient whose ipsilateral veins have been stripped or harvested previously, we do not hesitate to use ectopic limb veins placed in reversed or nonreversed (orthograde) configurations depending on the taper of the particular vein used.

SURGICAL TECHNIQUES

Once preoperative evaluation is completed, the patient is taken for operation. Epidural or spinal anesthesia is usually adequate, and may well be desirable in most cases. Loupe magnification and coaxial fiberoptic magnification are standard. After skin preparation and draping, papaverine (60 mg in 240 ml saline) is infused into the perivenous space around the below-knee segment of the greater saphenous vein in order to minimize venous spasm and its resultant endothelial injury.

A vertical, oblique, or transverse skin incision is made at the groin. After the superficial fascia is incised, the proximal saphenous vein is identified immediately below this layer and papaverine is again infused into the perivenous space. After the deep fascia is incised, the femoral arteries are isolated.

Unless preoperative venous imaging demonstrates a multiply branched double venous system in the thigh, making the use of the intraluminal valve cutter unsafe, a second incision is made immediately below the knee paralleling the saphenous vein. A short segment of vein is exposed to locate a small branch. If the outside diameter of the dilated thin-walled vein is less than 2.0 mm in diameter, then it is probably not suitable for use as an *in situ* bypass.

At this point, the patient is systemically heparinized (35 to 50 units per kg) and the vein divided at its proximal end. Given a more distal site for the proximal anastomosis, the vein may need simple division and ligation of the saphenofemoral junction. If a more proximal site for anastomosis is chosen, or if the saphenofemoral junction is relatively cephalad, the femoral vein may be tangentially clamped with a curved Cooley-type clamp and a patch of the femoral vein excised with the saphenous vein. The resultant linear femoral venotomy may be closed with fine continuous suture without fear of thrombosis or stenosis. Proximal branches of the saphenous vein are ligated with fine sutures and divided. A 5 cm to 8 cm length of vein is mobilized.

A 500-ml plastic solution bag of low molecular weight Dextran (av MW 40,000 Daltons) to which has been added 1,000 units of heparin and 120 mg of papaverine is pressurized to 150-200 mm Hg. A sterile standard IV set is connected between this solution and the operative field. A 6 or 8 Fr suction catheter is attached to the IV set and inserted into the proximal saphenous vein to dilate this segment. The most proximal valve leaflets may be tangentially excised with iris scissors. The remaining valve or valves within the proximal 3 cm to 5 cm may be incised with valve scissors and/or the valvulotome (Figs 37–2 and 37–3). A No. 3 Fogarty embolectomy catheter is inserted into the previously isolated and divided branch of the saphenous vein below the knee. This catheter is passed cephalad until it exits the proximal end of the saphenous vein. The catheter is then sharply and obliquely divided at either the 20 cm or 30 cm mark. If the thigh segment of the vein is large (> 4 mm OD), a 3 mm valve cutter is selected; a smaller, 2 mm cutter is appropriate in smaller veins. The cutter is screwed onto the cut end of the Fogarty catheter. The suction catheter is then attached to the proximal end of the cutter with a 15 mm to 20 mm loop of fine monofilament suture. The cutter blades are then carefully oriented to run perpendicular to the plane of valve closure, which is parallel to the plane of the skin (Fig 37–4). The cutter and the end of the suction catheter are drawn into the saphenous vein (Fig 37–5). A small silastic loop is used to form a watertight seal around the vein and enclosed suction catheter. The cutter is drawn down the remainder of the thigh segment of the vein by grasping both the distal end of the Fogarty catheter and the proximal end of the suction catheter. The cutter is internally rotated approximately 90 degrees as it passes down the vein in order to compensate for the change in the plane of valve closure as marked by the skin. This may be repeated to ensure valve incision. The cutter is then pulled out the proximal end of the vein and the Fogarty catheter transected immediately below the cutter. The catheter is removed from the vein.

After valve incision is completed, the proximal anastomosis is performed with

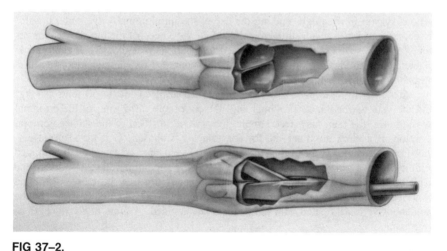

FIG 37–2.
Concept of valve incision. Blunted scissors are advanced to depths of valve sinus with leaflets in functionally closed position and valve leaflets cut.

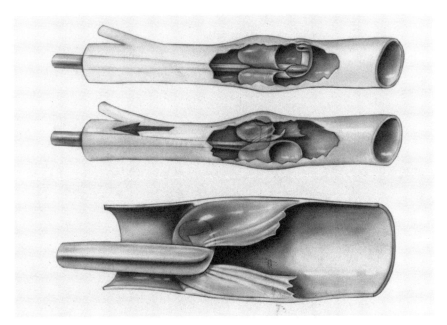

FIG 37–3.
Valve incision with valvulotome.

fine monofilament suture (usually 7–0 polypropylene). After completion of the anastomosis, the arteries are unclamped. Fistula flow in the thigh segment may be detected by the use of an 8–10 MHz pencil Doppler probe placed on the proximal vein with simultaneous occlusion of the vein at the knee.

If valves have successfully been incised and fistula flow is not overwhelming, there will be a palpable pulse at the knee. Because the proximal vein is now arterialized, endothelial ischemia is minimized.

If the peroneal artery is patent at the mid-calf level, as described in our patient, the calf incision is usually extended distally to this level. The saphenous vein is located, and the length of vein necessary to form a tension-free anastomosis is measured; this is usually the length of vein exposed by the skin incision. If available, an extra 1 cm to 2 cm of vein should be mobilized so that it may be discarded after manipulation.

If the peroneal artery is not patent or otherwise unsuitable for anastomosis, the anterior tibial artery would, in this case, be explored and used for *in situ* bypass. If the vein is adequate, the distal anastomosis may be carried as far distally as the dorsalis pedis or posterior tibial arteries in the foot, with excellent results.

After division of the vein at its distal mobilized end, the below-knee segment of vein is then dilated with the Dextran solution introduced into a side branch or the transected end of the vein via a 22-gauge plastic angiocath. If spasm is present,

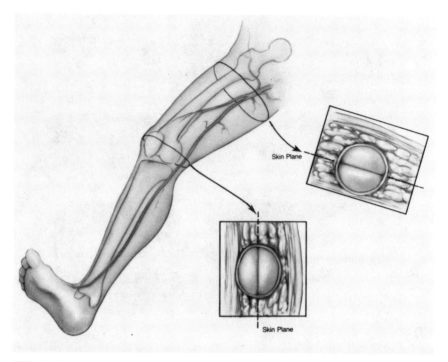

FIG 37–4.
Demonstration of plane of valve closure parallel to skin.

the vein must be dilated fully before any valve incision is undertaken; intraluminal instrumentation of the vein in spasm will produce circumferential endothelial injury with resultant formation of occluding platelet aggregates. The retrograde valvulotome is then used to incise valves in the distal segment. The valvulotome is introduced through the distal end of the vein or alternatively through a branch. After these steps are completed, the flow through the open end of the vein is examined. A constant strong stream is ideal. A diminishing or intermittent stream indicates that there is probably a residual valve present. A weak stream signifies the presence of a proximal stenotic lesion and/or a major amount of fistula flow proximally.

If flow through the bypass appears to be satisfactory, the outflow artery is clamped proximally and distally with Yasargil clips. Alternatively, an orthopedic tourniquet, applied above the knee, may be used, especially when dealing with heavily calcified arteries. Finally, the use of small Fogarty balloon catheters or other soft intraluminal occluders (Flo-Rester) are occasionally useful.

An arteriotomy is performed with a No. 11 scalpel blade and extended with small iris scissors. The arteriotomy is usually 4 mm to 8 mm long (1.5 – 2 x diameters of the larger vessel). The vein is brought into apposition with the arteriotomy

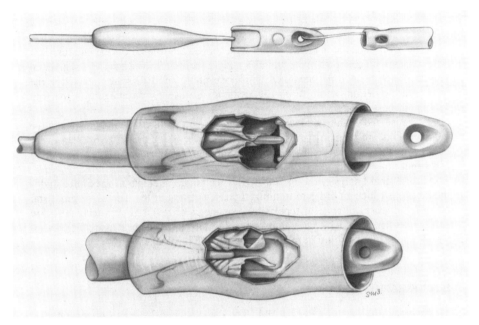

FIG 37–5.
Valve incision with valve cutter.

and then clamped proximally with a Yasargil clip. The vein is transected at the proper level and then opened along its vertical axis for the formation of the distal anastomosis. Generally, 8–0 polypropylene is used for anastomoses to tibial arteries. A continuous parachute technique is again employed. After completion, the clamps are removed.

With flow through the bypass established, the hand-held Doppler is used to estimate volume flow at and through the distal anastomosis. By holding the Doppler at the proximal vein segment, total bypass flow may be assessed. If the distal segment is then occluded, remaining flow through the proximal segment consists solely of fistula flow. Sequential digital compression of the bypass will reveal the location of any significant fistulae, which are marked on the skin, and provide an indication of their size.

At this point, a 22-gauge angiocath is inserted into the vein near the proximal anastomosis. Nineteen gauge hypodermic needles are taped onto the skin to provide a reference grid. Operative angiograms are then obtained. The angiogram is then examined for platelet aggregates (which require vein patch angioplasty of the affected segment) or technical problems at the distal anastomosis. Fistulae that have sufficient flow to opacify the deep venous system with contrast are marked on the skin, exposed through small incisions, isolated, and ligated in continuity. The Doppler will localize the fistula within the small skin incision plus or minus 1 mm to 2 mm, thus minimizing the amount of surgical dissection required to identify and control it. After the major fistulae are ligated, fistula flow and total bypass flow are checked again with the Doppler.

The groin incision is closed with two layers of interrupted fascial sutures. Staples are used to reapproximate the skin. Pulse volume recordings and segmental pressures are obtained the next day. Duplex scanning and PVRs are obtained in the postoperative period before discharge. Patients are usually discharged on the fifth to seventh postoperative day.

Because the majority of bypass failures occur within the first postoperative year, patients are seen in the office every eight weeks for the first year and every six months thereafter. At each visit, pulse volume recordings and duplex ultrasound assessment of resting and hyperemic bypass flow are obtained.

In the final analysis, the *in situ* bypass technique attempts to maximize endothelial preservation in order to optimize bypass patency in the face of severe distal occlusive disease. In spite of reports by proponents of reversed vein techniques, *in situ* bypass has been demonstrated by several groups to be the best available conduit for the long, low flow infrapopliteal bypass for limb salvage.

BIBLIOGRAPHY

1. Karmody AM, Leather RP, Shah DM, et al: Peroneal artery bypass: A reappraisal of its value in limb salvage. *J Vasc Surg* 1984; 1:809–816.
2. Leather RP, Karmody AM: In situ saphenous vein arterial bypass for the treatment of limb ischemia, in Mannick JA, et al (eds): *Advances in Surgery*, vol 19. Chicago, Year Book Medical Publishers, 1986, pp 175–219.
3. Leopold PW, Shandall AA, Corson JD, et al: Initial experience comparing B-mode imaging and venography of the saphenous vein before in situ bypass. *Am J Surg* 1986; 152:206–210.
4. Shah DM, Chang BB, Leopold PW, et al: The anatomy of the greater saphenous venous system. *J Vasc Surg* 1986; 3:273–281.

38 Limb-Threatening Ischemia and No Ipsilateral Greater Saphenous Vein— Alternative Choices

A 70-year-old woman is admitted with dry gangrene of the right second toe. Three months previously, occlusion of a prior right femoropopliteal graft done with the right greater saphenous vein had been documented. She is diabetic and gives a history of occasional angina pectoris. She has moderately severe claudication in the left leg. Repeat angiography shows a patent aortoiliac system, occlusion of the right femoropopliteal graft, and occlusion of the superficial femoral artery in both right and left legs. Both popliteal arteries are patent below the knee, with single vessel runoff.

Consultant: Frank J. Veith, M.D.

This patient's limb is clearly threatened and reintervention is unequivocally indicated despite the fact that she, like most patients with threatened limbs, has evidence of substantial coronary artery disease and diabetes. The previously failed saphenous vein femoropopliteal bypass should not preclude further efforts at limb salvage. In fact, late thrombosis of a substantial proportion of infrainguinal arterial reconstructions is to be expected with time. Such late graft failure can be due to intimal hyperplasia which involves the vein graft or its arterial anastomoses and usually manifests itself between two and 18 months after the initial operation. After that time failure is usually due to progression of the atherosclerotic disease process involving the inflow or outflow tracts of the vein graft.

FAILING GRAFT CONCEPT

It is unfortunate that the previous vein graft in this patient is occluded as documented arteriographically. Many, perhaps most, such grafts that are destined to fail with thrombosis go through a "failing graft" stage in which a flow reducing lesion develops in, proximal, or distal to the graft and yet the graft remains patent. Such lesions, if untreated, will cause eventual graft failure. However, if patients are followed at frequent intervals by their surgeon, with a careful pulse exam and perhaps noninvasive laboratory tests, it is usually possible to suspect the presence of such lesions before they cause graft occlusion. Accordingly, we recommend *urgent arteriography* in any patient with a previous arterial reconstruction who develops recurrent ischemic symptoms, a change in the pulse examination, or noninvasive indices distal to the previous bypass. If a lesion that is causing the failing state is detected, it can be corrected by a simple reintervention with sustained patency and limb salvage results that are far superior to those that can be obtained if the reintervention is delayed until graft thrombosis occurs. For example, we have found that percutaneous transluminal angioplasty has frequently been effective in correcting stenotic inflow or outflow lesions, or short stenoses within vein grafts. If long stenoses or occlusions are responsible for the failing state or the lesion is inaccessible for percutaneous angioplasty, a patch angioplasty or graft extension with vein or PTFE can be performed simply and with excellent late results. In this patient, it is possible that urgent arteriography three months ago, when graft occlusion was presumed, would have revealed a failing graft that could have been corrected easily with preservation of the autogenous vein graft, and would have avoided the more complex reoperation that will now be required because her original vein graft can not be salvaged.

REOPERATIVE STRATEGIES

Although this patient's aortoiliac segment is patent, it is important to exclude significant iliac artery stenoses. If present, these could have contributed to the failure of her previous bypass even though the ipsilateral femoral pulse is now normal. If an iliac artery stenosis is present and narrows the arterial lumen by more than 50%, it should be treated by percutaneous transluminal angioplasty even if the femoral artery pressure is normal. This is indicated since the increased iliac arterial flow resulting from the proposed new bypass may produce an iliac pressure gradient, though none presently exists. If such an inflow gradient (> 25 mm Hg) is detected *after* performance of the femoropopliteal bypass, an inflow procedure from the opposite femoral artery, the aorta or the axillary artery, will have to be performed.

Although acceptable mid-term and long-term patency and limb salvage rates can be expected after a secondary bypass performed with an expanded polytetrafluoroethylene (PTFE) graft to the below-knee popliteal artery, I believe that an autogenous vein graft would provide slightly better results in this setting. However, several other considerations would influence the choice of graft. Paramount among these would be the availability of a healthy segment of vein that was adequate in terms of length, diameter and freedom from recanalized thrombophlebitic segments. Venography and duplex ultrasonography of the superficial veins may be helpful in identifying suitable venous segments. We routinely perform these evaluations in any patient who has had a previous arterial reconstruction and requires operative reintervention. Because the results of PTFE femoropopliteal bypasses in terms of patency and limb salvage are as good as they are, I do not believe it is justified to harvest autogenous vein from the opposite lower extremity. This is particularly true if the patient has occlusive or stenotic arterial disease in the opposite limb, as in the patient under consideration. If vein were harvested from such a limb, the incisions might not heal and this opposite limb could be jeopardized. Even in the absence of arterial occlusion in the contralateral lower extremity, we would avoid use of its superficial veins for contralateral femoropopliteal bypass because of the symmetry of the disease process. Because of this, there is at least a 25% chance that these veins will be needed during the patient's lifetime to treat ischemia in this contralateral leg. The only circumstance that justifies use of vein from the contralateral lower extremity is the need to perform a bypass to an infrapopliteal artery. In this circumstance the patency rates of vein grafts are so far superior to those for PTFE grafts that contralateral vein harvest risks are acceptable.

What about use of upper extremity superficial veins? Unquestionably cephalic and basilic veins can sometimes be used as effective bypass conduits. However, these veins are thin walled, have many fine side branches, and are more difficult to use than are lower extremity veins. Moreover, I have found a high incidence of stenoses and occlusion in cephalic and basilic veins in limb salvage patients who have usually had multiple intravenous infusions and venipunctures. Because of all these considerations and the near comparable performance of vein and PTFE grafts to the popliteal artery, I only use upper extremity veins for infrapopliteal bypasses. If one uses cephalic vein in this or other settings, it is necessary to assure adequate luminal patency, and we have found that several segments must often be joined together end-to-end because of segmental scarring or occlusions.

Thus in the absence of an intact ipsilateral greater saphenous vein in a patient requiring a femoropopliteal bypass, I would restrict potential sources of autogenous vein to the ipsilateral lower extremity. Vein segments that might be available for use as a secondary bypass in a patient who has a failed primary greater saphenous femoropopliteal bypass include the lesser saphenous vein, accessory greater saphenous veins and the lower half of the greater saphenous vein, if only the upper portion was used for the primary operation. Before attempting to harvest any of these vein segments, it is essential to evaluate their length and diameter by venography or duplex ultrasonography to be sure a long enough segment of adequate diameter (≥ 3.5 mm) will be available for the planned secondary femoropopliteal bypass.

An important strategy to decrease the length of vein that will be required is to use the *most distal* patent, undiseased artery possible as the inflow site for the bypass. This *distal origin strategy* suggests that the superficial femoral and all parts of the deep femoral artery, including its distal two portions, may be used to provide inflow for the bypass if there is no proximal stenosis greater than 20% to 40% of the luminal diameter. For many years we have advocated use of these distal origin grafts and have shown that they work well. In fact there is recent evidence that such *short vein grafts* have better patency rates than comparable long vein grafts. Moreover, use of portions of the superficial and deep femoral arteries distal to their origins as secondary bypass inflow sites allows the surgeon to avoid dissection in scarred or previously infected groins. This *virginal approach strategy* shortens and simplifies the operation, minimizes the chances of infection that is particularly prone to develop in reoperated incisions and, as already noted, increases the ability to perform the secondary bypass with autogenous vein. To facilitate this virginal approach strategy, we have developed a variety of unusual approaches to infrainguinal arteries; these are described in several of the references included in the suggested reading list at the conclusion of this chapter. These also frequently facilitate use of shorter vein grafts and include a direct approach to the distal two thirds of the deep femoral artery and lateral approaches to the popliteal artery both above and below the knee.

PREOPERATIVE EVALUATION AND PREPARATION

In addition to the arteriography and venography already discussed, the patient should have baseline noninvasive assessment with Doppler determined segmental pressures and Doppler or plethysmographic pulse volume recordings. These will not influence the decision to operate but will provide a baseline to assess the postoperative result and monitor graft patency in a semiquantitative manner. Cardiologic evaluation should include a thorough examination to exclude congestive failure, some form of stress testing such as an exercise MUGA or radionuclide (Thallium) myocardial perfusion scan, preferably with intravenous Persantine stress. Some patients with marked abnormalities may benefit from coronary angiography and, if critical lesions are detected, even from coronary artery bypass prior to treating the foot ischemia. Determination of which patients should have this approach necessitates close collaboration between the vascular surgeon and the cardiologist and depends on the severity and urgency of the patient's cardiac status, as well as the rapidity of progression of the gangrene and any infection in the foot.

Before operation the patient should have a balloon catheter placed percutaneously in her pulmonary artery. Cardiac hemodynamics should be measured and optimized by appropriate fluid administration or diuretics. Intraoperatively, this monitoring of cardiac hemodynamics should be continued and serve as a guide to fluid management, blood replacement and use of inotropic agents.

USE OF PROSTHETIC GRAFT

If after all the alternative strategies to help find ipsilateral lower extremity autologous vein are considered and still a healthy vein segment of adequate length and diameter cannot be obtained, a prosthetic bypass conduit will have to be employed. Although some vascular surgeons have reported acceptable patency rates with externally supported Dacron fabric grafts used for below-knee femoropopliteal bypasses, experience with this graft is limited and no large prospective study comparing its performance to autogenous vein or PTFE grafts has been reported. Similarly, although human umbilical vein grafts have been used successfully in this setting, the high mid-term and late incidence of aneurysm formation probably precludes widespread use of this graft. This leaves the PTFE graft as the best suited, optimal alternative bypass conduit for use in patients who require below-knee femoropopliteal bypass and who do not have adequate autogenous vein. Acceptable late results in terms of both limb salvage and graft patency have been reported in such patients, even when this graft is used as a secondary bypass.

OPERATIVE DETAILS

Before operation the patient should be started on antiplatelet agents (0.3 gm aspirin, BID; dipyridamole 125 mg TID). Anesthesia, whether general or epidural, should be administered by an anesthesiologist experienced in the care of patients with extensive cardiac disease. On the operating table, care should be taken to prevent heel necrosis by placing padded support beneath both Achilles tendons.

Incisions should be planned to avoid previous operative scars and the virginal approach strategy used whenever possible, although with care and diligence it is possible to redissect arteries safely. The use of sharp (scalpel) dissection is particularly helpful in avoiding damage to scarred arteries. With blunt (scissors) dissection the easiest plane to enter is sometimes in the wall of the artery rather than around it. Other operative details are similar to those used for primary bypass operations on infrainguinal arteries. Heparin (7500 IU) should be given before arterial occlusion. Particular care must be employed to occlude these often diseased arteries as gently as possible. Gentle traction with silastic vessel loops, microclips or small atraumatic clamps gently applied are preferable to large vascular clamps firmly applied with crushing of the vessel wall. We believe the artery should be opened with a sharp scalpel, not scissors. In this way all layers of the arterial wall are cut cleanly. Endarterectomy should generally be avoided adjacent to the anastomotic sites since end points are difficult to arrive at or tack down securely. The anastomosis should be constructed with extreme care, employing fine suture bites and catching evenly spaced bites of all layers of the arterial wall. These points are particularly crucial for the distal anastomosis and when the popliteal artery is severely diseased as it often is. Good light and exposure are important to provide adequate visualization of every stitch both from within and outside the artery and the graft.

Intraoperative (completion) arteriography is only performed if the preoperative arteriogram is not adequate or some problem is suspected at the anastomosis or beyond. Certainly if clot must be removed from the popliteal artery lumen, we would perform a completion arteriogram. We do not use such arteriograms routinely in femoropopliteal reconstructions since they rarely visualize the entire reconstruction procedure and since false positive and false negative results can be obtained. After completion of the anastomoses, heparin is reversed with protamine and careful hemostasis is obtained. The wounds are closed meticulously. Hematoma and infection go together and both are more common in redissected wounds. If the toe gangrene is extensive or associated with infection, we would excise the toe along with any necrotic or infected tissue. The toe wound would then be left open.

Postoperatively, the patient should be maintained in an intensive care environment with suitable cardiac monitoring until perioperative myocardial infarction has been ruled out. Objective evidence of graft patency should also be monitored. If graft occlusion occurs, the patient should be subjected to urgent reoperation and the problem corrected according to guidelines which are beyond the scope of the present chapter. (See chapter 46.)

CONCLUSION

With meticulous attention to operative and perioperative details and with use of some of the principles outlined, there is a high likelihood of successful limb salvage in this patient even though she is already a treatment failure and even though she has widespread arteriosclerosis.

BIBLIOGRAPHY

1. Ascer E, Collier P, Gupta SK, et al: Reoperation for PTFE bypass failure: The importance of distal outflow site and operative technique in determining outcome. *J Vasc Surg* 1987; 5:298–310.
2. Nunez A, Veith FJ, White-Flores S, et al: Direct approach to the second and third portions of the deep femoral artery for secondary bypass origin or insertion. Manuscript in preparation.
3. Veith FJ, Ascer E, Gupta SK, et al: Tibiotibial vein bypass grafts: A new operation for limb salvage. *J Vasc Surg* 1985; 2:552–557.
4. Veith FJ, Ascer E, Gupta SK, et al: Lateral approach to the popliteal artery. *J Vasc Surg* 1987; 6:119–123.
5. Veith FJ, Ascer E, Nunez A, et al: Unusual approaches to infrainguinal arteries. *J Cardiovasc Surg* 1987; 28:58.
6. Veith FJ, Gupta SK: Femoral-distal artery bypasses, in Bergan JJ, Yao JST (eds): *Operative Techniques in Vascular Surgery*. New York, Grune & Stratton, 1980, pp 141–150.
7. Veith FJ, Gupta SK, Ascer E, et al: Six-year prospective multicenter randomized comparison of autologous saphenous vein and expanded polytetrafluoroethylene grafts in infrainguinal arterial reconstructions. *J Vasc Surg* 1986; 3:104–114.
8. Veith FJ, Gupta SK, Daly V: Management of early and late thrombosis of expanded polytetrafluoroethylene (PTFE) femoropopliteal bypass grafts: Favorable prognosis with appropriate reoperation. *Surgery* 1980; 87:581–587.

9. Veith FJ, Gupta SK, Samson RH, et al: Progress in limb salvage by reconstructive arterial surgery combined with new or improved adjunctive procedures. *Ann Surg* 1981; 194:386–401.
10. Veith FJ, Gupta SK, Samson RH, et al: Superficial femoral and popliteal arteries as inflow sites for distal bypasses. *Surgery* 1981; 90:980–990.
11. Veith FJ, Weiser RK, Gupta SK, et al: Diagnosis and management of ailing lower extremity arterial reconstructions. *J Cardiovasc Surg* 1984; 25:381–384.

39 Combined Superficial Femoral Artery Disease and Profunda Disease: Profundaplasty versus Distal Bypass

A 72-year-old man is admitted with ischemic rest pain in the right foot. He has a good right femoral pulse but absent distal pulses on the affected side. There is a prominent right femoral bruit. Angiography demonstrates good inflow, a tight proximal profunda femoris stenosis, and a lengthy superficial femoral artery occlusion with reconstitution of the distal popliteal artery and two-vessel runoff to the foot.

Consultant: Jonathan B. Towne, M.D.

PROFUNDA ANATOMY

The profunda femoris is a major artery in an extensive chain of longitudinal anastomosing vessels of the lower extremity and a key component of a collateral network that extends from the internal iliac to the tibial vessels. It usually arises 2 cm to 4 cm below the inguinal ligament, passing posterolaterally to the superficial femoral artery. The medial and lateral circumflex arteries diverge from the proximal profunda to form the major collaterals to the internal iliac. However, frequent variations in the origin of the proximal profunda and circumflex arteries occur. These should be noted on preoperative arteriograms and looked for during surgical dissection.

The main profunda trunk gives off three to four perforating arteries that pass posterolaterally into the adductor musculature to join with the descending branch of the lateral circumflex femoral artery, forming an extensive intramuscular vascular arcade. The profunda terminates in the adductor magnus muscle with distal muscular branches communicating with the popliteal and tibial arteries to complete the collateral network.

PATTERNS OF ARTERIAL DISEASE

Patients with symptomatic ischemia of the lower extremity most commonly have atherosclerotic involvement of the aortoiliac and/or femoropopliteal segments. Although the patterns of arterial involvement are quite variable, severe stenosis of both the superficial femoral artery and the profunda is uncommon. In the majority of patients with superficial femoral artery occlusive disease, the profunda system is relatively spared. However, Beales reported evidence of some profunda disease in 59% of ischemic extremities studied by biplanar angiography. Martin, in a similar study, found the atherosclerotic disease to be localized in the proximal profunda segment in 74% of affected limbs and to the profunda orifice alone in 55%. Fortunately, when atherosclerosis involves this artery, it is generally localized to the proximal portion of the vessel.

Nonvisualization of the profunda by angiography occurs in 4% to 6% of cases and is usually associated with aortoiliac obstruction and common femoral artery occlusion. However, complete profunda obliteration is rare. The distal trunk is almost always patent and profundaplasty is routinely employed successfully to provide arterial outflow to the leg.

SURGICAL OPTIONS

In patients with critical limb ischemia and combined disease of both the superficial femoral artery and profunda artery, there are two options for management—femoral-distal bypass, preferably using autogenous tissue, and profundaplasty. In special circumstances, a combination of both profundaplasty with distal bypass is used. Each procedure has its relative advantages and disadvantages. Femoral-distal bypass requires autogenous material, if the best short- and long-term results are to be obtained. In patients who have had prior reconstructive procedures, or who have had coronary artery bypass, a saphenous vein may not be available for use. The distal bypass procedures are usually lengthy, requiring either continuous or multiple incisions down the leg. With autogenous tissue the results are excellent, with early patency rates and limb salvage generally being greater than 90% in well-selected patients. These excellent results hold up well over the first three to five years. Profundaplasty, on the other hand, is usually done through a single groin incision, usually not greater than six to eight inches in length. The amount of autogenous tissue necessary for a vein patch is much less, rarely exceeding 10 cm to 12 cm. The results with profundaplasty are not as good as they are with distal bypasses. Taking into account all patients with limb salvage ischemia, there is approximately a 50% success rate. When one breaks down critical limb ischemia into ischemic ulcers, rest pain, and gangrene, the results likewise vary, with the best result of isolated profundaplasty being in patients who have ischemic ulcers followed by rest pain, and the worst results in patients with gangrene. These success rates range from 53% for ischemic ulcer, decreasing to 30% for rest pain and ischemic necrosis.

PATIENT SELECTION

The most important aspect in selecting patients for profundaplasty alone as treatment for critical limb ischemia are those factors related to the extent and distribution of the occlusive disease. First, one must determine that there is no significant inflow occlusive disease. Clinically, qualitative data is provided by grading of femoral pulses, palpation for thrills, and auscultation for bruits. More important is careful inspection of the angiograms. If in doubt about the physiologic significance of any inflow lesions, pressure measurements may be performed either at the time of angiography or intraoperatively to determine if there is any significant inflow disease. The resting femoral artery pressure should be equal to or greater than the brachial pressure, and following injection of papaverine, the pressure should not drop more than 10 mm Hg.

Hemodynamic stenosis of the profunda that narrows that arterial lumen to less than 50% of its normal diameter must be present. It is most accurately assessed angiographically by oblique projections. Atherosclerotic plaque is frequently present on the posterior arterial wall and may not be visualized in anteroposterior projection alone. Suspected profunda stenosis may be diagnosed intraoperatively by directly measuring the resting and papaverine-augmented common femoral and profunda femoral pressures, or by sizing the profunda orifice with an arterial dilator.

The clinical presentation in limb salvage patients should also be considered, since it affects the ultimate success of profunda revascularization. In general, profundaplasty frequently heals chronic ischemic ulcers, but is less successful in abolishing rest pain, and does not reliably heal areas of ischemic gangrene.

The most important determinants of the success of isolated profundaplasty are the adequacy of the profunda-popliteal collateral network around the knee and the severity of tibial arterial occlusive disease. Angiographic criteria that reliably predict the successful outcome include: minimal occlusive disease of the distal profunda, well-developed profunda-thigh collaterals, patent popliteal artery, and minimal tibial occlusive disease. Segmental Doppler pressure measurements can reliably locate and determine the extent of occlusive disease in each limb segment by providing an estimate of the resistance in each collateral bed. Resistance across the knee joint is the most important determinant of profundaplasty success. It can be evaluated by the measurement of the profunda-popliteal collateral index, the PPCI, which is calculated from the formula:

$$\frac{(\text{Above-knee pressure}) - (\text{Below-knee pressure})}{(\text{Above-knee pressure})}$$

An index greater than 0.45 implies high resistance across the knee joint as a result of poor development of collateral vessels, and is associated with profundaplasty failure in almost all cases. A PPCI less than 0.19 usually results in limb salvage, as this indicates there is excellent collateral development between the distal profunda and the patent popliteal artery. Evaluation of our patients undergoing isolated profundaplasty for limb salvage in patients whose PPCI was 0.19 or less shows limb salvage was obtained in 10 of 11 patients, as opposed to no patients with a PPCI of greater than 0.45 obtaining limb salvage.

Another noninvasive test which helps us select patients for profundaplasty is the use of the ankle-brachial index (ABI). Patients in the critical limb ischemia category generally do well with profundaplasty when they have lesser degrees of ischemia as indicated by ABIs which are at higher levels (0.30 or 0.40). The mean preoperative ABI on our patients who underwent isolated profundaplasty for limb salvage that was successful was 0.42, compared to 0.27 in patients in whom profundaplasty was unsuccessful. With the severe forms of vascular occlusive disease, profundaplasty is just not sufficient for salvaging extremities. There is a direct correlation with the extent of tibial occlusive disease and preoperative AB index. Patients who have combined superficial femoral and profunda occlusive disease, and who have severe coexisting tibial occlusive disease, are more likely to have very low ankle-brachial indices. I think it is important to identify these patients, because profundaplasty is not likely to help them.

A group of patients that generally does well with profundaplasty are those who have common femoral artery occlusion, and whose occlusive process extends into the orifices of the profunda artery. Generally, the occlusive process in the profunda femoris artery rarely extends to the first perforator in these patients. Common femoral endarterectomy with profundaplasty will significantly augment blood flow to the lower extremity. Other factors related to the selection of profundaplasty for patients with combined profunda-superficial femoral disease are those related to the conduit. Some patients have absence of suitable autogenous tissue, either because of previous stripping or ligation of saphenous veins for venous insufficiency, use of veins for coronary artery bypass, or previous attempts to perform lower extremity bypass surgery. Another group of patients in whom profundaplasty is an excellent alternative are those who have groin sepsis. This is most commonly seen in patients who have infected femoral-distal artificial conduit in place. The infectious process mandates removal of all foreign material. Profundaplasty with patch closure with autogenous tissue, with the addition of muscle coverage with either sartorius or gracilis muscle, is an excellent way to extract oneself from a very difficult and potentially limb- and life-theatening clinical situation.

OPERATIVE TECHNIQUE

In patients with adequate aortoiliac inflow, restoration of the profunda collateral system is the primary goal. A vertical groin incision is made over the common femoral artery at the level of the inguinal ligament and extended 10 cm distally. Following control of the common femoral artery, the superficial femoral artery is freed enough to facilitate exposure of the profunda, which usually courses laterally and posteriorly. The large circumflex femoral vein crosses the profunda within 1 cm to 2 cm of its origin and is ligated in continuity and divided. The anterior surface of the profunda is exposed distally until normal artery is encountered. This is ascertained by palpation of the vessel and reference to the arteriogram. The atherosclerotic plaque almost always ends at a profunda branch. Following systemic heparinization, the common femoral artery and its branches are clamped. The profunda branches are controlled with Heifitz clips, double looped 0-silk ties, or silastic loops. A vertical incision is made anteriorly in the common femoral artery and carried down onto the profunda to approximately 1 cm distal to the disease. In cases in which early arborization of the profunda occurs, the arteriotomy is extended distally into the largest branch. Care is taken to avoid the crotch of the common femoral branches and the major branches. Endarterectomy of the atheromatous plaque is performed if the luminal surface is irregular or ulcerated or if it occludes profunda branches. If the profunda is only thickened and the branches are patent, an endarterectomy is not necessary. During endarterectomy, most occluded profunda branches are easily opened by careful plaque removal since the occlusive disease rarely involves more than the branch orifices. If a clean intimal break point is not obtained, the distal intima must be tacked down with 6-0 sutures to prevent dissection of the artery. Rarely is a profunda orifice atheroma encountered and it is easily removed by simple endarterectomy and tack-down of the distal intima. The length of profundaplasty and type of disease present determine how the profunda arteriotomy is closed. An orifice atheroma may sometimes be removed and the short profunda arteriotomy closed longitudinally. When a short segment of both profunda and superficial femoral artery is diseased, endarterectomies are performed, and the common femoral bifurcation is moved distally by sewing the profunda and the superficial femoral arteries together. The majority of cases require patch angioplasty. It is important that a narrow patch is used so that the final repair approximates the size of the normal artery in order to provide the best flow characteristics.

Autogenous tissue is the preferred patch material because of its greater long-term patency and resistance to infection. The authors preferentially use an endarterectomized segment of the occluded superficial femoral artery to patch the arteriotomy. It is easily prepared, performs as well as saphenous vein, and preserves the vein for later use in distal arterial bypass or coronary revascularization.

RESULTS

The results following profundaplasty alone for critical limb ischemia are reasonable. We obtained 30-day limb salvage in 75% of our patients. Both the patency and limb salvage had decreased to 50% by 36 months postoperatively. The efficacy and durability of profundaplasty are primarily determined by the pattern of atherosclerotic disease and the operative indications. In patients with critical limb ischemia with normal arterial inflow into the groin, there is often significant involvement of the entire collateral system as well as coexistent tibial occlusive disease. Cumulative limb salvage in this group is only 36% at five years. When profundaplasty was performed for nonhealing ulceration, rest pain, or ischemic gangrene, the results indicated a five-year cumulative patency of 30%. Survival for limb salvage patients was 35% at five years, with the majority of deaths directly attributable to atherosclerotic disease. Of interest is that at 24 months postoperatively, the limb salvage patient began a significant acceleration in both mortality and graft occlusion rates. This demonstrates a more rapid progression of the atherosclerotic disease process in this group.

MANAGEMENT OF THIS CASE

Based on the above criteria, I would recommend profundaplasty alone for the patient described in this case if the profunda origin stenosis appeared severe in good quality arteriograms with multiple projections, especially if profunda collaterals appeared well developed on the arteriograms and the profunda-popliteal collateral index suggested good collateralization across the knee. The two-vessel runoff described is also encouraging. Isolated profundaplasty would be particularly appropriate if the patient did not have a good saphenous vein or was otherwise not a good candidate for distal bypass. If those factors are not present, I would likely proceed with femoropopliteal bypass, probably correcting the orificial profunda stenosis at the same time, if anatomically feasible.

BIBLIOGRAPHY

1. Beales JSM, Adcock FA, Frawley JS, et al: The radiological assessment of disease of the profunda femoris artery. *Br J Radiol* 1971; 44:854–859.
2. Boren CH, Towne JB, Bernhard VM, et al: Profundapopliteal collateral index: A guide to successful profundaplasty. *Arch Surg* 1980; 115:1366–1372.
3. Cotton LT, Roberts VC: Extended deep femoral angioplasty: An alternative to femoro-popliteal bypass. *Br J Surg* 1975; 62:340–343.
4. David TE, Drezner AD: Extended profundaplasty for limb salvage. *Surgery* 1978; 84:758–763.
5. Malone JM, Goldstone J, Moore WS: Autogenous profundaplasty: The long-term patency in secondary repair of aortofemoral graft occlusion. *Ann Surg* 1978; 188:817–823.
6. Martin P, Frawley JE, Barabas AP, et al: On the surgery of atherosclerosis of the profunda femoris artery. *Surgery* 1972; 71:182–189.
7. Mitchell RA, Bone GE, Bridges R, et al: Patient selection for isolated profundaplasty. Arteriographic correlates of operative results. *Am J Surg* 1979; 138:912–919.
8. Peace WH, Kempczinski RF: Extended autogenous profundaplasty and aortofemoral grafting: An alternative to synchronous distal bypass. *J Vasc Surg* 1984; 1:455–458.
9. Rollins DL, Towne JB, Bernhard VM, et al: Isolated profundaplasty for limb salvage. *J Vasc Surg* 1985; 2:585–589.
10. Towne JB, Bernhard VM, Rollins DL, et al: Profundaplasty in perspective: Limitations in the long-term management of limb ischemia. *Surgery* 1981; 90:1037–1046.
11. Towne JB, Rollins DL: Profundaplasty: Its role in limb salvage. *Surg Clin North Am* 1986; 66:403–414.

40 Isolated Popliteal Segment vs Direct Tibial Bypass Grafting

An elderly patient is admitted with a nonhealing painful ischemic ulcer of the left foot. There is a history of prior stroke and several myocardial infarctions, the most recent six months ago. Arteriography demonstrates satisfactory aortoiliac vessels, occlusion of the superficial femoral artery, reconstitution of an isolated popliteal artery segment which reoccluded at the level of the distal popliteal artery, and visualization of a tibial vessel in the calf.

Consultant: Herbert Dardik, M.D.

This case presents a number of challenges that require a clear analysis of the clinical and angiographic components, as well as an appreciation of hemodynamic and pathologic factors. The scenario is compounded by the risk factors that include the patient's age, prior CVA and several myocardial infarctions. A satisfactory inflow simplifies the problem by obviating the need for balloon angioplasty or a surgical procedure.

Mannick and his associates first demonstrated the efficacy of bypass to an isolated popliteal segment, that is, one having total occlusion of the superficial femoral artery, segmental reconstruction of the popliteal artery and total distal popliteal arterial occlusion with no direct tibial runoff. Other investigators have also compared the patency of vein bypasses to isolated popliteal segments in one group of patients with vein bypass to tibial arteries in another group. Although the groups were often not entirely comparable, these studies did provide support for the concept of bypass to an isolated popliteal segment.

In 1972, DeLaurentis and Freidman described the successful application of the sequential graft concept in which a prosthetic graft from the femoral artery to an isolated popliteal segment was augmented by a vein bypass from the latter to an isolated distal tibial artery. Over the ensuing years, these authors and others confirmed the validity of this concept and extended it to sequential grafting to any of the crural arteries in the absence of an isolated popliteal segment (Figs 40–1 and 40–2).

266

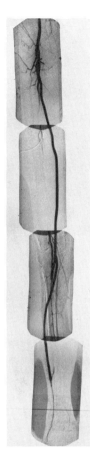

FIG 40–1.

A postoperative composite digital arteriogram depicting a femoral sequential bypass whose upper distal anastomosis terminated at the tibioperoneal trunk. Because of the high resistance at this level, a sequential jump was also employed, which originated from the distal newly placed graft, passed through the interosseous membrane, and terminated in the distal anterior tibial artery. (From Dardik H: *Arterial Reconstruction in the Lower Extremity,* McGraw Hill, New York 1986. Used by permission.)

Review of the early literature on this subject indicates the initial superiority of isolated popliteal segments for maintaining graft patency compared to grafts extending to the tibials. However, after five years comparable patency rates were noted. Similar conclusions were drawn with respect to limb salvage rates. Sixty-eight percent of patients undergoing sequential grafting achieved limb salvage compared to more than 80% of patients undergoing bypass to an isolated popliteal segment. It is important to recognize, however, that these studies were not randomized and that the superior results of isolated popliteal bypass over tibial bypass or sequential grafting are, in fact, more indicative of favored case selection. In other words, patients with lesser degrees of ischemia were generally submitted for isolated popliteal segment bypass, whereas those with advanced pregangrene or tissue loss underwent complex distal procedures, frequently in the absence of a patent popliteal segment.

The choices presented by the patient described in this case thus include bypass

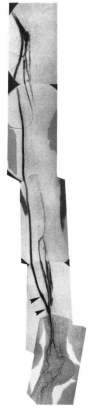

FIG 40–2.
A postoperative digital study depicting a lower limb graft originating from the distal portion of a previously placed axillofemoral bypass graft. The graft is in a subcutaneous position and distally (darkened area at arrows) has sequential components to the peroneal and anterior tibial arteries, both constructed with distal arteriovenous fistulas. Perfusion into the distal arterial runoff and the venous return circulation from the fistulas is noted. (From Dardik H: *Arterial Reconstruction in the Lower Extremity*, McGraw Hill, New York 1986. Used by permission.)

to the isolated popliteal segment alone, bypass directly from the femoral to the tibial artery, and bypass to both of these segments in the form of a sequential reconstruction. These theoretic approaches are, in fact, limited by consideration of risk factors, angiographic appearance of the runoff vessels, and the graft material(s) available. In general, most surgeons prefer to minimize the time expended and the complexity of the procedure in those patients presenting with one or more significant risk factors. Nevertheless, it must be appreciated that the morbidity of lower limb revascularization procedures is generally associated with how the procedure is performed rather than its duration. It is obvious that a smooth procedure performed with minimal blood loss and tissue trauma will fare much better than a less well-executed operation, no matter how short the operative time. These considerations, along with the use of epidural anesthesia, have contributed enormously to improved patency rates and minimized morbidity.

The extent or degree of ischemia is the most critical clinical factor in any consideration for limiting the distal graft implantation to an isolated popliteal segment or for establishing a more remote anastomosis. The absence of trophic lesions in the presence of an isolated popliteal segment suggests adequacy of collateral runoff from the popliteal segment to the distal circulation. Conversely, the presence of ischemic lesions suggests poorly developed collaterals from the popliteal segment. In this situation a distal anastomosis is desirable to allow direct flow to the foot without passage through high-resistance collateral vessels. The availability of autologous vein also enters the formula. In its absence, and in a patient at good risk with an end-stage limb, consideration should be given to using both runoff sites in a sequential reconstruction.

Angiographic criteria for the selection of an isolated popliteal segment versus a tibial artery becomes frustrating only when both are of comparable morphologic quality. Superiority of one or the other obviously favors that particular site for bypass. If both vessels are of reasonably good quality, we would be guided by the clinical presentation of the patient. In this circumstance, reconstruction to an isolated popliteal artery will usually suffice, in that the presence of end-stage ischemic lesions is unlikely in association with good quality vessels at both popliteal and crural levels. If the quality of artery at both of these levels is poor, serious consideration should be given to primary amputation if the ischemic state is far advanced and autologous vein is unavailable. In some of these cases we perform distal prosthetic reconstruction with adjunctive arteriovenous fistulae. The rationale for this procedure is based on the need to reduce the overload to the distal circulatory bed with high resistance and limited capacitance. Despite the considerable negativism for this concept and procedure by most vascular surgeons, we still find its use valuable in maintaining patency of prosthetic bypass grafts to crural vessels. Additionally, the perioperative thrombectomy rate is reduced from 22% to less than 8%.

Intraoperative exploration and assessment of resistance may be necessary in an occasional patient. Again, the site of initial exploration will be dictated by clinical and angiographic considerations. Although sophisticated technology is available to quantitate runoff, the simple technique of injecting saline into the circulatory bed and assessing one's tactile response to it will suffice. A highly resistant circuit will require consideration of a sequential reconstruction, use of a distal arteriovenous fistula or even abandoning the proposed reconstruction in favor of amputation.

The challenge of an ideal graft material for lower limb reconstructions, as exemplified by the above case, has taxed the imagination of many surgeons for decades. Virtually all vascular surgeons attest to the superiority of autologous saphenous vein. Current differences of opinion do exist with regard to the claimed superiority of the *in situ* method compared to the reversed technique, but it is clear that the former method has expanded utilization of the saphenous vein, which, in other circumstances, would be considered too small to use at the reversed proximal end. In the presence of an adequate saphenous vein we would favor reconstruction to a tibial artery over the use of a blind popliteal segment and would additionally favor the *in situ* method. The Albany group has documented a very low incidence for need of the isolated popliteal segment and has reserved this site for cases in which the saphenous vein is absent or of inadequate length.

The availability of prosthetic material does provide for various alternative approaches to correcting ischemic states in the presence of isolated popliteal segments and reconstituted crural runoff. Polytetrafluoroethylene (PTFE) has enjoyed wide usage but has been disappointing with regard to the need for repetitive thrombectomy and low patency rates, particularly in the infrageniculate position. Glutaraldehyde-stabilized umbilical vein grafts have enjoyed better patency rates, but have the disadvantage of a high rate of biodegradation after implant periods exceeding five years. Thus the choice of prosthetic involves consideration of life expectancy and potential for reoperation. Our experience with umbilical veins to isolated popliteal segments has been favorable. Patency rates, though not statistically different from those performed to popliteal segments with direct tibial runoff, tend toward the lower level of popliteal reconstructions and approach the results obtained with umbilical vein reconstruction to good quality tibials. I now advocate the use of an adjunctive distal arteriovenous fistula with all prosthetic reconstructions to distal crural arteries.

The case in point is characterized by the need for limb salvage in the face of multiple risk factors. The optimal procedure would be an *in situ* saphenous vein reconstruction to the tibial artery. We would proceed in this direction given the presence of a satisfactory vein and would perform this operation under epidural anesthesia. In the absence of a suitable ipsilateral saphenous vein, one could consider a two-team approach and employ contralateral or upper extremity veins by reversed or nonreversed methods. We would be reluctant to apply this method in the case presented because of the multiple risk factors and limited life expectancy. We would prefer the secondary choice of an umbilical vein graft to the popliteal artery and limit the procedure at this level if one could demonstrate a low resistance runoff. High resistance runoff would dictate a sequential component using autologous vein, if possible, or umbilical vein to the tibial with a fistula at this level. In the presence of an adequate tibial and a good venae concomitant system, the popliteal component could be abandoned and the procedure simplified by bringing the reconstruction directly to the tibial artery using an adjunctive fistula. Although PTFE can be used satisfactorily for obligatory above-knee isolated popliteal segments, our choice for infrageniculate bypass is the umbilical vein graft, particularly, as in this patient, where reoperations need to be avoided and where life expectancy is limited so that concern for graft biodegradation can be minimized.

In conclusion, the approach to the patient with an isolated popliteal segment and a patent tibial vessel requires consideration of the clinical presentation and extent of ischemia, risk factors, angiographic patterns, intraoperative assessment of arterial quality and resistance, and finally, the available graft material. A simplistic approach to this problem based on a single factor is not possible. The experienced vascular surgeon will consider the multiple facets of these challenging cases and employ that procedure from his repertoire that will maintain patency and which can be performed expeditiously. Complex procedures including sequential components and distal arteriovenous fistulae are required infrequently and only where a direct simpler approach would predictably fail. Finally, all vascular surgeons should consider primary amputation in favor of multiple attempts at limb salvage procedures in which the likelihood of failure is predictable; such failures might result in a higher amputation level and increased patient morbidity and mortality.

BIBLIOGRAPHY

1. Brewster DC, Charlesworth PM, Monahan JE, et al: Isolated popliteal segment vs. tibial bypass for limb salvage: Comparison of hemodynamic and clinical results. *Arch Surg* 1984; 119:775–779.
2. Dardik H, Sussman B, Ibrahim IM, et al: Distal arteriovenous fistula as an adjunct to maintaining arterial and graft patency for limb salvage. *Surgery* 1983; 94:478–486.
3. Dardik H: The use of an adjunctive arteriovenous fistula in distal extremity bypass grafts with outflow obstruction, in Kempczinski RF (ed): *The Ischemic Leg.* Chicago, Year Book Medical Publishers, 1985, pp 463–484.
4. Davis RC, Davies WT, Mannick JA: Bypass vein grafts in patients with distal popliteal artery occlusion. *Am J Surg* 1975; 129:421–425.
5. DeLaurentis DA, Friedmann P: Sequential femoropopliteal bypasses: Another approach to the inadequate saphenous vein problem. *Surgery* 1972; 71:400–404.
6. Edwards WS, Gerety E, Larkin J, et al: Multiple sequential femoral tibial grafting for severe ischemia. *Surgery* 1976; 80:722–728.
7. Friedmann P, DeLaurentis DA, Rhee SW: The sequential femoropopliteal bypass graft. *Am J Surg* 1976; 131:452–456.
8. Kaminski DL, Barner HB, Dorighi JA, et al: Femoropopliteal bypass with reversed autogenous vein. *Ann Surg* 1973; 177:232–236.
9. Mannick JA, Jackson BT, Coffman JD, et al: Success of bypass vein grafts in patients with isolated popliteal artery segments. *Surgery* 1967; 61:17–25.
10. Purdy RT, Bole P, Makanju W, Munda R: Salvage of the ischemic lower extremity in patients with poor runoff. *Arch Surg* 1974; 109:784–786.

41 Acute Postoperative Thrombosis of Femoropopliteal Bypass Grafts

You perform a femoropopliteal bypass graft for severe intermittent claudication in a 61-year-old truck driver. The procedure goes well, and a completion arteriogram appears satisfactory. Six hours postoperatively, the foot appears ischemic and pulses cannot be felt.

Consultant: John W. Hallett, Jr., M.D.

DISCUSSION

This case scenario represents the most common early complication of a femoropopliteal bypass: acute graft occlusion. The cause of early thrombosis may not be apparent at first, as it may not have been in this case where pedal pulses were initially present after operation (Fig 41–1). Consequently, you must have a strategy for preventing and treating acute femoropopliteal graft thrombosis.

In this discussion, prevention and intraoperative detection and correction of technical errors will be emphasized. Technical mishaps remain the primary cause of early thrombosis. In a recent prospective study, we identified correctable technical problems in the operating room in 8% of femoropopliteal or tibial bypasses. Intraoperative correction of these problems assured postoperative patency in every case. In an additional 3.5% of patients, acute postoperative thrombosis was detected after the patient left the operating room. The cause was poor runoff combined with clot accumulation at the distal anastomotic site. Thrombectomy and anticoagulation salvaged most of these grafts.

PREVENTION

Prevention encompasses assurance of three key ingredients to a successful femoropopliteal bypass: Adequate aortoiliac inflow to assure long-term patency, sufficient

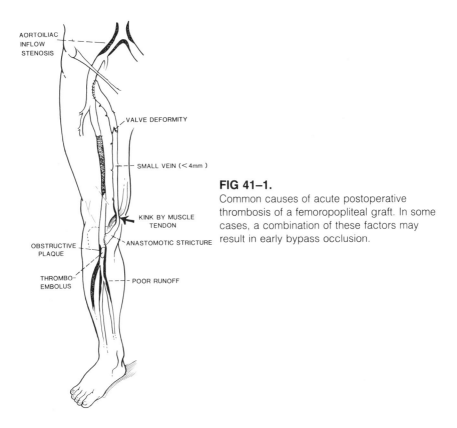

FIG 41–1.
Common causes of acute postoperative thrombosis of a femoropopliteal graft. In some cases, a combination of these factors may result in early bypass occlusion.

distal runoff, and proper selection and placement of a graft. Less common causes of postoperative graft occlusion include low-flow states due to impaired cardiac output from acute myocardial infarction, thromboembolism due to atrial fibrillation, or hypercoagulability.

Adequate Aortoiliac Inflow

Early and late femoropopliteal graft patency depends on adequate aortoiliac inflow pressure and flow rates. The simplest sign of good inflow remains a strong femoral pulse without bruits. Of course, the lack of significant aortoiliac stenosis on aortography is an essential prerequisite before distal bypass. Biplane views may be necessary to reveal important posterior plaques not seen on anterior-posterior projections. If femoral pulses are marginal, we measure a femoral artery pressure (FAP). Significant aortoiliac disease is suspected if the FAP is 10 mm less than central arterial pressure or drops more than 15% after reactive hyperemia.

Sufficient Distal Runoff

Poor distal runoff is commonly associated with acute femoropopliteal graft occlusion.

Patients with claudication, like our case example, generally have a superficial femoral artery occlusion with a patent popliteal artery and good runoff. Although an above-knee segment of popliteal artery may be available for anastomosis, you must be certain that this segment is not diseased and that the mid and distal popliteal artery does not have any significant stenosis.

Patients with more severe ischemia (e.g. rest pain, foot ulcer, or gangrene) usually have some tibial occlusive disease. If the distal anastomosis is made to the popliteal artery, you must be certain that the openings into the tibial arteries are not compromised by atherosclerotic plaque. Gently insinuating an appropriately sized coronary dilator (2.5 mm to 3.0 mm) down the tibial branches is one method of checking for adequate runoff. If runoff from the popliteal artery is diseased, a distal sequential bypass from the hood of the popliteal anastomosis to another tibial artery should be considered.

Graft Selection and Placement

Since the primary purpose of this chapter is to discuss management of early postoperative graft occlusion, we will focus on problems involving the graft and its placement that are preventable or correctable.

Autogenous vein, because of its durability, remains the best choice for femoropopliteal bypass. However, the size and quality of the vein must be adequate to prevent early thrombosis. For reversed saphenous vein grafts, we prefer at least a 4 mm vein, with no thickening due to previous phlebitis. Nonreversed or *in situ* vein grafts may perhaps succeed with smaller luminal size (2.5 mm to 3.5 mm), but we caution that some early *in situ* vein failures are probably due to too small a vein with slow flow rates (<50 cc per min). If the vein size or condition is questionable and no other suitable vein is available, a synthetic graft is preferable to a marginal vein. Adequate size for prosthetic grafts is 6 mm to 8 mm, since smaller diameters have generally had poor early and late patencies.

Positioning the graft is critical to early patency since kinking or extrinsic compression can quickly cause thrombosis. To prevent twisting of the graft during tunneling, you should mark a line on the graft with a vital dye or use the line already on some prosthetic grafts to assure proper orientation. You must avoid passage of the graft through muscle fibers that may constrict the graft once the patient is awake and moving. In particular, you must avoid impingement by the sartorius and heads of the gastrocnemius muscle. If a medial subcutaneous route is used, the medial knee tendons can kink the graft as it dips into the below-knee popliteal space. The semimembranosus, semitendenosus, and gracilis muscles can be detached to prevent such kinking. Before cutting the graft, the knee should be extended and the graft measured to the distal anastomotic site. In the case example, a problem with tunneling or kinking of the graft would have to be strongly considered since pedal pulses were initially present and then were lost.

Finally, anastomotic mistakes are a primary cause of early graft thrombosis. Anastomotic problems are usually caused by an inadequate arteriotomy, local atherosclerotic plaque, constricting suture placement, or a thrombotic or atherosclerotic embolus. The length of the arteriotomy should be at least twice the arterial diameter to assure a gentle, less turbulent anastomotic angle. Local atherosclerotic plaque must be avoided, removed by local endarterectomy, or tacked down to prevent elevation. Sutures must be placed to assure an adequate inflow lumen as well as outflow lumen. Sometimes interrupted sutures are necessary at the distal "toe" of the anastomosis to prevent constriction. We also find it helpful to pass an appropriately sized coronary dilator (2.5 mm to 4.0 mm) through the anastomotic site before final suture closure. Since a satisfactory anastomosis can be acutely obstructed by a thrombo- or atheroembolus, the graft and proximal arteries must be carefully flushed and irrigated as clamps are opened. Such emboli can be a cause of early postoperative thrombosis of apparently successful femoropopliteal grafts. Such a thromboembolus is another possible cause of acute thrombosis in our 61-year-old truck driver.

Anticoagulation

During femoropopliteal reconstructions, we heparinize patients with an intravenous bolus of 2,500 to 5,000 units. If operation exceeds three hours, an additional 1,000 units is administered for each subsequent hour of operation. After operation, low molecular weight dextran is started in the recovery room with a 100 cc bolus followed by 20 cc per hour for a total of 500 cc in the first 24 hours. Dextran-40 appears to significantly reduce early postoperative thrombosis following difficult lower extremity bypasses, according to data from Rutherford's study. Whether continued use of antiplatelet drugs or anticoagulants improves long-term patency remains controversial. We generally administer enteric-coated aspirin 325 mg bid for vein grafts and add dipyridamole 50 mg bid for synthetic grafts.

RECOGNITION OF PROBLEMS

Despite an apparently good technical insertion of a femoropopliteal graft, 5% to 10% of bypasses will thrombose in the operating room or recovery area. Early recognition of a problem obviously enhances the chance of successful correction. Delay leads to progressive ischemia and often makes complete thrombectomy more difficult as thrombus propagates and organizes.

Intraoperative Monitoring

After completion of a femoropopliteal bypass, you should use some method to ascertain that it is patent, that the foot is adequately perfused, and that there are no technical problems that might cause thrombosis after the patient leaves the operating room. We use a combination of methods to check both the anatomic and functional results (Fig 41–2).

Graft patency can be ascertained by a palpable pedal pulse, an arteriogram, a biphasic Doppler signal over the graft and the pedal arteries, an improved distal

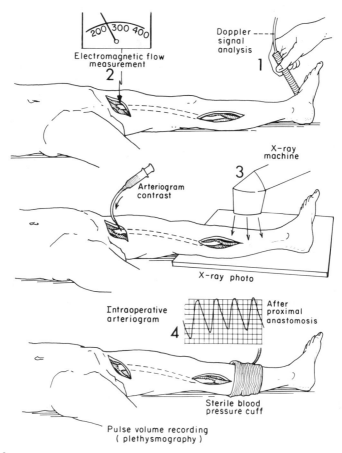

FIG 41–2.
Methods of intraoperative assessment of femorodistal bypass. Doppler signal analysis *(1)* with a sterile probe is the simplest method after pulse check to assure distal flow. Electromagnetic flow measurement *(2)* is useful for vein grafts but cannot be done over PTFE synthetic conduits since PTFE is an electrical insulator. An operative arteriogram *(3)* is the "gold standard" way to check the anatomy of the distal anastomosis and runoff. Finally, we use a sterile blood pressure cuff to check a distal pulse volume recording. (From Hallett JW Jr, Brewster DC, Darling RC: *Patient Care in Vascular Surgery*, ed. 2, Boston, Little, Brown, and Co, 1987. Used by permission.)

segmental plethysmograph (Pulse Volume Recorder^R or Vasograph^R), or electro-magnetic-measured flow rates (100 to 300 cc per min). An arteriogram remains the simplest method to inspect the graft, distal anastomosis, and runoff. When pedal pulses are not palpable, a sterile Doppler probe can be used in the operative field to auscultate pedal arterial signals. We also find that a good pulse volume tracing below the distal anastomosis provides additional assurance of adequate flow (Fig 41–3). We have primarily used electromagnetic flow measurements to inspect *in situ* vein bypasses. We measure a proximal and distal flow over the graft and look for a drop-off in distal flow that may indicate a patent arteriovenous (AV) fistula. Such an AV fistula can usually be identified on arteriography, by direct inspection of the exposed vein, or by a Doppler probe.

We consider foot perfusion adequate if a pedal pulse is present, the foot has good capillary refill, and a biphasic Doppler signal is present at the ankle. Absence of a pedal or ankle Doppler signal usually indicates inadequate revascularization. It is best to correct any technical problem with the graft at this time and not wait until the patient "warms up" in the recovery room.

Technical problems include anastomotic problems, valve deformities, graft kinks, or distal emboli. An arteriogram remains the simplest means to identify these problems. Poor Doppler signals or flow rates are usually present, too. Recently, angioscopes have allowed direct visualization of venous valves, anastomotic sites, and distal vessels, especially in construction of *in situ* vein bypasses. B-mode ultrasonography is another imaging method but is currently more cumbersome and expensive than plain arteriography.

Postoperative Monitoring

Most acute postoperative femoropopliteal graft occlusions occur within six hours. Consequently, graft patency should be checked hourly during this critical period. If the patient is still sedated or has continuous epidural catheter analgesia, he may not become symptomatic if the bypass occludes. Thus, pulses and Doppler ankle signals must be checked. Any ischemic symptoms (e.g., pain, paresthesia, or cool-

CALF PLETHYSMOGRAPH

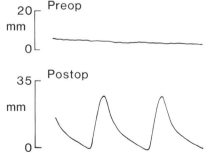

FIG 41–3.
Segmental calf plethysmograph (Pulse Volume Recording or Vasograph^R). In the operating room, a sterile blood pressure cuff can be used before and after bypass grafting to ascertain arterial perfusion at the calf or ankle level. A good arterial wave form after graft insertion is a dependable functional sign of success.

ness), loss of palpable pulses, or deterioration of ankle Doppler signals or pulse volume recordings indicate a failing or occluded graft.

TREATMENT

Once graft occlusion is suspected, the treatment plan must be designed to preserve limb function, but not at the expense of life. Since graft occlusion usually means reoperation, the patient's general condition must be stable enough for a return to the operating room. A quick check of vital signs with special attention to cardiac status is essential. If the patient is unstable or has sustained a perioperative myocardial infarction, reoperation may not be advisable. Generally, however, most patients can return immediately to the operating room. We do not delay for a preoperative arteriogram since that study can be performed in the operating room. As the operating room is being readied, we administer a bolus of heparin (5,000 units) to prevent clot propagation and administer another dose of antibiotics.

In the operating room, the abdomen and both lower limbs are prepared since an inflow procedure or harvest of a contralateral leg vein may be necessary. If an epidural catheter is still in place, it is simply reinjected to establish regional anesthesia.

The distal anastomotic site is exposed first. A longitudinal opening is made over the distal anastomosis. A Fogarty balloon catheter is passed proximally to remove thrombus from the graft and ensure good inflow. If good inflow is not reestablished, the proximal anastomosis is reexposed. Distal thromboembolectomy by means of a balloon catheter is performed, and the outflow tract is gently irrigated with heparinized saline. Intraoperative low-dosage fibrinolytic therapy (e.g. streptokinase 20,000 to 100,000 units or urokinase) can be used as an adjunct to Fogarty catheter thromboembolectomy if an intraoperative arteriogram reveals that the balloon catheter has not completely retrieved all of the thrombus lodged in the tibial arteries.

Any anastomotic problem is corrected. Correction may require removal or tacking of an atherosclerotic plaque, resuture of a strictured anastomotic site, application of an anastomotic patch, or extension of the graft by a sequential bypass to a more distal anastomotic site. If the graft cannot be satisfactorily cleared of thrombus and flow reestablished, the graft may have to be replaced by a new one.

Once flow is reestablished, an arteriogram is performed to check the graft and distal arteries. An arteriogram is especially important for *in situ* vein bypasses which have a propensity for problems at valvular sites. An angioscope may be another useful tool for inspecting such failed grafts.

The heparin is not reversed. Either low-dose continuous intravenous heparin or low molecular weight Dextran-40 is continued after operation. Generally, an oral anticoagulant such as Coumadin is used for six to eight weeks as graft healing is occurring, or indefinitely if a coagulation problem is identified.

Hypercoagulability

Coagulation abnormalities are usually suspected when multiple recurrent graft or other arterial thromboses occur. Their hematologic evaluation should include platelet count, antithrombin III level, Factor VIII activity, and platelet aggregation studies. Heparin-induced thrombosis is associated with a falling platelet count and platelet antibodies. Heparin must be stopped and dextran administered. Antithrombin III deficiency can be corrected by infusion of fresh frozen plasma. Dextran infusion can be used to correct Factor VIII abnormalities. Platelet aggregation problems can be alleviated by administration of an aspirin suppository.

RESULTS

The early results of reoperation for acute femoropopliteal bypass thrombosis are encouraging. Immediate graft thrombectomy and revision restore patency and achieve limb salvage in 70% to 85% of patients. However, late graft patency following acute perioperative thrombosis has been poor, regardless of the type of conduit. One-year patency for reoperated reversed saphenous veins was only 30% in Craver's report. Our recent experience for early reoperation of PTFE graft occlusions achieved immediate patency in 82%, but two-year patency was only 18%. Likewise, immediate failure of *in situ* vein grafts has been associated with successful restoration of flow in most patients. Nonetheless, close hemodynamic surveillance has been necessary to detect failing vein grafts and revise them before occlusion. Such prophylactic revision *before* thrombosis has significantly boosted late patencies from 50% to 60% at 36 months to 80% to 90% according to Bandyk's data. These encouraging results with *in situ* vein graft revision support a program of frequent hemodynamic testing in the perioperative period and during later follow-up, with an aggressive approach to reoperation for correction of mechanical problems.

CONCLUSION

In summary, acute postoperative thrombosis will occur in 5% to 10% of femoropopliteal bypass grafts. Some technical error is the primary cause of most occlusions. Consequently, prevention of this discouraging complication depends on precise operative technique, as well as intraoperative detection and correction of any technical mishaps. Poor distal runoff is also commonly associated with acute graft thrombosis. Perioperative use of low molecular dextran appears to enhance early patency in such difficult reconstructions. If postoperative occlusion occurs, early reoperation can usually restore graft patency and maintain limb function.

BIBLIOGRAPHY

1. Bandyk DF, Cato RF, Towne JB: A low flow velocity predicts failure of femoropopliteal and femorotibial bypass grafts. *Surgery* 1985; 98:799–808.
2. Brewster DC: Early complications of vascular repair below the inguinal ligament, in Bernhard VM, Towne JB (eds): *Complications in Vascular Surgery,* ed 5. Orlando, Grune & Stratton, Inc, 1985, pp 37–54.
3. Craver JM, Ottinger LW, Darling RC, et al: Hemorrhage and thrombosis as early complications of femoropopliteal bypass grafts: Causes, treatment, and prognostic implications. *Surgery* 1973; 74:839–845.
4. Quinones-Baldrich WJ, Zierler E, Hiatt JC: Intraoperative fibrinolytic therapy: An adjunct to catheter thromboembolectomy. *J Vasc Surg* 1985; 2:319–326.
5. Rutherford RB, Jones DN, Bergentz SE, et al: The efficacy of dextran 40 in preventing early postoperative thrombosis following difficult lower extremity bypass. *J Vasc Surg* 1984; 1:765–773.
6. Seeger JM, Abela GS: Angioscopy as an adjunct to arterial reconstructive surgery: A preliminary report. *J Vasc Surg* 1986; 4:315–320.

42 Late Failure of Femoropopliteal Bypass Grafts

A 54-year-old woman presents with a six-hour history of severe recurrent right foot ischemia. Two and one-half years previously she underwent a right femoropopliteal vein graft, with relief of ischemic rest pain. Examination reveals a normal right femoral pulse, absent distal pulses, and a cold mottled right foot.

Consultant: Anthony D. Whittemore, M.D.

An increasingly complex array of reconstructive arterial procedures provides effective palliation for disabling claudication and significant limb salvage in patients with arterial insufficiency of the lower extremity. The majority of such limbs are compromised by superficial femoral arterial occlusions necessitating infrainguinal revascularization. The reversed autogenous saphenous vein has withstood the test of time as an effective conduit for restoring blood flow to ischemic limbs since its introduction in 1948 by Kunlin. The recent popularization of the *in situ* nonreversed autogenous saphenous vein graft may yet provide superior results, particularly for patients requiring distal infrapopliteal reconstruction and for those with small caliber vein where the reversed technique would not otherwise be attempted. The five-year patency rates for these autogenous vein grafts range between 65% and 85%. Yet, as exemplified by the patient presented, a significant minority of such grafts continue to fail.

CAUSES OF GRAFT FAILURE

Management of patients with failed grafts requires some understanding of the mechanisms responsible for thrombosis. Although such mechanisms remain obscure in approximately one third of these patients, the most likely cause for graft failure can be determined in the majority and secondary reconstruction carried out. Early failures occurring during the first 30 days postoperatively, and usually within 72 hours, have frequently been associated with technical defects consisting of narrowed anastomoses, intimal flaps, residual thrombus, vein of inadequate caliber or quality, and a variety of mechanical difficulties such as twists or kinks. These have been considered in more detail in Chapter 41. As such defects have been recognized with the routine use of completion arteriography and therefore immediately corrected, a group of patients with hypercoagulopathies, hyperviscosity syndromes, and embolic difficulties become of increasing importance. An additional small group of early failures result from distal arterial spasm, usually encountered in younger patients, and from inadequate distal runoff associated with advanced disease.

Late graft failure as has occurred with this patient, however, usually results from either of two pathologic entities: progression of atherosclerosis or fibrous intimal hyperplasia. In our experience, and as illustrated in Fig 42–1, stenotic lesions resulting from fibrous intimal hyperplasia tend to occur within the two-year interval

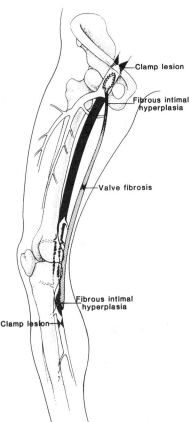

Vein Graft Stenosis

Clamp lesion

Fibrous intimal hyperplasia

Valve fibrosis

Fibrous intimal hyperplasia

Clamp lesion

FIG 42–1.
Approximately 25% of vein graft failures result from intrinsic vein graft stenoses occurring within the 6 to 24 month interval following bypass.

while failures beyond this two-year period occur increasingly from progressive arteriosclerosis. Vein graft aneurysms are exceedingly rare and usually occur as anastomotic pseudoaneurysms. Stenotic lesions resulting from fibrous intimal hyperplasia occur most commonly at the proximal anastomosis in reversed vein grafts and at the distal anastomosis of *in situ* vein grafts, both occurring within the narrowest segment of the original vein. Less often, vein graft stenoses occur at the site of a fibrotic valve or phlebitic segment in the midportion of the graft. In those grafts failing beyond two years, the responsible lesion results from progression of atherosclerosis in the distal runoff bed, or less commonly in the distribution of the proximal inflow (Fig 42–2). Regardless of the underlying etiology, however, the vast majority of patients with late failures initially operated on for limb salvage will require major amputation unless secondary reconstruction is successfully undertaken.

Progression Of Atherosclerosis

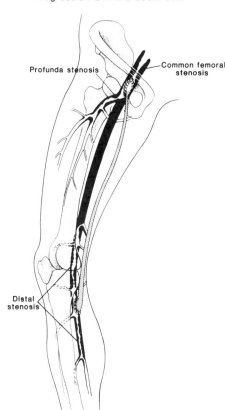

Profunda stenosis

Common femoral stenosis

Distal stenosis

FIG 42–2.
Progression of atherosclerosis in native vessels is responsible for 15% of vein graft failures and becomes more frequent beyond two years.

MANAGEMENT

Considered in the generic sense, secondary reconstruction results in a 50% five-year cumulative limb salvage rate in patients with thrombosed vein grafts with an associated 2% to 3% operative mortality. This result appears to apply to all such patients regardless of atherogenic risk factors and regardless of the number of secondary reconstructions required. The secondary five-year patency rate for thrombosed vein grafts approximates 35%, however, depending on the method used to approach the specific causative lesion.

An important principle underlying our current approach toward secondary reconstruction is illustrated by the subgroup of patients with short-segment, well localized stenotic lesions. Restoration of patency is most easily effected with simple vein patch angioplasty. For patients with recurrent ischemic symptoms or diminished Doppler ankle pressures resulting from a patent but stenotic vein graft following infrainguinal revascularization, simple patch angioplasty results in an 80% to 85% five-year secondary patency rate. In contrast, those patients with a thrombosed graft resulting from the same short-segment stenotic lesion require initial catheter thrombectomy prior to similar patch angioplasty and demonstrate a significantly lower 28% five-year patency rate. It was hypothesized, therefore, that the balloon catheter removes a significant portion of the luminal endothelium, initiating a cascade of events that ultimately results in fibrous intimal hyperplasia and subsequent recurrent failure.

The advent of thrombolytic therapy, however, provided a means of avoiding this initial endothelial damage, thereby improving results with subsequent secondary intervention. Preliminary results using initial thrombolysis, as opposed to catheter thrombectomy are encouraging, but far from conclusive; yet an initial attempt at thrombolytic therapy in patients with thrombosed vein grafts is warranted where time permits.

This patient's graft failure, in all probability, resulted from progressive atherosclerotic disease or fibrous intimal hyperplasia, although an obvious embolic etiology needs to be ruled out, if possible. The initial critical decision concerns the timing of intervention which, to a certain extent, determines the mode of intervention. If neuromuscular function in the affected extremity is deteriorating rapidly, restoration of adequate perfusion within four to six hours becomes imperative. This time frame may preclude angiography with initial thrombolysis and mandate immediate surgical thrombectomy in the operating room. If the clinical course has been less abrupt and the limb is not immediately threatened, initial angiography is recommended prior to either thrombolytic therapy or surgical thrombectomy. In either case, preoperative angiography is advisable to assess the status of native vessels proximal and distal to the occluded graft, which may shed some light on the mechanism of failure and aid in operative management. Many causative lesions, particularly those compromising proximal inflow, may not be apparent at the time of surgical exploration. In addition, angiography allows the opportunity for initial thrombolysis which, as mentioned previously, has several inherent advantages.

First, with satisfactory dissolution of thrombus the causative lesion may be better determined preoperatively and the appropriate procedure undertaken more expeditiously. Second, if distal runoff vessels have been compromised by embolization of thrombus, reperfusion may be established with successful thrombolysis. Third, successful thrombolysis obviates the necessity for using an embolectomy catheter, thereby minimizing both endothelial damage and residual adherent thrombus within the original graft.

Our current thrombolytic protocol requires the initial passage of a guidewire through the entire length of the occluded graft, if possible. Following subsequent passage of a small infusion catheter, a loading dose of 50,000 to 100,000 units of urokinase is injected throughout the length of the thrombus as the catheter is withdrawn and repositioned within the proximal 2 cm or 3 cm of thrombus. Urokinase infusion is then initiated with a decreasing dosage schedule of 240,000 units per hour for two hours, 120,000 units per hour for the next two hours, followed by a constant infusion of 60,000 units per hour until the next interval arteriogram routinely obtained every 12 hours. In an effort to minimize catheter-induced thrombosis, a simultaneous infusion of heparin is administered to maintain the partial thromboplastin time at 1.5 to 2.0 times normal. If little progress is made during the initial 24 hours or in the event of a hemorrhagic complication, thrombolysis is terminated and operative intervention pursued after six to 12 hours. If, at any time, the patient's foot becomes imminently threatened, it is important to continue thrombolytic therapy since, in all probability, this has resulted from embolization of proximal thrombus. Continued thrombolytic therapy will usually digest such distal thrombus and restore satisfactory perfusion.

Surgical Treatment

In the event that thrombolytic therapy is unavailable or unsuccessful, or in cases where neuromuscular function is obviously deteriorating, urgent revascularization is required and the patient should be taken without hesitation to the operating room. Under regional anesthetic, and after preparing both groins and lower extremities to ensure availability of the contralateral vein, the ipsilateral groin is reincised and the proximal common femoral artery dissected free and controlled. The superficial and deep femoral arteries with the proximal vein graft are similarly isolated, but if scarring is dense and dissection either time-consuming or hazardous, internal control can be secured with Fogarty embolectomy catheters. Following systemic heparinization and proximal control, the vein graft is thrombectomized through a transverse incision in the hood of the proximal anastomosis. Proximal anastomotic stenosis may be obvious and, if so, is patched open with autogenous vein. Otherwise, following satisfactory thrombectomy, the small incision is closed, clamps released and an intraoperative arteriogram obtained. In the case of a nonreversed *in situ* graft, while it is technically feasible to thrombectomize from either a proximal, mid or distal incision, intraoperative arteriography remains mandatory, and it therefore seems wise to utilize an initial groin incision as well.

Arteriography may then delineate one of three general mechanisms of vein graft failure. The first consists of the aforementioned localized stenosis, characteristically more common at the proximal anastomosis in a reversed vein graft and at the distal anastomosis in the nonreversed *in situ* graft (Fig 42–3). Localized stenoses may also be found in the midsection of the graft, perhaps at the site of a fibrotic valve, particularly in the reversed configuration. Although simple patch angioplasty of thrombectomized grafts with the localized lesion seems logical and is probably effective for vein grafts of otherwise adequate caliber, the five-year secondary patency rate, in our experience, has been slightly lower than that observed when a longer segment of graft is replaced. It would appear, therefore, that angiography tends to underestimate the degree of disease present in a vein graft and it may prove wiser to replace a longer length of the graft if suitable vein is available.

Following initial thrombectomy, arteriography may in fact demonstrate a more diffusely diseased segment of the vein graft and, if possible, the entire graft should probably be replaced with contralateral autogenous saphenous vein. If saphenous vein is not available, however, acceptable results may be achieved using a segment of autogenous vein from either arm or lesser saphenous systems to bypass the diffusely diseased portion of graft to or from the otherwise adequate original vein graft. Distal extension grafts are also useful when failure results from progression

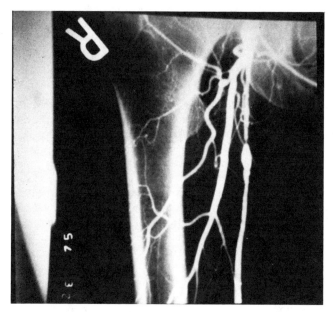

FIG 42–3.
Intraoperative arteriogram following thrombectomy of a failed vein graft illustrates proximal vein graft stenosis with poststenotic dilatation.

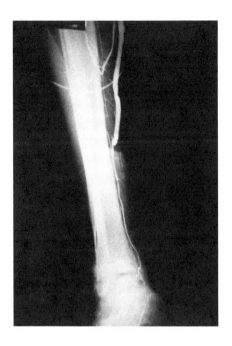

FIG 42–4.
The original femorotibial vein graft illustrated in this intraoperative completion arteriogram failed, due to progression of atherosclerosis in the posterior tibial artery distal to the original anastomosis. A segment of basilic arm vein has been used as an extension graft from the original vein graft proximally to the mid-posterior tibial artery distally bypassing the intervening diseased segment.

of atherosclerosis in the distal outflow bed (Fig 42–4). Such extension grafts, either proximally or distally, are associated with a 35% five-year patency rate and a 50% limb salvage rate.

If suitable lengths of vein are not available, shorter segments may prove adequate by utilizing an endarterectomized superficial femoral artery or the distal profunda/femoris as alternate sites for proximal anastomosis. Our experience using prosthetic material has been uniformly dismal, with none remaining patent beyond three years when used in this secondary reoperative setting. We have carried out delayed amputation for most patients in whom we have exhausted all sources of autogenous tissue. For the majority of patients with failed vein grafts, however, aggressive secondary reconstruction may achieve significant continued limb salvage.

BIBLIOGRAPHY

1. Brewster DC, LaSalle AJ, Robison JG, et al: Femoropopliteal graft failures: Clinical consequences and success of secondary reconstructions. *Arch Surg* 1983; 118:1043–1047.
2. Graor RA, Risius B, Young JR, et al: Peripheral artery and bypass graft thrombolysis with recombinant human tissue-type plasminogen activator. *J Vasc Surg* 1986; 3:115–124.

3. Koltun WA, Gardiner GA, Harrington DP, et al: Thrombolysis in the treatment of peripheral arterial vascular occlusions. *Arch Surg* 1987; 122:901–905.
4. Stept LL, Flinn WR, McCarthy WJ, et al: Technical defects as a cause of early graft failure after femorodistal bypass. *Arch Surg* 1987; 122:599–603.
5. Szilagyi DE, Elliott JP, Hageman JM, et al: Biologic fate of autogenous vein implants as arterial substitutes. *Ann Surg* 1973; 178:232–246.
6. Whittemore AD, Clowes AW, Couch NP, et al: Secondary femoropopliteal reconstruction. *Ann Surg* 1981; 193:35–42.
7. Zwolak RM, Adams MC, Clowes AW: Kinetics of vein graft hyperplasia: Association with tangential stress. *J Vasc Surg* 1987; 5:126–136.

43 Recurrent Symptoms and Vein Graft Stenosis — The Failing Graft

A 67-year-old man is seen for recurrent left calf claudication of six weeks duration. Seven months previously he had undergone a left femoropopliteal vein bypass graft for ischemic rest pain, with a successful outcome. Examination reveals an intact femoral pulse and faintly palpable popliteal and dorsalis pedis pulses. Repeat arteriography reveals a patent graft with a significant segmental stenosis in the upper third of the bypass.

Consultant: Robert W. Hobson, II, M.D.

This case report exemplifies the importance of identifying the "failing" graft prior to occlusion. Femoropopliteal and femoral distal bypasses are among the most commonly performed vascular reconstruction, and yet graft occlusion during the early postoperative period occurs in 5–30% of cases. In review of our results with revascularization of the lower extremity, the five-year patency for femoropopliteal bypass using reversed autogenous saphenous vein was 74%, with graft occlusion during the first postoperative year accounting for a major portion of the loss in patency. Identification of the "failing" graft in a symptomatic patient indicates arteriography and provides an opportunity in this case for revision by localized operative or interventional radiologic techniques.

An ideally planned program of postoperative graft surveillance should allow detection of pathophysiological mechanisms responsible for graft occlusion in larger numbers of cases, including asymptomatic patients. Common causes of early graft failure include operative technical errors such as vascular clamp injuries, undetected intimal flaps, graft kinking or entrapment problems, and strictures or technically inadequate anastomoses. Later graft failures may be due to valvular hypertrophy, neointimal fibroplasia, progressive proximal or distal atherosclerosis, structural abnormalities within the vein graft, or deficiencies of the prosthetic material utilized in performing the bypass. Regardless of the etiology of the graft failure, identification of a predisposing cause prior to graft occlusion would then allow selective use of postoperative arteriography and revision of the confirmed deficiency.

Localized stenoses as demonstrated in this case report should be repaired expeditiously. Although it is tempting to consider balloon dilatation of these stenoses in autogenous vein bypasses, localized operation and patch angioplasty has been so successful that I regard it as the preferred technique. Valvular hypertrophy or vascular clamp injuries have accounted for most of these localized stenoses. Successful repair can be anticipated in virtually all cases. However, in instances of stenotic lesions developing just proximal or distal to PTFE prostheses, transluminal balloon angioplasty has been reported as effective in the majority of cases which confirms our clinical experiences.

PREVENTION OF EARLY POSTOPERATIVE
GRAFT OCCLUSION

The prevention of early postoperative occlusion begins in the operating room with utilization of precise surgical techniques as well as intraoperative arteriography for detection of unsuspected technical errors. Although their incidence has become less in experienced surgical practices, confirmation of a technically adequate arteriographic result is essential and performed routinely. Anastomotic stricture, retained thrombus, intimal irregularities or entrapped grafts as well as anticipated difficulties with distal run-off can be identified by aggressive use of intraoperative arteriography. Prebypass operative arteriography is also valuable in decisions regarding anastomotic placement, particularly when distal run-off is not well defined on preoperative arteriography.

Although intraoperative arteriography has been the most commonly applied method for detection of localized technical deficiencies or anastomotic stenoses, its limitations in the usual one plane operative view are well known. This has stimulated several clinicians to explore use of intraoperative and postoperative duplex scanning. Most surgeons have adopted routine measurement of segmental Doppler arterial pressures in patients following infra-inguinal vascular reconstructions. However, one limitation in use of Doppler pressure measurements has been the difficulty encountered in interpretation of results during the first several postoperative hours, particularly when run-off is poor. Early postoperative improvement in Doppler systolic pressures may be delayed because of reactive hyperemia and early elevation in run-off resistance caused by the operative event. As a generalization, however, improvement in systolic pressures and reappearance of peripheral pulses should occur within the first few hours after operation. Absence of an improved ankle to arm index postoperatively should prompt consideration for re-operation. Although auscultation of Doppler signals over the graft and at the ankle can provide useful qualitative information, quantification of these observations though duplex scanning warrants further consideration as discussed in one of the following sections.

FREQUENCY OF POSTOPERATIVE EVALUATIONS

Patients with infra-inguinal bypasses should be examined two to three weeks postoperatively, at which time peripheral pulses are evaluated and recorded. Doppler segmental systolic pressure measurements are obtained and an ankle to arm index compared with the preoperative values. Lower extremity wounds are examined for adequacy of healing and an impression of the patient's improvement in symptomatology is obtained. Thereafter, examinations at three-month intervals for the first eighteen months postoperatively and at six month intervals thereafter constitutes our current practice, as one attempts to identify the greatest number of patients at risk for graft occlusion. Any historical evidence of recurrent symptomatology as noted in this case report prompts consideration for arteriography and appropriate intervention. Frequently, this is accompanied by a decrease in the ankle/brachial systolic pressure index, which if present and exceeds 0.1–0.15 indicates arteriography in the symptomatic or asymptomatic patient. Unfortunately, changes in these resting indices may not be significant and yet occlusion of the graft or prosthesis observed. Although repeat Doppler pressure measurements after provocative testing including reactive hyperemia or treadmill exercise may be useful in patients with autogenous or prosthetic bypasses, routine evaluation has not been adopted due to more lengthy time requirements for testing as well as medical concerns for treadmill exercise in elderly patients. Consequently, expanding use of these provocative techniques is not a realistic answer to detection of a greater number of reconstructions at risk in the minimally symptomatic or asymptomatic patient. However, newer noninvasive duplex scanning may offer that opportunity.

DUPLEX SCANNING FOR GRAFT SURVEILLANCE

Several authors have reported the value of utilizing duplex scanning for the evaluation of infra-inguinal vascular reconstructions. Bandyk reported that 25% of the "failing" in situ grafts in his clinical experience would not have been identified by the measurement of resting Doppler segmental pressures alone. Since use of duplex scanning has become a standard part of our noninvasive evaluation of carotid occlusive disease, extension of these methods to the surveillance of infra-inguinal bypasses should be encouraged, dependent upon availability of trained technical support. Anatomical description of anastomoses or suspected bypass stenoses can be obtained from B-mode ultrasonography and combined with hemodynamic information regarding flow velocity within the bypass. New diagnostic criteria (Table 43–1) will need to be evaluated prospectively in other laboratories and cost effectiveness measured against the potentially increased diagnosis of the "failing" graft.

TABLE 43–1.

Categories of Graft Flow Patterns

DUPLEX CATEGORY	VELOCITY SPECTRA CHARACTERISTICS
Normal, high PVR	Triphasic waveform configurations, peak systolic velocity greater than 45 cm/sec. No spectral broadening
Normal, low PVR	Biphasic waveform configuration, end-diastolic flow velocity greater than zero, peak systolic flow velocity greater than 45 cm/sec. No spectral broadening
Abnormal, low flow velocity high PVR	Triphasic or monophasive waveform configuration, no diastolic forward flow velocity less than 45 cm/sec. No spectral broadening
Abnormal, low flow velocity low PVR	Biphasic waveform, diastolic forward flow greater than zero, peak systolic flow velocity less than 45 cm/sec. No spectral broadening
Wall irregularity, less than 20 percent DR	No increase in peak systolic velocity in relation to proximal arterial segment but showing spectral broadening during systole.
20–49 percent DR	Greater than 30 percent increase in peak systolic velocity with respect to site just proximal to stenosis. Spectral broadening throughout the entire pulse cycle.
50–99 percent DR	Loss of reverse flow with 100 percent increase in peak systolic velocity in relation to segment proximal to stenosis. Uniform spectral broadening throughout pulse cycle with simultaneous reverse flow components.
Total occlusion	No flow signal from visualized segment.

DR = diameter reduction; PVR = peripheral vascular resistance. (From Bandyk DF: Perioperative use of the duplex scare, in Bergan JJ, Yao JST (eds): *Arterial Surgery: New Diagnostic and Operative Techniques:* Orlando, Grune & Stratton, 1988, 467–82.

BIBLIOGRAPHY

1. Bandyk DF: Perioperative use of the duplex scan, in Bergan JJ, Yao ST (eds): *Arterial Surgery: New Diagnostic and Operative Techniques.* Orlando, Grune & Stratton, 1988, 467–82.
2. Blackshear WM, Thiele BL, Strandness DE Jr: Natural history of above and below-knee femoropopliteal grafts. *Am J Surg* 1980; 140:234.
3. Brewster DC: Early complications of vascular repair below the inguinal ligament, in Bernhard V, Towne J (eds): *Complications in Vascular Surgery.* Orlando, Grune & Stratton, 1986, 37–49.
4. Hobson RW, Lynch TG, Jamil Z, et al: Results of revascularization and amputation and severe lower extremity ischemia: a five year clinical experience. *J Vasc Surg* 1985; 2:174–85.
5. Johnson WC, Logerfo FW, Corson JD, et al: The prognostic value of preoperative and postoperative Doppler ankle systolic pressures in vein bypass grafts in the lower extremity, in Diethrich ED (ed): *Noninvasive Cardiovascular Diagnosis.* Littleton, MA, PSG Publishing Co., 1981, 175–84.

6. Kohler TR, Strandness DE Jr: Duplex scanning of peripheral arteries: practical application, in Bergan JJ, Yao ST (eds): *Arterial Surgery: New Diagnostic and Operative Techniques*. Orlando, Grune & Stratton, 1988, 437–46.
7. Veith FJ, Weiser RK, Gupta SK, et al: Diagnosis and management of failing lower extremity arterial reconstructions. *J Cardiovasc Surg* 1984; 25:381.

PART FOUR

Trauma

44   Acute Carotid Injury

A 23-year-old male is brought to the emergency room with a gunshot wound to the neck after a barroom incident. He has been drinking heavily. Examination reveals an entry wound in the lower left neck and prominent left cervical swelling. He is intoxicated, but responsive, and appears to have mild right-sided weakness.

Consultant: Malcolm O. Perry, M.D.

ETIOLOGY

Most vascular injuries are the result of aggressive acts of violence, usually from knives or bullets traveling at low velocities. The injuries therefore are mainly confined to the wound tract, but if firearms that generate high velocities are used there may be considerable damage from the blast effects. Blunt trauma is often more difficult to diagnose and manage, and the superficial evidence of injury is scanty. Moreover, patients involved in motor vehicle accidents or falls may have blunt trauma to the head and neck which causes other problems because of the combination of injuries.

EVALUATION OF THE PATIENT

In patients with penetrating trauma to the neck, it is helpful to divide the neck into the three zones as described by Monson, Saletta and Freeark. Zone I extends from 1 cm above the clavicle down to include the base of the neck and the thoracic outlet; Zone II from 1 cm above the clavicle to the angle of the mandible; and Zone III from the angle of the mandible to the base of the skull. Although important neurovascular structures traverse all three zones, their relationships to each other and to the surrounding structures vary in each zone, and these differences require specialized diagnostic maneuvers.

It is the author's practice to recommend exploration of all penetrating wounds of the neck that pierce the platysma muscle. This remains controversial and in the absence of the specific identification of a major vascular injury, some trauma surgeons will defer surgery for a period of observation. During this time various tests can be performed to rule out injury to the vascular structures, or to the aerodigestive tract. In patients who have clear evidence of penetration of the aerodigestive tract (subcutaneous air, drainage) surgical exploration will be required. Adjunctive methods to rule out penetration of the aerodigestive tract (endoscopy, esophageal contrast studies) all have a significant incidence of false negative results and cannot be relied on to exclude damage to the trachea, esophagus or hypopharynx.

In the evaluation of carotid injuries it is helpful to divide the patients into three groups. The first and largest group consists of those patients who have a penetrating injury to the carotid arteries, but have no neurologic deficit. In general, their outlook is quite good and one can anticipate that surgical repair will be successful. The second group contains those patients who have a mild neurologic deficit as manifested by monoparesis, hemiparesis, or transient episodes of cerebral ischemia. Repair of carotid injuries in these patients also can be expected to have a successful outcome. Group 3 consists of those patients who have a severe neurologic deficit in association with a carotid injury. This group has a much poorer outlook overall, and in fact, it appears that in most of these patients the eventual outcome is directly related to the extent and severity of the neurologic deficit prior to surgical treatment. Most trauma surgeons recommend that all penetrating carotid injuries in patients in Group 1 and Group 2 be repaired, but controversy continues to surround selection of patients in Group 3 for repair of an injured carotid artery. Many surgeons recommend repair of carotid wounds in the patients in this group as well, if prograde arterial blood flow is uninterrupted, and if the patient does not have an acute severe stroke with coma.

Because of the close relationship of the brachial plexus, the cervical plexus, and other cranial nerves, a thorough and careful neurological examination is necessary in all of these patients. Detection of a Horner's syndrome, for example, suggests that a wound at the base of the neck may have injured other structures. In addition, injuries to cranial nerves or the brachial plexus should be identified prior to the operation, not only to determine the extent of the injury, but also to alert the surgeon to the possibility of accidental injury to these structures during exploration. The status of the vocal cords should be known as well. If this cannot be ascertained by the preoperative examination, at the time of induction of anesthesia the vocal cords can be inspected, and their function and position recorded. The exact status of all the neurologic problems should be carefully recorded prior to operation.

ADJUNCTIVE STUDIES

Although plain radiographs may not disclose a major vascular injury, biplane films of the neck, chest, and head are important, particularly in the treatment of patients with gunshot wounds. The vagaries of bullet trajectories are well known, and one cannot simply draw a line between the site of entrance and the final resting place of the missile. Nevertheless, some estimation of the direction and path of the bullet needs to be determined preoperatively in order to guide the extent of the exploration. All of the important structures in the wound tract between the entry site and the final resting place or exit of the missile should be inspected. The detection of a wide mediastinum, the presence of subcutaneous or mediastinal emphysema, elevation of the diaphragm, and deviation of the trachea or esophagus suggest injury of vascular structures and perhaps the aerodigestive tract.

In stable patients with penetrating injuries to the neck, a four-vessel arteriogram with biplane intracranial films can be very helpful (Fig 44–1). These patients should also have a CT scan of the head, especially if there is a neurologic deficit present. The neurologic deficit may be related to the penetrating trauma to the neck, but in patients who have multiple injuries there may be closed head trauma. Also, there may be congenital or acquired intracranial malformations that can have a bearing on the eventual outcome. In older patients with hypertension and diffuse atherosclerosis, intracranial hemorrhage can be a factor; this can be detected by CT scan.

TREATMENT

Most trauma surgeons recommend that patients who have injuries in Zone I and Zone III and all who have a neurologic deficit, have biplane cervical and intracra-

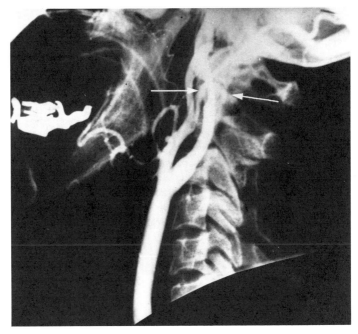

FIG 44–1.
This injury to the internal carotid artery was not detectable on examination *(arrows)*.

nial arteriograms. Even those patients who have penetrating trauma restricted to Zone II may benefit from preoperative arteriography since the planning of the operation is simplified if the extent and number of wounds are known.

Recent reports by Fry and others have suggested that vertebral artery injuries may be more common than suspected. One would anticipate that a four-vessel study prior to operation would expose these potentially dangerous lesions, and permit their assessment and proper repair at the time of the initial operation.

Patients who are unstable should not be sent to the radiology suite, but should be taken immediately to the operating room where abbreviated studies can be performed while preparation is being made for surgical exploration. Carotid arteriography can be performed in the operating room by simple techniques. Utilizing an 18-gauge Courmand needle, a puncture can be made in the common carotid artery and biplane films exposed after injection of approximately 10 cc of a 60% radiographic contrast medium. This was a standard method of performing arteriograms for many years, and with proper timing one can visualize the entire cervical and intracranial carotid in a single injection, although it may be necessary to make two injections to get anterior-posterior and lateral views. The same technique can be used for completion arteriography following repair of the carotid artery. These studies are especially important when the patient has a neurologic deficit since distal thromboembolism may already have occurred.

Associated Injuries

Trauma patients frequently have more than one injury, even though a simple penetrating wound to the neck may be what brought them to the emergency room. Injuries in Zone I may result in mediastinal wounds, or perhaps in penetration of the chest there may be a hemopneumothorax. If a patient has a hemopneumothorax, a closed thoracostomy tube should be put in place prior to the induction of pressure assisted ventilation since this will increase the air leak and perhaps cause a tension pneumothorax. Several intravenous access lines should be obtained; at least one should be placed in an uninjured extremity and reserved for the administration of fluid and blood, and not used for administration of antibiotics or drugs. If blood loss does occur, the requirement for blood may be substantial and one line should be reserved for such resuscitation. Patients are generally initially given an electrolyte solution such as lactated Ringer's, but blood loss is replaced with blood.

Prior to the operation, it is prudent to prepare and drape the saphenous vein at the ankle so that it can be used for patch graft material or as a replacement of an injured carotid artery. On occasion, some surgeons have used the external jugular vein for a patch graft, but for the most part cervical veins are too fragile for use in the arterial system.

Operative Management

The entire neck, including both anterior triangles and supraclavicular areas, and the chest down to the nipples should be prepped and draped into the operative field.

Although the carotid artery can be exposed satisfactorily by the standard sterno-mastoid incision, it may be necessary to extend this incision into a medial sternotomy in patients who have injuries at the root of the neck in Zone I. In fact, some trauma surgeons recommend median sternotomy in any patient who has a suspected vascular injury below the cricoid bone (or in Zone I). Preliminary control of the great vessels in such cases reduces the chance of exsanguinating hemorrhage.

Prior to exposing the injury, the common carotid artery is approached and encircled with a soft tape. Then the hematoma is carefully removed. In most cases bleeding from the carotid artery can be controlled by gentle pressure with the finger for the remainder of the exposure. It is important to avoid fragmentation of the clot, reducing the chances of distal thromboembolism. In older people who have athero-sclerotic arteries it is especially important to remember, as Wylie said, "to dissect the patient away from the artery." Such gentleness in handling these vascular wounds will reduce the possibility of cerebral embolism. Once the wound is identified and the common, internal and external arteries are controlled with soft vascular clamps, clots are evacuated and the area examined. In most cases there is a puncture or small laceration, but on occasion there can be complete transection. Backflow from the internal carotid artery is evaluated by releasing the distal occluding clamp. Brisk, bright red, pulsatile backflow is satisfactory evidence of adequate cerebral perfusion, and in these situations shunts should not be required. If there is a question as to the adequacy of the backflow, stump pressures can be measured. If the ICA pressure exceeds 60 mm Hg one can proceed with repair without the insertion of a shunt. There are no controlled data that give firm guidelines as to whether shunting is needed or not. Most surgeons use a dilute heparin solution for local irrigation, but if the patient has only an isolated vascular wound and no other trauma to the eyes or central nervous system, heparin may be given during the period of temporary carotid occlusion.

The methods of repair include standard vascular techniques. It is necessary to debride only that portion of the vessel which is visibly damaged unless the injury is caused by high velocity bullets. In these cases it is advisable to debride 3 mm to 4 mm beyond the apparent damage. Although lateral suture repair may be possible in arteries of this size, resection and anastomosis are favored in most cases unless the wound is only a small puncture. Autogenous patch graft angioplasty utilizing the saphenous vein from the ankle can be used to repair larger defects. After resection, if an anastomosis without tension is not possible, one can either transpose the proximal external carotid for inflow if it is uninjured (Fig 44–2), or interpose an autogenous saphenous vein graft to repair the injured ICA segment (Fig 44–3). Although not essential in every case, it is often best to perform these repairs with interrupted 6–0 monofilament sutures. The vessels are smaller in diameter during the repair than they will be when full arterial pressure is restored. Moreover, the interrupted suture technique prevents suture line stenosis at a later date. Although it is usually easy at the time of operation to determine if the repair is satisfactory (examination of the distal pulse in the internal carotid artery, and confirming the presence of adequate flow with a sterile Doppler probe), many surgeons recommend that all of these patients have a completion arteriogram. As described above, this

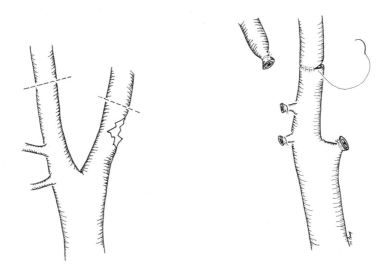

FIG 44–2.
If the ICA is severely damaged it may be possible to restore flow by substituting the external carotid artery.

can be done simply by inserting an 18-gauge needle into the common carotid artery and injecting approximately 10 cc of 60% Conray.

Most surgeons believe that the only patients who might require ligation of the internal carotid artery are those in whom there is complete carotid occlusion and a severe neurologic deficit associated with coma, or patients in whom the distal internal carotid artery cannot be cleared of clots. Repair of the carotid artery is indicated in those patients who have continued prograde flow and no distal obstruction.

RESULTS

A successful outcome can be anticipated in most of the patients in Groups 1 and 2 if the injury can be repaired (Table 44–1). A patient who has a severe stroke and coma is not likely to be benefited by operation, particularly if the internal carotid artery is completely occluded as a result of blunt trauma.

MANAGEMENT OF THIS PATIENT

Based on the initial findings of an entry wound at the base of the neck and an obvious cervical hematoma, it seems clear that this patient has had a major vascular injury. If vital signs are unstable or active ongoing blood loss is present, the patient

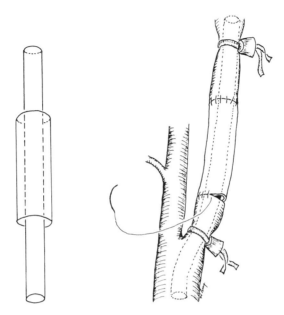

FIG 44–3.
Occasionally a saphenous vein graft and temporary inlying shunt may be needed. The
method shown here is useful in such cases.

should be taken directly to the operating room. If urgent operation were required in
such an unstable patient with an entry wound at the base of the neck (Zone I), I
would certainly begin operative exploration with a median sternotomy to ensure
proximal control and allow complete evaluation of the great vessels within the mediastinum. If necessary, intraoperative carotid arteriography can be performed as
previously described.

 If the patient were clinically stable, I would proceed with emergency angiog-

TABLE 44–1.
Results of Treatment

	NUMBER OF PATIENTS	DIED	RESIDUAL NEUROLOGIC DEFICIT
Group 1 No Deficit	49	0	1
Group 2 Mild Deficit	8	1	0
Group 3 Severe Deficit	15	5	8

raphy, due to the high likelihood of major vascular injury as well as the apparent neurologic deficit. Further surgical management would be guided by the arteriographic findings. Since a marked neurologic deficit is not described in our patient, I would proceed with repair of an injured carotid vessel, especially if prograde flow was still present. If the injured vessel were totally occluded or transected by the gunshot wound, I would still attempt repair if good backbleeding was evident when clot was removed from the injured segment. I believe this would offer the best chance of successful recovery.

BIBLIOGRAPHY

1. Flint LM, Snyder WH, Perry MO, et al: Management of major vascular injuries in the base of the neck. *Arch Surg* 1973; 106:407–417.
2. Fry RE, Fry WJ: Extracranial carotid artery injuries. *Surgery* 1980; 88:581–587.
3. Monson DO, Saletta JD, Freeark RJ: Carotid vertebral trauma. *J Trauma* 1979; 9:987–999.
4. Perry MO: *The Management of Acute Vascular Injuries*. Baltimore, Williams and Wilkins, 1981.
5. Roon AJ, Christensen N: Evaluation and treatment of penetrating cervical injuries. *J Trauma* 1979; 19:391–397.
6. Thal ER, Snyder WH, Hays RJ, et al: Management of carotid artery injuries. *Surgery* 1974; 76:955–962.

45 Gunshot Wound to the Groin

A 32-year-old man is brought in by ambulance to the emergency room after a hunting accident. He has sustained a gunshot wound to the right groin when a nearby hunter tripped and his gun discharged. He is hypotensive, with vigorous bleeding from the femoral area being controlled by direct pressure applied by the paramedics.

Consultant: Norman M. Rich, M.D.

Unfortunately, this clinical situation is being seen with increasing incidence in our civilian emergency rooms. Urban hostilities and terror have escalated considerably over the past 15 years in the United States. Increasingly sophisticated weaponry is being utilized, making many of the extremity wounds more like the higher velocity and more destructive military wounds. Hunting accidents occur during each hunting season in certain areas of the United States. Both the weapons utilized and the missiles fired by hunters frequently are more destructive than many civilian gunshot wounds where lower velocity and less destructive handguns are utilized.

The obvious emergency is that this individual is hypotensive with vigorous bleeding, therefore, immediate control of the bleeding and appropriate resuscitation are imperative. There are a number of important questions that need to be resolved and additional information would be helpful. From the history given, it would appear that this is a single gunshot wound; nevertheless, it is important to rule out additional bullet wounds or other associated injuries as soon as possible. Typically, this accident occurs in a young man whom we can assume has been healthy and vigorous prior to this incident. From numerous wars in this century we have learned that the chance of survival is excellent when the wounded individual reaches the emergency room in a definitive surgical center alive. Consequently, we will concentrate on the right lower extremity challenge. We are not informed about the time of the accident nor the location, and this information would be helpful. We do not know whether or not the patient is responsive.

PREOPERATIVE ASSESSMENT AND MANAGEMENT

The patient has hemorrhagic shock. The bleeding is controlled by direct pressure in the femoral area and this direct pressure should be continued in order to control the hemorrhage. Two upper extremity large-bore intravenous lines should be started immediately with Ringer's lactate infused rapidly. This should have an immediate response in restoring the patient's intravascular volume to a more appropriate level. During the infusion of crystalloid and repeated monitoring of vital signs, it will be possible to insert a urinary catheter into the bladder to decompress the bladder, to ensure that there is no hematuria and to provide further monitoring. Baseline hematologic studies should be requested, and the patient's blood should be typed and cross-matched for at least four units of whole blood. Consideration for infusion of 0-negative blood might be warranted. If the patient's vital signs respond appropriately, additional valuable information could be obtained by X-rays in two views to locate retained foreign bodies (missiles) and to determine whether or not there is an associated fracture of the femur. This should be accomplished in the emergency room. All of this rapid activity is in preparation to transfer the patient to the operating room.

A question that is discussed repeatedly is one regarding the merit of tourniquet control of hemorrhage in the extremities. Tuffier of the French Army in 1915 demanded that all tourniquets be removed from the ambulances because of the associated complications from improper use. Proper use of a tourniquet is mandatory. There is probably inadequate space proximal to the wound to consider using a tourniquet in this patient and direct pressure control has been effective anyway.

INTRAOPERATIVE MANAGEMENT

As soon as the patient's general resuscitation is satisfactory, the patient should be moved to the operating amphitheater. Obviously, appropriate lighting, instruments, and type-specific blood should be available. After appropriate preparation, a longitudinal incision should be utilized to gain proximal and distal control of the femoral vessels. This will probably be possible without crossing the femoral crease or going above the inguinal ligament. Up to this point we do not know whether or not the bleeding has been arterial or venous, or both. However, this might have been determined by bright red spurting blood from an arterial wound or steady pooling of darker blood from a venous wound. Because the femoral artery and vein are in close proximity, a wound of both vessels is highly probable. Atraumatic vascular clamps should be applied to the vessels above and below the area of injury. The injury can range from a small perforation or incomplete transection to a complete transection with retraction of the vessel ends. Location of the wounds in the common or in the superficial femoral area should be determined, as well as the status of the deep femoral vessels and the greater saphenous vein. In most circumstances with very minor vessel wounds lateral suture repair might be possible. Venous patch grafts might be utilized to eliminate stricture of the vessel at the repair site. In the vast majority of arterial injuries, however, the injury will usually be significant enough that resection of the area of injury is indicated. An end-to-end anastomosis may be possible without undue tension or sacrifice of major collaterals, even with the loss of 1 cm to 1.5 cm of artery. If an arterial substitute is required, the greater saphenous vein provides an acceptable interposition conduit. Prosthetic material should be avoided if at all possible in contaminated wounds. Monofilament vascular suture should be utilized. Remembering the adage of "life over limb," ligation of the injured artery may be required if the patient's general status deteriorates. It should be emphasized that this is a lifesaving measure only. The World War II statistics must be remembered noting that acute ligation of the superficial femoral artery has a 55% amputation rate and acute ligation of the common femoral artery has an associated amputation rate of 81%. Collateral arterial circulation is important in those not requiring amputation.

If there is a concomitant venous injury the decision-making is more complicated and controversial. Frequently, a lateral venous repair, prior to the arterial repair, is helpful in controlling hemorrhage and easier to do than mobilization of the vein for ligation. The venous anatomy has considerably more anomalies than arterial anatomy; consequently, experience has suggested that venous injuries can be ligated with less sequelae in general than can ligated injured arteries. Yet, with massive destruction of soft tissue and lymphatics, as well as interruption of the majority of the venous return, there can be significant long-term problems associated with chronic venous hypertension that should be avoided if at all possible. End-to-end venous anastomosis can be successfully utilized in some cases. If an interposition graft is required this can be fashioned as a panel graft from a segment of the contralateral greater saphenous vein. The ipsilateral greater saphenous vein should be utilized only if it is injured. If intact, the ipsilateral saphenous vein may provide a vital pathway for venous return and thus should not be electively interrupted for use in a vascular reconstruction for trauma. Prostheses should be avoided in the venous system. Debridement of the wound is very important, with removal of devitalized tissue and as much foreign material as possible. This will assist in preventing a wound infection that could be disastrous. Copious irrigation with saline solution is helpful. If there is an associated femoral fracture immobilization should be accomplished. This can usually be accomplished fairly rapidly by external means either before or after the vascular repair, depending on the exact circumstances. If there is going to be a considerable delay in effecting arterial repair, the possible temporary utilization of a shunt might be considered. Associated nerve injuries should be identified; however, there should be no consideration for primary nerve repair.

Another controversial area is related to the use of fasciotomies in the compartments of the leg. Fasciotomies should be considered and utilized if the wound involves both the artery and vein, if there has been more than a six-hour delay in repair, or if there is an indication that there is elevated compartmental pressure. Measuring compartment pressures can be helpful. The fascial compartments of the thigh will be released with exposure of the femoral vessels. Coverage of the vascular repairs with viable tissue is mandatory. The sartorius muscle can be utilized most often for this purpose. In contaminated wounds it is always safer to leave the wound open with a light dressing. Inspection of the wound in four or five days can be followed by delayed primary closure of the wound if there is no evidence of infection, with essentially the same healing time and strength of the wound at the end of three weeks.

RESULTS

Limb salvage should be possible in the vast majority of injuries. Early thrombosis of the vascular repair can be corrected with prompt recognition and treatment. Infection remains the bane of existence for both the patient and the vascular surgeon and this is best avoided if at all possible. If there is delayed hemorrhage with associated infection, ligation of the vessel may be required at that time. Doppler ultrasound over the pedal vessels may be helpful in determining whether or not there is adequate collateral circulation for limb viability. Later arterial reconstruction may be possible, and also venous reconstruction may be indicated in an unusual situation; however, this is an area of remaining challenge.

SUMMARY

Successful management of the vascular injury in this patient should be anticipated and accomplished. There are several remaining controversies, particularly those involving the management of the venous injury and the appropriate utilization of fasciotomy. Management of concomitant fractures remains another area of controversy. There is adequate recent experience to emphasize that there are differences in managing civilian gunshot wounds from those in the military experience. The weapon utilized in hunting will determine whether the wound is similar to the civilian wound or to the military wound, with the latter usually associated with more massive soft tissue injury.

BIBLIOGRAPHY

1. DeBakey ME, Simeone FA: Battle injuries of the arteries in World War II: An analysis of 2,471 cases. *Ann Surg* 1946; 123:534–579.
2. Feliciano DV, Bitondo CG, Mattox KL, et al: Civilian trauma in the 1980's: A 1-year experience with 456 vascular and cardiac injuries. *Ann Surg* 1984; 199:717–724.
3. Hobson RW II, Rich NM, Wright CB: *Venous Trauma-Pathophysiology, Diagnosis and Surgical Management.* Mount Kisco, Futura Publishing, 1983.
4. Rich NM, Spencer FC: *Vascular Trauma.* Philadelphia, WB Saunders Co, 1978.

46 Blunt Popliteal Artery Injury

A 29-year-old motorcycle rider is brought to the emergency room after a highway accident. There is obvious deformity and instability in the area of the left knee, and the left foot is noted to be cold and pulseless.

Consultant: James O. Menzoian, M.D.

Morbidity following popliteal artery injuries is high. Early experience during World War II showed a 70% amputation rate with ligation of the popliteal artery. This was improved to some degree in the Korean conflict as well as in the Vietnam experience, but reports of a 20% to 30% amputation rate for popliteal injuries are not uncommon. Extreme force is required to dislocate or fracture the knee. The popliteal and proximal tibial vessels are intimately opposed to the posterior joint capsule and are firmly anchored above by the adductor muscles and below by the gastrocnemius and soleus muscles. The popliteal artery is also anchored by the geniculate arteries. Anterior dislocation of the knee will likely result in stretching over a long length of artery. Posterior dislocation usually results in a clean, short, intimal fracture due to the cutting effect of the sharp edged tibia.

Upper tibial fractures are usually due to a hyperextension injury which can also dislocate the knee, resulting in a popliteal artery injury. One should suspect a popliteal artery injury in all tibial fractures, but especially with upper tibial fractures. In short, a high index of suspicion for a popliteal or proximal tibial injury should be maintained in all patients with orthopedic injuries in this area.

INITIAL ASSESSMENT AND MANAGEMENT

After an initial thorough examination of the patient to assure that vital signs are stable and there are no life threatening injuries, attention should be directed to the left leg. Evaluation of the injured extremity should follow the framework of inspection, palpation, and auscultation, with assessment including color, temperature, sensation, motor function, and examination of peripheral pulses. Inspection reveals a pale extremity. Palpation reveals a cool extremity as well as absent pulses below the femoral artery. Sensation in the area of the toes is diminished, and motor function is impaired. Auscultation with the stethoscope reveals a bruit in the region of the popliteal artery. Doppler assessment of the extremity includes the detection of diminished blood flow, a decreased ankle/brachial index, and abnormal wave form analysis. Although some of these findings may be related to direct musculoskeletal injury, they also provide presumptive evidence for an arterial injury.

The probability of an arterial contusion and thrombosis is high with this type of injury. With these findings, intravenous heparin should be given at systemic doses to prevent clot propagation and thrombosis of collateral blood vessels, assuming that no other significant injuries or active bleeding contraindicate heparin administration.

After appropriate external stabilization of the extremity, X-rays should be obtained. These may reveal dislocation of the knee and/or fractures. The dislocation may be anterior, although posterior dislocation occurs more commonly (Fig 46–1). Fractures may include supracondylar fractures of the femur as well as those of the tibial plateau and proximal fibula. In some instances X-ray evidence of dislocation or fracture is lacking, but one must consider that a dislocation may have been present which subsequently reduced.

Once the orthopedic injury has been evaluated, determination of the cause of arterial insufficiency is indicated. In some instances, reduction of a knee dislocation

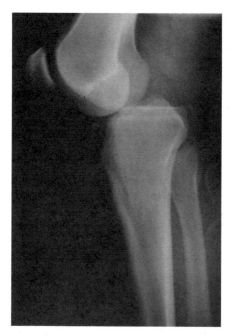

FIG 46–1.
Lateral X-ray of the left knee showing posterior dislocation of the knee.

or fracture may result in the return of pulses. Even in such cases, arteriography is recommended since approximately 30% of knee dislocations result in popliteal artery injury. The most common arterial injury is contusion with subsequent thrombosis, requiring operative repair (Fig 46–2).

If the viability of the limb is not in imminent jeopardy, preoperative arteriography is indicated even in obvious vascular injuries to delineate the exact nature and location of the injury. In addition to the popliteal artery, injury may involve the tibioperoneal trunk and the proximal tibial vessels. If threatened limb viability, evidenced by loss of sensation, poor motor function and pallor, precludes the option of preoperative angiography, the patient should be brought directly to the operating room for intraoperative arteriography or direct exploration of the vessels.

OPERATIVE PROCEDURE

Contrary to traditional teaching, evaluation of a suspected vascular injury should take precedence over operative stabilization of the fracture in patients with combined injuries. Early reversal of tissue ischemia can greatly decrease the risk of permanent neurologic dysfunction, myonecrosis, and amputation. An alternative

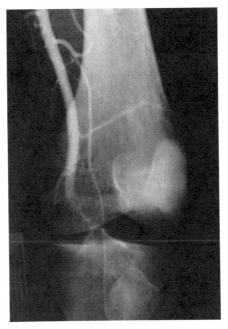

FIG 46-2.
Angiogram revealing thrombosis of the popliteal artery.

but less ideal approach is identification of the vascular injury and placement of an intraluminal shunt across the injury to allow adequate perfusion of the extremity during orthopedic stabilization.

A medial incisional approach allows easy access to the distal femoral artery, popliteal artery, and all tibial vessels. If at the time of operative exploration it is felt that compartmental pressures are increased, this can be verified by standard techniques for measuring compartmental pressures. In addition, at the time of surgical exploration if there is obvious bulging of ischemic muscle, then prompt fasciotomy should be done as a first procedure. The possibility of a compartment syndrome should again be reconsidered at the completion of the surgical procedure. Our own preference for fasciotomy is through multiple full-length skin and fascial incisions. Once the vascular injury is identified, standard techniques for repair are employed. If the injury is a local contusion, resection with end-to-end anastomosis can be considered. This is often extremely difficult because the popliteal and tibial vessels are tethered by geniculate branches as well as the adductor magnus proximally and the gastrocnemius and soleus muscles distally, precluding adequate mobilization for end-to-end anastomosis (Fig 46–3). Ligation of geniculate vessels for purposes of mobilization is not recommended since this will decrease blood supply to an already critically ischemic limb.

Our preference is to use the saphenous vein from the opposite extremity or the cephalic or basilic veins from the arm for interposition bypass grafting. Use of the ipsilateral greater saphenous vein should probably be avoided, if possible, as associated injuries to the ipsilateral deep venous system may make superficial venous collateral routes more important. The use of prosthetic material such as PTFE can be considered in those few patients who do not have adequate autogenous veins. Prior to completion of the arterial repair, embolectomy catheters should be passed proximally and distally to remove thrombus that may have developed during the period of ischemia. The presence of back bleeding from the distal vessel should not be taken as sufficient evidence that there is no distal thrombosis. In addition, irrigating the distal vessels with a solution containing 500 cc plasmalyte, 2000 u heparin and 60 mg papaverine will help to diminish peripheral vasospasm.

In those patients with concomitant popliteal vein injuries, we strongly recommend repair of the popliteal vein. Although a subject of some controversy, the work of Rich and others has clearly shown that patients with combined popliteal artery and vein injuries suffer a much higher morbidity, and they thus advocate direct venous repair. Our experience at Boston University confirms that venous repair reduces this morbidity to some degree. Popliteal vein injuries can be managed by the usual techniques which include removal of thrombus, resection of contused vein with end-to-end anastomosis if possible, or interposition vein grafting. Some would recommend repairing the popliteal vein prior to the repair of the popliteal artery.

Once the vascular repair is complete, completion angiography is essential (Fig 46–4). This will assure the technical adequacy of the repair and assess for evidence of distal thrombosis. In addition, evidence of poor tibial vessel perfusion may indicate increased compartmental pressure and the necessity for fasciotomy.

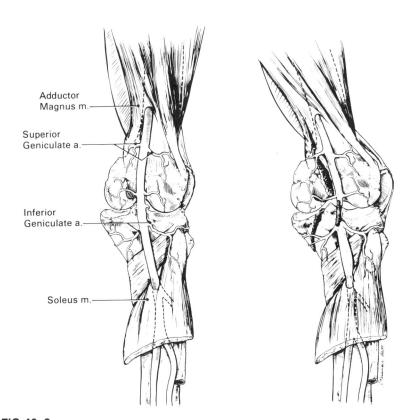

FIG 46–3.
On the left a posterior view of the popliteal fossa. The popliteal and tibial vessels are tethered by the geniculate branches and the adductor magnus proximally and the gastrocnemius and soleus muscles distally. On the right an oblique view showing possible fractures and dislocation with resultant popliteal injury.

Orthopedic stabilization is now undertaken. This may include repair of the disrupted knee capsule and collateral ligaments, as well as fracture alignment and stabilization by internal or external fixation. In many instances external fixation is preferred, especially in those patients with significant soft tissue injury. This allows for excellent stabilization and direct access to these complex soft tissue wounds for daily management. Throughout the period of orthopedic stabilization, it is especially important to assess circulatory adequacy to assure that the recent vascular repair is still intact.

Once orthopedic stabilization is complete, it is again essential to assess compartment pressures. If pressures exceed 40 mm Hg or if there is obvious muscle

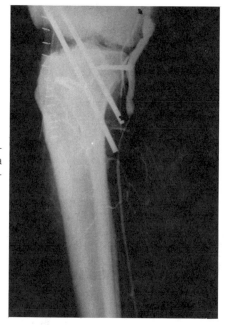

FIG 46–4.
Completion angiogram following a saphenous vein graft interposition to repair a thrombosed popliteal artery shown in Figure 46–2.

swelling, then fasciotomy should be performed. The soft tissue wounds can next be attended to. In patients with significant edema and fasciotomy, the skin wounds may be left open. It is important, however, to mobilize viable tissue over any exposed nerves, blood vessels, and vascular bypass grafts. A standard dressing is then applied. Open wounds should be kept moist to prevent tissue dessication. After a period of 48 to 72 hours when tissue edema is subsiding, delayed primary closure or split thickness skin grafting is performed.

POSTOPERATIVE MANAGEMENT

Following arterial repair, the patient should be frequently evaluated for the presence of pulses, sensation and motor function, as well as the degree of edema of the extremity. Postoperative management should also include limb elevation to diminish edema as well as physical therapy to the degree permitted by the injury itself. In those patients with a popliteal vein repair without extensive soft tissue injury, full heparinization is recommended to prevent thrombosis of the repair. In addition, extrinsic intermittent venous compression of the calf is recommended to increase flow through the venous repair and prevent deep vein thrombosis. Postoperative deep vein thrombosis, especially in those patients with venous injuries, is a well-known complication.

SUMMARY

Prompt and thorough evaluation of these patients should include evaluation of the pulses, sensation, and motor function. Preoperative angiography is extremely helpful in delineating the extent of the injury as well as demonstrating very early contusion or intimal fracture injuries prior to thrombosis. Prompt operative intervention with vascular reconstruction, appropriate orthopedic stabilization, and fasciotomy, if necessary, can result in excellent limb salvage and preservation of function. Long-term morbidity following such injuries may include persistent sensory loss due to nerve injury as well as long-term edema related to concomitant venous injury and the possibility of subsequent venous thrombosis and venous insufficiency.

BIBLIOGRAPHY

1. Alberty RE, Goodfried, G, Boyden AM: Popliteal artery injury with fractural dislocation of the knee. *Am J Surg* 1981; 142:36–40.
2. Bishara RA, Pasch AR, Lim LT, et al: Improved results in the treatment of civilian vascular injuries associated with fractures and dislocations. *J Vasc Surg* 1986; 3:707–711.
3. Dart CH, Jr, Braitman HE: Popliteal artery injury following fracture or dislocation at the knee. *Arch Surg* 1977; 112:969–973.
4. Downs AR, MacDonald P: Popliteal artery injuries: Civilian experience with sixty-three patients during a twenty-four year period (1960 through 1984). *J Vasc Surg* 1986; 4:55–62.
5. Lim LT, Michuda MS, Flanigan DP, et al: Popliteal artery trauma. *Arch Surg* 1980; 115:1307–1313.
6. Menzoian JO, Doyle JE, LoGerfo FW, et al: Evaluation and management of vascular injuries of the extremities. *Arch Surg* 1983; 118:93–95.
7. Menzoian JO, Doyle JE, Cantelmo NL, et al: A comprehensive approach to extremity vascular trauma. *Arch Surg* 1985; 120:801–805.
8. Settembrini PG, Spreafico G , Zannini P: Popliteal artery injuries associated with knee dislocation. Three cases treated with successful outcome. *J Cardiovasc Surg* 1981; 22:135–140.
9. Snyder WH III, Watkins WL, Whiddon LL, et al: Civilian popliteal artery: An eleven year experience with 83 injuries. *Surgery* 1979; 85:101–108.

47 Brachial Artery Occlusion Following Cardiac Catheterization

A 62-year-old woman is seen in consultation for loss of her right radial pulse two hours after transbrachial cardiac catheterization to evaluate symptomatic angina pectoris. The procedure was uneventful, but the floor nurses have been uncertain of the presence of a radial pulse since her return from the cath lab. The patient complains of slight numbness in the hand and fingers, and the hand is cool but clearly viable.

Consultant: Patrick J. O'Hara, M.D.

In this clinical setting, the most likely diagnosis is brachial artery thrombosis following cardiac catheterization, particularly if the patient has no prior history of upper extremity arterial ischemic symptoms and has been documented to have a normal radial and ulnar pulse examination prior to the cardiac catheterization. Another possible diagnosis is embolization to the upper extremity. However, this is much less likely especially if the patient is not in atrial fibrillation and has no other obvious embolic source, such as ventricular mural thrombus.

Transbrachial cardiac catheterization was first described in 1962 at the Cleveland Clinic. It continues to be the preferred route of vascular access by many cardiologists because it requires a shorter, more easily maneuvered catheter than the transfemoral route.

The incidence of iatrogenic brachial artery injury following cardiac catheterization has been reported to range from 0.3% to 28%. In a series reported from the Cleveland Clinic, the incidence of brachial artery occlusion requiring repair was 1.5% of 73,750 cardiac catheterizations from 1965 through 1980.

RELEVANT ANATOMY

The usual anatomy of the distal brachial artery is illustrated in Figure 47–1A. It is superficial from the midhumerus to the bend of the elbow where it descends into

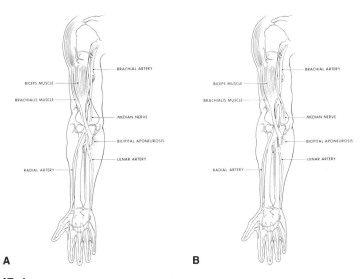

FIG 47–1.
A, Usual anatomy of the brachial artery, with bifurcation distal to the elbow into the radial and ulnar arteries. **B,** Common variation of brachial artery anatomy. Note its bifurcation proximal to the elbow.

the antecubital fossa and divides, approximately 1 cm to 2 cm distal to the elbow crease, into the radial and ulnar arteries. Its distal part is covered by the bicipital aponeurosis, whose fibers usually must be divided to expose the origins of the radial and ulnar arteries. The median nerve crosses the brachial artery from its lateral to medial aspects at the midhumeral level and lies medial to the brachial artery at the elbow. In approximately 19% of limbs the brachial artery bifurcates into its radial and ulnar branches proximal to the elbow as illustrated in Figure 47–1B. A well-developed collateral network consisting of superior and inferior ulnar collateral and profunda brachial arteries proximally supply the radial and ulnar arteries via the radial and interosseous recurrent and anterior and posterior ulnar recurrent arteries distally. Because of this collateral network, the optimal site for the cardiac catheterization arteriotomy is proximal to the elbow crease in the brachial artery distal to the inferior ulnar collateral artery. Ligation of the brachial artery distal to the collateral branch origins is reported to result in amputation in only 3% to 4% of patients. Because of this rich collateral network, occlusion of the distal brachial artery after cardiac catheterization may not result in resting ischemic symptoms in many patients. Commonly, a palpable collateral ulnar or radial pulse may be detected in the presence of total occlusion of the distal brachial artery, an observation that may lead to an error in diagnosis.

CAUSES OF OCCLUSION

The mechanism of occlusion is probably a combination of intimal injury from abrasion by the angiographic catheter and stenosis of the artery in the region of the arteriotomy closure leading to slow blood flow and brachial thrombosis. Intimal injury releases local tissue factors inciting platelet deposition and thrombosis. Larger intimal flaps or dissected atherosclerotic plaques may mechanically obstruct blood flow causing stasis and thrombosis (Fig 47–2A). Distal emboli, consisting of thrombotic or atherosclerotic debris, may originate from the catheter or stenosed arteriotomy site and obstruct distal palmar arch or digital vessels, further jeopardizing hand viability.

A common method of arterial closure employed following cardiac catheterization utilizes a purse string suture placed around the brachial arteriotomy site. The suture is tied as the angiographic catheter is removed and may distort or narrow the brachial artery especially if it is small or the suture bites are generous (Fig 47–2B).

Several factors have been reported to be associated with an increased risk of brachial artery thrombosis following cardiac catheterization (Table 47–1). These include lengthy procedures lasting more than four hours, particularly if multiple catheter changes are required. Severe abrasion of the arterial intima is more likely to occur among women who, in general, have smaller caliber arteries. Arterial spasm probably increases the severity of intimal abrasion, although this factor is difficult to quantify. Finally, relative inexperience of the cardiac catheterization team in precise arterial closure techniques may predispose to arterial stenosis and thrombosis, especially among patients with small arteries. Surprisingly, little association has been demonstrated between the incidence of brachial thrombosis and the

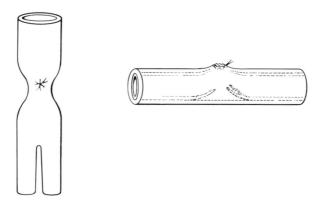

FIG 47–2.
A, Intimal injury and flap formation in the brachial artery. **B,** Stenosis of the brachial artery caused by the purse string arteriotomy closure.

TABLE 47–1.
Factors Influencing Brachial Artery
Thrombosis Following Transbrachial
Cardiac Catheterization

INFLUENTIAL
1. Length of study
2. Number of catheter changes
3. Sex of patient
4. Size of artery
5. Experience of catheterization team

NONINFLUENTIAL
1. Recatheterization
2. Cardiac output
3. Hemoglobin concentration

need for recatheterization, the presence of diminished cardiac output or hemoglobin concentrations of more than 15 mg%.

PREOPERATIVE ASSESSMENT

The diagnosis of brachial artery occlusion is usually established by the history and physical examination. In the Cleveland Clinic series, 68% of patients had no resting ischemic symptoms when a diminished or absent radial pulse was noted following cardiac catheterization. Twenty-six percent of patients described the sensation of coolness or paresthesias in the hand and only 6% had ischemic rest pain. Ninety percent had absent radial and ulnar pulses while 10% had weak collateral pulses which would disappear after forearm and hand exercise. Most patients had either cyanosis of the fingertips or pallor and poor capillary filling with elevation of the hand. On occasion, segmental Doppler arterial blood pressures and pulse volume recordings were used to document a resting or exercise-induced gradient across the brachial artery catheterization site.

Although distal brachial artery occlusion rarely causes limb threatening ischemia, many unrepaired patients will subsequently develop troublesome claudication upon resumption of normal activity. Preservation of brachial artery patency has the practical advantage of preserving radial artery inflow to facilitate subsequent radial artery catheterization for blood pressure monitoring, arterial blood gas sampling, or hemodialysis. Furthermore, the brachial artery is preserved as a site for subsequent cardiac catheterization, if necessary. Early brachial repair may also eliminate intimal injury as a potential source of irretrievable distal emboli.

Early exploration, thrombectomy and arterial repair can usually be performed under local anesthesia and is generally a technically uncomplicated procedure limited to the antecubital area with uniformly good results when performed within 24 hours of injury. Arterial spasm of clinical significance is unusual and is not easily diagnosed without angiography or exploration. The Cleveland Clinic experience has suggested that simple thrombectomy and repair alone is not usually successful if attempted more than three weeks after injury because of thrombus organization and adherence to the arterial wall. If brachial repair is inordinately delayed, more extensive reconstructions requiring arterial bypasses may be necessary.

For these reasons, it has been the practice at the Cleveland Clinic to recommend early brachial artery thrombectomy and reconstruction once the diagnosis of brachial artery thrombosis is established. Under the circumstances of extreme cardiac instability, brachial repair is deferred until the cardiac status permits safe intervention.

In the absence of indications of proximal arterial disease, the pathology is usually confined to the brachial arteriotomy site. Preoperative angiography has not been routinely obtained because the yield of useful information is usually insufficient to justify the delay required for its completion. Rarely, however, it may be necessary if the coronary angiographer suspects proximal occlusive disease or dissection because of difficulty with catheter manipulation or visualization of an intimal flap on the cine study. Furthermore, intraoperative arteriography can usually be easily obtained if indicated.

OPERATIVE MANAGEMENT

The primary objective of brachial artery repair is restoration of normal limb perfusion. The procedure is best performed in the operating room on the same day as cardiac catheterization, although it may be delayed overnight in the asymptomatic patient. Local anesthesia and careful cardiac monitoring are employed. The principal intraoperative considerations are removal of the local thrombus, establishment of adequate arterial inflow and outflow, and local repair and closure of the artery. Antibiotics are not routinely utilized and systemic heparin anticoagulation is not administered unless the patient has experienced recurrent thrombosis following a previous brachial thrombectomy.

The brachial arteriotomy is exposed through the same transverse incision utilized for cardiac catheterization and is located approximately 1 cm proximal to the elbow crease. Additional proximal or distal exposure may be obtained by longitudinal extension from the corners of the transverse incision. The brachial artery is isolated over silastic vessel loops and dissected proximally and distally to allow application of vascular clamps. Care is taken to avoid injury to the median nerve. The bicipital aponeurosis may require division to expose the distal brachial or proximal ulnar and radial arteries. The previously placed purse string suture is removed and the arteriotomy is extended transversely. Local thrombus is removed to identify the arterial lumen, and a No. 3 Fogarty embolectomy catheter, inflated with air rather than saline, is inserted proximally to recover propagated thrombus. The catheter is gently passed until brisk inflow is achieved and no further thrombus is obtained. Local anticoagulation is achieved by instilling a dilute (5 units per cc) intraarterial heparinized-saline solution prior to the application of the proximal vascular clamp. The same steps are repeated for thrombectomy and heparinization of the distal arterial segment. Individual isolation of the radial and ulnar arteries may sometimes be necessary to allow selective thrombectomy of these vessels. A No. 2 Fogarty embolectomy catheter is useful when the radial or ulnar artery is small. The catheter is gently passed until no more thrombus is recovered and back bleeding is brisk. If inflow or outflow is inadequate, an intraoperative arteriogram can be performed through the arteriotomy, although this is rarely required. Gentle dilatation of the proximal and distal brachial arterial segments may be necessary if significant arterial spasm is present, but care must be taken to avoid further intimal injury. Local papaverine solution (10 mg to 20 mg per 100 cc saline) applied to the adventitial surface of the artery may help to alleviate spasm. Local inspection of the lumen is undertaken and, if necessary, the arteriotomy is extended proximally and distally to the extent of significant intimal injury. Arterial reconstruction is carried out utilizing local repair, segmental resection with end-to-end anastomosis, or interposition vein grafting as the situation requires.

If insignificant intimal damage is present, local arteriotomy debridement and transverse closure with interrupted 6–0 or 7–0 polypropylene sutures is sufficient (Fig 47–3A).

However, if significant intimal abrasion, disruption or flap formation is observed, segmental resection of all the severely damaged intima is required. The arterial ends are spatulated to minimize stenosis along the suture line and end-to-end anastomosis is accomplished using either interrupted or running 6–0 or 7–0 polypropylene suture as required (Fig 47–3B). Usually end-to-end anastomosis can be carried out if only 1 cm to 2 cm of brachial artery requires resection. Mobilization proximally and distally with interruption of one or two small side branches, and bending the elbow slightly, may facilitate completion of the anastomosis without significant tension.

If the ends of the brachial artery cannot be approximated without excessive tension, an autogenous vein graft can be used to bridge the resulting gap (Fig 47–3C). Although cephalic vein may be locally available and adequate for this purpose, reversed saphenous vein from the lower leg usually better approximates the diameter of the brachial artery and is more substantial.

The optimal end point of brachial artery reconstruction is the recovery of a well-perfused hand with normal wrist pulses. Although restoration of both radial and ulnar pulses is preferable, the presence of either pulse has generally ensured a satisfactory result.

If the brachial artery is small, as commonly observed among female patients, has undergone rethrombosis, or exhibits extraordinary intimal damage or spasm, a continuous intravenous heparin infusion is administered postoperatively for 12 to 24 hours. Thrombolytic therapy is only rarely required to treat irretrievable, severe distal arterial thrombus and has been associated with hemorrhage from the antecubital incision.

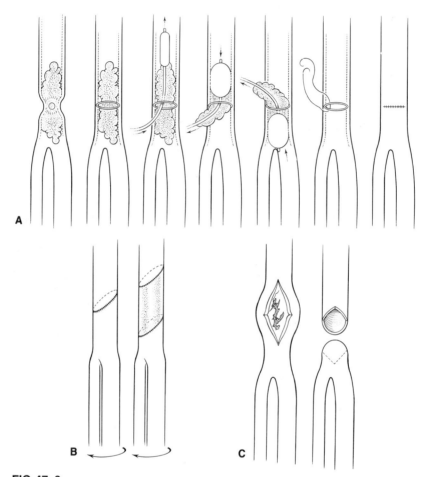

FIG 47–3.
A, Technique of brachial thrombectomy and local arterial repair utilizing transverse arteriotomy closure. **B,** If occluded brachial artery segment has severely damaged intima, the arteriotomy is extended, the injured brachial artery resected, and end-to-end reanastomosis performed. **C,** Brachial artery reconstruction utilizing end-to-end anastomosis *(left)* or an autogenous interposition graft *(right)*.

RESULTS

In the Cleveland Clinic series, 87% of patients undergoing thrombectomy and repair of brachial artery thrombosis following cardiac catheterization had successful early results. Seventy-five percent of the patients had both normal wrist pulses palpable postoperatively, whereas 12% had either a normal radial or normal ulnar pulse restored. Thirteen percent of the patients in the series experienced recurrent brachial thrombosis despite early repair, and normal pulses were restored in all 11 patients who underwent reoperation. The one patient who refused reoperation and the other patient, whose unstable cardiac status precluded safe reoperation, both experienced early claudication symptoms. Variables thought to influence the incidence of early recurrent brachial thrombosis are summarized in Table 47–2. The only statistically significant finding was the increased incidence of early rethrombosis among women, presumably related to the smaller diameter of the brachial artery.

Late follow-up (mean, 26 months) results revealed that 80% of those patients available for analysis were asymptomatic and had no signs suggestive of brachial rethrombosis, whereas 20% had symptoms or signs suggesting late reocclusion. Fifty-eight percent of these patients had symptoms of claudication or vasospasm, while 42% demonstrated an asymptomatic blood pressure discrepancy between the two arms. One patient in the series required ligation of an infected pseudoaneurysm at the brachial artery repair site but remained asymptomatic. Variables thought to influence the incidence of late recurrent brachial thrombosis are summarized in Table 47–3. A statistically significant increase in the incidence of late recurrent brachial thrombosis was demonstrated among women and among those patients who required early reoperation because of early recurrent thrombosis.

TABLE 47–2.
Variables Influencing the Incidence of Early Recurrent Brachial Thrombosis Following Brachial Thrombectomy and Repair

VARIABLE	MEN	WOMEN	P
Sex	6%	25%	<0.02
	Yes	No	
Postoperative heparin	0%	15%	N.S.
Previous catheterization	6%	14%	N.S.

TABLE 47–3.
Variables Influencing the Incidence of Late Recurrent Brachial Thrombosis Following Brachial Thrombectomy and Repair

VARIABLE	MEN	WOMEN	P
Sex	12%	35%	0.02
	Yes	No	
Preoperative heparin	7%	22%	N.S.
Previous catheterization	14%	21%	N.S.
Early reoperation	73%	13%	<0.001

SUMMARY

Brachial thrombosis following cardiac catheterization is best managed by early thrombectomy and arterial reconstruction under local anesthesia within 24 hours of the iatrogenic injury. In most instances, an early repair can be accomplished locally and can provide a durable functional result. Early operation is indicated to maintain brachial artery patency, prevent forearm claudication, provide brachial access for subsequent cardiac catheterization, allow blood pressure monitoring by means of radial artery catheterization and preserve potential forearm angioaccess sites. Experience suggests that resection of the brachial artery segment sustaining intimal damage and subsequent end-to-end anastomosis probably yields the most durable long-term result. Furthermore, intravenous heparin infusion for 12 to 24 hours following brachial reconstruction may enhance late patency rates among patients with small caliber brachial arteries.

BIBLIOGRAPHY

1. Cole CW, Machleder HI: Extremity arterial iatrogenic catheter injury, in Ernst CB, Stanley JC (eds): *Current Therapy in Vascular Surgery*. Toronto, BC Decker Inc, 1987, pp 273–276.
2. Gray H: *Anatomy of the Human Body* Goss CM (ed). Philadelphia, Lea & Febiger, 1967, pp 618–621.
3. Holleman JH, Hardy JD, Williamson JW, et al: Arterial surgery for arm ischemia: A survey of 136 patients. *Ann Surg* 1980; 191:727–737.
4. Kitzmiller JW, Hertzer NR, Beven EG: Routine surgical management of brachial artery occlusion after cardiac catheterization. *Arch Surg* 1982; 117:1066–1071.
5. McCollum CH, Mavor E: Brachial artery injury after cardiac catheterization. *J Vasc Surg* 1986; 4:355–359.
6. Mills JL, Wiedeman JE, Robison JG, et al: Minimizing mortality and morbidity from iatrogenic arterial injuries: The need for early recognition and prompt repair. *J Vasc Surg* 1986; 4:22–27.
7. Nicholas GG, DeMuth WE: Long-term results of brachial thrombectomy following cardiac catheterization. *Ann Surg* 1976; 183:436–438.
8. Orcutt MB, Levine BA, Gaskill HV, et al: Iatrogenic vascular injury. *Arch Surg* 1985; 120:384–385.
9. Ricotta JJ, Scudder PA, McAndrew JA, et al: Management of acute ischemia of the upper extremity. *Am J Surg* 1983; 145:661–666.
10. Whitehouse WM Jr: Direct revascularization for forearm and hand ischemia, in Bergan JJ, Yao JST (eds): *Evaluation and Treatment of Upper and Lower Extremity Circulatory Disorders*. Orlando, Grune & Stratton, 1984, pp 231–248.

48 Acute Leg Ischemia Secondary to Intraaortic Balloon Pump Insertion

A 67-year-old male is admitted to the coronary care unit with an acute myocardial infarction and hypotension. An intraaortic balloon pump is inserted percutaneously via the left femoral artery in an attempt to stabilize his condition, with initial benefit. Four hours later the patient complains of pain in the left foot, which is noted to be mottled and cold, and you are consulted.

Consultant: Bruce S. Cutler, M.D.

The intraaortic balloon pump (IAB) is the most widely used left ventricular assist device. Approximately 10,000 are inserted annually. It is primarily useful in two clinical situations: first, in stabilizing patients in cardiogenic shock who are refractory to pharmacological treatment following myocardial infarction and second, in weaning patients from cardiopulmonary bypass following cardiac surgery. Because of the intraarterial location of the IAB, vascular complications are not uncommon.

INCIDENCE

It is difficult to obtain an accurate estimate of complications caused by counterpulsation. Reported rates vary from 5% to 50%. Prospective series that have employed strict definitions of complications and which include both reversible and nonreversible deficits in all patients (not just survivors) have reported morbidity rates approaching 50%. Since the IAB is inserted through the femoral artery it is not surprising that limb ischemia accounts for 70% of the morbidity.

Initially, counterpulsation required surgical insertion of the IAB into the common femoral artery. Recently developed techniques for percutaneous placement have greatly simplified insertion and are now in widespread use. It was hoped that percutaneous insertion would be associated with fewer vascular complications than was the surgical method. However, two recently published prospective comparisons between the two techniques have both concluded that although the technical ease and success rate for insertion of percutaneous intraaortic balloon pumps was greater than that for open surgical methods, the incidence of vascular complications was also greater. These studies also found that the intravascular portion of the IAB was frequently covered with an adherent thrombus, and that an occlusive clot was often found in the common and superficial femoral arteries. The authors speculated that the reason for a lower complication rate in surgically removed IAB was that the thrombus encasing the IAB was removed at the time of operation. It would therefore appear that the surface of the IAB is thrombogenic and is a potential contributing factor to limb ischemia.

As mentioned earlier, counterpulsation is frequently employed when pharmacological measures fail to reverse cardiogenic shock following myocardial infarction or following cardiopulmonary bypass. In these situations, a number of factors conspire to produce limb ischemia: cardiac output and systemic blood pressure are both decreased which lowers the velocity of blood flow around the balloon; the IAB obscures most or all of the lumen of the femoral artery which may already be narrowed by atherosclerosis, thereby slowing blood flow; and lastly, in the postoperative patient anticoagulant and antiplatelet drugs are discontinued and fresh blood products including platelets are frequently administered to promote hemostasis. In light of the foregoing, it is surprising that ischemic complications are not the *inevitable* consequence of counterpulsation.

RISK FACTORS

It is useful to know which clinical factors are most likely to be associated with complications of IAB therapy. Using multivariant analysis, Gottlieb, et al, found that the female gender and a history of peripheral vascular disease were the most significant predictors. Other studies have confirmed that the incidence of complications in women may be as high as 32%, prompting the theory that disproportionately small arteries for body size may be a sex-linked characteristic. Other risk factors of significance are insulin dependent diabetes and a history of hypertension. Surprisingly, neither the indication for counterpulsation, its duration, nor the age of the patient influence the incidence of complications. Although the physician cannot have the luxury of selecting patients who are free of the above mentioned risk factors, knowledge of them does provide a basis for recommending earlier catheterization and surgery in patients in whom they are present.

MONITORING CIRCULATION

Limb ischemia may develop at any time after placement of IAB. It is therefore crucial that the peripheral circulation be objectively monitored on a regular basis and that the observations be recorded for later comparison. Such observations may be easily overlooked in the patient requiring intensive treatment for cardiogenic shock. Frequent vascular assessment is particularly important in the patient who is heavily sedated or unconscious since such a patient cannot complain of ischemic rest pain.

In the cooperative patient, the preservation of peripheral pulses, normal motion, and sensation is assurance that peripheral perfusion is adequate. In practice, however, pedal pulses are frequently absent following IAB insertion. In this case it is important to obtain an ankle pressure using a portable ultrasonic flow detector (Doppler) and to calculate the ankle/arm index. Indices greater than 0.4 combined with normal motion and sensation indicate adequate peripheral perfusion. When arterial signals are no longer audible at the ankle by Doppler (corresponding to an ankle/arm index less than 0.3) severe ischemia is present and will lead to tissue necrosis, if not promptly reversed.

MANAGEMENT

Acute limb ischemia may occur at any time after initiation of counterpulsation. However, it is most likely to occur at one of the three following times: immediately after placement of IAB; following decreases in cardiac output, especially if accompanied by increases in inotropic support; and immediately postoperatively. Some degree of ischemia occurs in many patients during counterpulsation and is well tolerated and reversible when the IAB is removed. Therefore, the initial management of limb ischemia, particularly if it appears to be mild, is conservative (Fig 48–1). Improvements in cardiac output, systemic blood pressure, and weaning from alpha adrenergic agents such as epinephrine or Levophed will often improve pe-

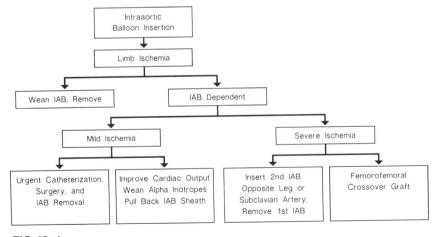

FIG 48–1.
Algorithm of patient management.

ripheral circulation. Sliding the insertion sheath back, out of the femoral artery, may also improve perfusion past the catheter.

Severe ischemia is indicated by the absence of an arterial signal at the ankle by Doppler examination and requires active intervention. The patient with ischemic heart disease should be considered for urgent cardiac catheterization and coronary revascularization, with plans to rapidly wean and remove the IAB after surgery. If coronary angiography and surgery are not indicated or feasible, or if the ischemia is sufficiently severe that the circulation must be improved promptly to prevent tissue necrosis, transfer of the IAB to the opposite limb is the most expeditious solution in the IAB dependent patient. Even if ischemia subsequently develops on the second side, it may "buy enough time" to establish adequate pharmacologic support of the circulation to proceed with cardiac catheterization and surgery. Ischemia of the second side is most likely to occur in females with preexisting peripheral vascular disease.

If IAB transfer to the opposite side is not desirable or is unsuccessful, a femorofemoral crossover graft may be used to restore peripheral perfusion. This procedure employs an extraanatomic bypass graft from the contralateral common femoral to the ipsilateral superficial femoral artery. The femorofemoral graft can be performed in the intensive care unit under local anesthesia, but the procedure is more easily performed and the infection rate is lower if carried out in the operating room. Although a relatively minor procedure, it may require one to two hours to perform and may be poorly tolerated by the unstable patient. The procedure is highly successful in restoring limb circulation, and the graft may be left in place when the IAB is removed.

Femoral insertion of the IAB is not possible due to aortoiliac disease in approximately 3% of patients. Although there have been reports of successful placement of IAB via the subclavian or axillary artery, the experience with this technique is so limited that it must be considered experimental at the present time. Intraaortic balloons have also been inserted directly into the aortic arch or in the abdominal aorta through a retroperitoneal incision. These routes require a surgical procedure for both insertion and removal. As a result, these approaches are usually reserved for patients with severe aortoiliac disease who require counterpulsation for separation from cardiopulmonary bypass. The final option for the balloon dependent patient is to accept the possibility of future amputation and to leave the device in place. Usually this choice is made only in the patient whose chances for survival are considered to be extremely poor.

It is important to recognize that toxic end products of anaerobic metabolism may be released into the systemic circulation from an ischemic limb following reperfusion. This is most likely to occur from a limb that has advanced ischemia as evidenced by anesthesia, muscle rigor, and absent ankle Doppler signals for an hour or more. Hyperkalemia and acidosis can occur within seconds of restoration of circulation and may lead to ventricular arrythmia or cardiac arrest. Rhabdomyolysis from ischemic muscle releases free myoglobin into the circulation that can cause acute renal failure. Intravenous hydration and alkalinization, together with prompt and aggressive debridement or amputation of dead tissue may be necessary to preserve life under these circumstances.

CONCLUSIONS AND RECOMMENDATIONS

At our institution, the vascular surgical service monitors the peripheral circulation of all patients during counterpulsation. The vascular service assesses the peripheral circulation prior to IAB placement and under most circumstances, recommends that the IAB be placed in the limb with the best peripheral perfusion. Thereafter, the peripheral circulation is periodically monitored both clinically and by Doppler ankle/arm indices. In the presence of ischemia, the vascular surgical service works with both cardiology and cardiac surgery to establish the best strategy for restoring peripheral circulation.

Because of the intraarterial location of the IAB, some degree of vascular compromise is the inevitable consequence of counterpulsation. The incidence of severe complications such as foot drop, ischemic neuritis, and amputation can be minimized by limiting the use of counterpulsation to well-accepted indications, by using meticulous insertion technique and by careful monitoring of limb circulation following implantation.

BIBLIOGRAPHY

1. Alderman JD, Gabliani GI, McCabe CH, et al: Incidence and management of limb ischemia with percutaneous wire-guided intraaortic balloon catheters. *JACC* 1987; 9:524–530.
2. Collier PE, Liebler GA, Park SB, et al: Is percutaneous insertion of the intra-aortic balloon pump through the femoral artery the safest technique? *J Vasc Surg* 1986; 3:629–634.
3. Cutler BS: The intraaortic balloon and counterpulsation, in Rippe JM, et al (eds): *Intensive Care Medicine.* Boston, Little, Brown & Co, 1985, pp 104–114.
4. Friedell MK, Alpert J, Parsonnet V, et al: Femorofemoral grafts for lower limb ischemia caused by intra-aortic balloon pump. *J Vasc Surg* 1987; 5:180–186.
5. Gold JP, Cohen J, Shemin RJ, et al: Femorofemoral bypass to relieve acute leg ischemia during intra-aortic balloon pump cardiac support. *J Vasc Surg* 1986; 3:351–354.
6. Goldberg JM, Rubenfire M, Kantrowitz A, et al: Intraaortic balloon pump insertion: A randomized study comparing percutaneous and surgical techniques. *JACC* 1987; 9:515–523.
7. Gottlieb SO, Brinker JA, Borkon AM, et al: Identification of patients at high risk for complications of intraaortic balloon counterpulsation: A multivariate risk factor analysis. *Am J Cardiol* 1984; 53:1135–1139.
8. Kantrowitz A, Wasfie T, Freed PS, et al: Intraaortic balloon pumping 1967 through 1982: Analysis of complications in 733 patients. *Am J Cardiol* 1986; 57:976–983.
9. Todd GJ, Breman D, Voorhees AB, et al: Vascular complications associated with percutaneous intra-aortic balloon pumping. *Surgery* 1983; 118:963–964.

PART FIVE

Venous

49   Symptomatic Venous Varicosities

A 37-year-old hairdresser is seen in the office for varicose veins. These have been present for 15 years, slowly enlarging in size. She complains increasingly of their appearance and burning discomfort and aching in the legs at work. Examination reveals moderate superficial varicosities of both thighs, as well as medial and posterior aspects of both calves.

Consultant: David S. Sumner, M.D.

This case presentation is typical of many patients who come to the vascular surgeon seeking advice concerning the treatment of varicose veins. It is likely that her varicosities are of the primary variety—that is, they are not associated with deep venous disease.

ETIOLOGY

Despite years of research, the etiology of primary varicose veins continues to be debated. One theory holds that they develop in response to the thrust of blood from incompetent perforating veins. Another suggests that they are caused by multiple small arteriovenous fistulae. A third theory attributes venous enlargement to increased compliance of the venous wall, which in pregnant patients may represent a hormonal influence. Thus, the frequent onset of varicose veins during pregnancy is logically explained by the combination of increased venous compliance and increased lower limb venous pressure caused by extrinsic compression by the gravid uterus. A final theory attributes varicose veins to the congenital absence of functioning valves in the common femoral or more proximal veins. When the subject stands, coughs, or strains the full weight of the column of blood from the right atrium to the groin impinges on the valve at the upper end of the greater saphenous vein; with time the vein stretches and the valve becomes incompetent. This process is repeated in serial fashion down the leg until all of the greater saphenous valves become incompetent. As a result, the superficial tributaries of the saphenous vein are subjected to increased pressure; their valves become incompetent; and they assume the characteristics of varicose veins. The observations that varicose veins are hereditary and that they are aggravated by prolonged standing are consistent with the descending valvular imcompetence theory. None of the hypotheses are completely satisfactory. Since they are not mutually exclusive, it is probable that more than one mechanism plays a role.

Secondary varicose veins represent enlarged collateral channels that develop in response to deep venous valvular incompetence, a condition that may be postthrombotic, congenital, or of unknown etiology. Much less frequently, traumatic or congenital arteriovenous fistulae are responsible for the appearance of secondary varicosities, the superficial venous channels having expanded to accommodate the increased blood flow. Developmental abnormalities of the venous system, such as the Klippel-Trenaunay syndrome, are relatively rare causes of varicose veins.

PATHOPHYSIOLOGY

Because of the absence of functioning valves in the superficial veins, some of the blood forced upward during calf muscle contraction refluxes down the superficial system when the leg relaxes, entering the deep system through perforating veins. This creates an inefficient recirculation of blood within the leg. The normal reduction in ambulatory venous pressure is not observed; and, with relaxation, pressures quickly return to preexercise levels. Since resting venous pressures are largely determined by the length of the hydrostatic column of blood to the heart, average pressures in venous varicosities exceed those normally observed in superficial veins. This, coupled with increased venous capacity, results in an increased volume of blood in the dependent portions of the extremity and may explain why patients with varicose veins often complain of aching, swelling, and heaviness of the legs. It also explains why elevation of the legs and elastic stockings afford relief.

Although limbs manifesting venous stasis changes in the gaiter area (pigmentation, induration, and ulceration) commonly have varicose veins as well, the reverse is seldom true. Stasis changes are rare in the absence of concomitant incompetence of the deep or perforating veins. Primary varicose veins are (in my experience) a benign condition. Even patients with massive, rope-like varicosities may have no symptoms, little edema, and normal skin. Complications, such as superficial venous thrombosis and bleeding, do occur; but they are rarely serious.

HISTORY AND PHYSICAL EXAMINATION

In the initial workup of a patient with varicose veins, the surgeon should attempt to ascertain the etiology (primary or secondary), identify the involved veins, and determine whether the condition is actually responsible for the symptoms. Onset following an operation or trauma or a history of deep venous thrombosis, severe edema, pigmentation, or ulceration strongly suggests the secondary variety. On the other hand, a long history of varicose veins that have gradually increased in size with little or no skin changes, a positive family history, and an onset during pregnancy points toward the primary variety. When there has been a previous attempt at therapy, it is important to find out what was done (ligation, stripping, or sclerotherapy) and whether the procedure was initially successful. An initially satisfactory result implies that the treatment focused on the underlying pathology and supports the diagnosis of primary varicose veins. A poor result suggests secondary varicose veins.

Patients often complain of pain, burning, aching, or swelling. If the symptoms are increased by standing and relieved by elevation or elastic support, it is likely that varicose veins are indeed the culprit. Complications, such as superficial thrombophlebitis or bleeding from an eroded varix, may be reported and are consistent with primary varicose veins.

Careful inspection and palpation of the limbs is most informative. The presence of severe edema, induration, stasis pigmentation, or ulceration suggests associated deep venous disease. Palpable "cords" just under the skin confirm the history of previous superficial thrombophlebitis. Defects in the fascia may identify sites of incompetent perforating veins. With the patient standing, the location of the varicosities is noted. Those distributed along the medial aspect of the thigh and calf are usually related to incompetence of the greater saphenous vein; whereas those located on the posterior-lateral aspect of the calf implicate incompetence of the lesser saphenous vein. Although they are seldom visible, palpation in these cases frequently reveals a dilated greater or lesser saphenous vein. Varicosities beginning in the upper posterior-medial thigh communicate with pudendal or obturator veins and are a manifestation of pelvic venous incompetence. They usually extend downward and laterally across the back of the thigh.

While other more complicated examinations, such as the Trendelenberg and Perthes tests, may be performed, they are often difficult to interpret and are being replaced by noninvasive evaluation.

OBJECTIVE TESTS

Noninvasive tests serve two major purposes: to detect deep venous disease and to determine the location of superficial venous incompetence. This information is helpful, not only for planning a rational therapeutic approach, but also for predicting the patient's prognosis.

A brief but carefully performed survey of the limbs with the Doppler flow detector usually provides sufficient information. Absence of flow or departures from the normal spontaneous or augmented flow patterns in the deep veins is indicative of previous deep venous thrombosis. Reflux in the superficial femoral, popliteal, or posterior tibial veins, detected when the limb is compressed or when the patient performs a Valsalva maneuver, is diagnostic of deep venous incompetence. Reflux in the common femoral vein is found in about 15% of otherwise normal limbs and is commonly detected in limbs with primary varicose veins—especially in association with incompetence of the greater saphenous vein. The greater saphenous vein should be examined in the thigh and calf, both in the supine and standing positions. Even when varicosities are in the appropriate distribution, the entire greater saphenous vein is involved in only 65% of the limbs. In about 25%, the below-knee saphenous vein remains competent; and in others, all or part of the above-knee saphenous vein may be competent. Similarly, the lesser saphenous vein should be studied to establish its competence, especially in legs with varicosities of the posterior calf. This examination is facilitiated by the use of a duplex scanner, which permits signals arising from the popliteal vein to be distinguished from those arising from the closely approximated lesser saphenous vein with greater accuracy than is possible with the Doppler alone.

The photoplethysmograph (PPG) can be used to measure the time required for cutaneous veins at the ankle level to refill with blood following calf muscle exercise. With the patient sitting, venous refilling times (VRT) exceed 20 seconds in legs with competent veins. Since the VRT will be abnormally short when either the superficial or distal deep system is incompetent, it is necessary to repeat the test, compressing the superficial veins with tourniquets applied to the thigh, upper calf, and ankle. Normalization of the VRT with the thigh tourniquet indicates incompetence of the greater saphenous vein; with the calf tourniquet, incompetence of the lesser saphenous vein; and with the ankle tourniquet, incompetence of the perforating veins. Failure to attain a normal VRT with the tourniquet at the ankle implies deep venous incompetence.

Phlebograms are not a part of the routine workup of patients with varicose veins. They may, however, be helpful for establishing the presence of deep venous disease when noninvasive tests are equivocal and for locating incompetent perforating veins. Because the anatomy of the lesser saphenous vein in the popliteal fossa is so variable, some surgeons advocate intraoperative phlebography when this vein is to be removed.

MANAGEMENT

It is likely that the patient whose case is being considered has incompetence of the greater saphenous vein, both in the calf and thigh, and possibly lesser saphenous incompetence as well. This is suggested by the distribution of the varices. Although she has symptoms which are compatible with varicose veins, the varicosities are not large. Since no skin changes are mentioned, it is probable that there is no associated deep venous incompetence. There are four general approaches to her problem:

(1) *Do nothing at all.* After all, she has had the condition for 15 years and the risk of her developing significant complications is slight. In fact, if she were

asymptomatic, this approach would be entirely reasonable. Certainly, if the patient were elderly, had a limited life expectancy, or had other problems that would make treatment hazardous, therapy limited to elevation of the legs and skin care would be the treatment of choice. It must be remembered that varicose veins are benign; there is no associated mortality and no major morbidity. Moreover, they can be treated at any time.

(2) *Elastic support.* Wearing good quality, properly fitted, elastic support stockings that provide graded compression from the ankle to the knee, will in most cases afford relief of symptoms. Unless the varicosities above the knee are symptomatic, there is no need for a long-leg or leotard-type stocking. Patients with no cosmetic concerns who do not object to wearing elastic stockings may prefer this method of treatment. They are appreciative of the relief provided by stockings and are content to wear them indefinitely. The only disadvantages of this approach are the expense of replacing the stockings and the trouble involved in putting them on and keeping them clean.

(3) *Sclerotherapy.* Injecting a sclerosing agent to obliterate the venous lumen has proved to be an effective treatment for small isolated varices; but recurrences are more frequent than with surgery and the method is not applicable when varices are large and extensive. The procedure is technically demanding, requiring the services of an experienced sclerotherapist to achieve good results. Intravenous clots and staining of the skin may occur, both of which compromise the cosmetic result. Although complications are uncommon, they can be serious. These include allergic reactions, gangrene following inadvertent arterial injection, peripheral nerve injection with associated pain, and ascending thrombophlebitis. The requirement that the legs be bandaged for two to six weeks and the fact that injections may have to be repeated on several occasions to completely eradicate the varices are relative disadvantages of sclerotherapy.

(4) *Surgery.* High ligation and stripping of the saphenous veins and all superficial varicosities is the most effective and enduring treatment for varicose veins. Removal of major incompetent veins interrupts the hydrostatic column that predisposes to dilatation of the superficial veins; thus, the premise on which this mode of therapy is based is physiologically sound. Most recurrences are due to incomplete ligation of tributary veins at the saphenofemoral or saphenopopliteal junction or represent varicosities that were overlooked at the time of operation. Some, however, are unavoidable since it is impossible to eradicate all possible communications with incompetent pelvic veins. Although recurrences are a nuisance, they are not serious or threatening in any way (we are not dealing with cancer or preventing limb loss); and they can usually be treated as an outpatient with a limited operation or sclerotherapy. Enthusiasm for radical surgery should be tempered by these considerations. Furthermore, to achieve good results, it is necessary to excise only those veins or portions of veins that are demonstrably incompetent. In many cases, removal of the entire saphenous vein is not required. The desire to preserve the saphenous vein for use as a graft in coronary artery or peripheral vascular opera-

tions has prompted a more conservative approach to varicose vein surgery. While this has—perhaps more than anything else—served to decrease the number of unnecessary varicose vein operations and has encouraged the development of more limited procedures, it must be remembered that a truly dilated varicosed saphenous vein is an unsuitable conduit for arterial revascularization. Thus, there is no reason to avoid removal of grossly involved veins. There are many advantages to surgical therapy and few disadvantages. Properly performed, it is safe, effective, and expeditious. Symptoms are relieved, cosmetic results are excellent, and elastic support is no longer required.

Before deciding on a plan of management, the surgeon should determine what aspects of the condition are perceived as most troublesome. Is the primary concern cosmesis, symptoms, or potential complications? Many patients, unfortunately, have received conflicting information from friends, magazine articles, TV or radio, or even other physicians regarding the etiology, prognosis, and optimal management of the condition. They may have heard tales of ulcers, phlebitis, and of clots going to the lungs or heart. Having no firm concept of the difference between arteries and veins, patients may even confuse diseases of the two systems. They may have acquaintances with "poor circulation" who have lost legs to gangrene. Some may be apprehensive that removal of veins will compromise limb blood flow and will deprive them of veins that might be needed in the future, should a coronary bypass be required.

It is the duty, therefore, of the vascular surgeon to understand the patient's concerns, to explain the nature of the disease, to erase popular misconceptions, and to offer alternative forms of therapy. Although the patient whose case is being discussed could elect to embark on any of the plans of management previously outlined, I would favor the surgical approach. Since she is symptomatic, young, presumably healthy, and working on her feet, doing nothing is not an attractive option. Having to wear elastic stockings for the rest of her working life would not only be inconvenient but would also be expensive. Sclerotherapy would not be applicable to the thigh varicosities and the calf veins might require repeated injections. Ligation and stripping of the varicose veins, on the other hand, should be well tolerated and allow her to return to work quickly without the need for repeated therapy or elastic support.

OPERATION

The surgeon should tailor the operation precisely to the pathophysiology, removing only those portions of the saphenous veins that are demonstrably incompetent. A carefully designed operation will be sufficiently delicate to ensure a pleasing cosmetic result, yet thorough enough to minimize recurrences and alleviate symptoms. When the upper part of the saphenous vein is involved, the incision is made above and parallel to the skin fold at the groin, beginning about 2 cm lateral and an equal distance distal to the pubic tubercle and extending laterally for about 5 cm. This incision, which lies directly over the saphenofemoral junction in the pubic hair region, not only provides excellent access to the tributary veins but also has the added advantage of being covered by a bikini. Prior to operation, the surgeon must carefully mark the skin overlying all superficial varices, tracing out their entire course with indelible ink. A No. 11 knife blade is used to make multiple short (2 mm to 3 mm) longitudinal incisions over the marked varicosities. (Longitudinal incisions cause less scarring than horizontal incisions.) The underlying vein is grasped with the tip of a fine mosquito clamp, pulled to the surface, and with a combination of traction, spreading, and rolling of the vein on the clamp, as much length as possible is extracted. No attempt is made to ligate the varicosities; they are simply avulsed. The incisions are closed with steristrips or one or two 5–0 nylon sutures. With the leg elevated, elastic bandages are applied firmly but with diminishing pressure from the base of the toes to the upper thigh. If the varices are bilateral but not too extensive, both legs may be operated on at the same time; otherwise, they are best treated on separate occasions.

The patient is kept at strict bedrest in the Trendelenberg position overnight. On the following morning, dressings are removed and replaced with simple gauze sponges. Elastic bandages are reapplied to the lower leg only; the patient is discharged and instructed to rewrap the leg at least twice a day. Normal activities are permitted but no strenuous exercise is allowed. The sutures are removed in one week. Unless there is some edema, no further elastic support is required, and within a few months, the scars become almost invisible.

SUMMARY

Although primary varicose veins may be cosmetically unappealing and cause mild symptoms, the condition is benign and seldom associated with significant complications. Treatment should be based on these considerations and on the patient's perception of his or her disability. Elastic support or sclerotherapy often suffice, but surgical therapy, limited to excision of incompetent veins, is more expeditious, more effective, and, in the long run, less expensive.

BIBLIOGRAPHY

1. Hobbs JT: A new approach to short saphenous vein varicosities, in: Bergan JJ and Yao JST (eds): *Surgery of the Veins*. Orlando, Grune & Stratton, 1985, pp 301–321.
2. Hobbs JT: Can we prevent recurrence of varicose veins? in: Greenhalgh RM, Jamieson CW, and Nicolaides AN (eds): *Vascular surgery: Issues in Current Practice*, Grune & Stratton, 1986, pp 355–373.
3. Koyano K, Sakaguchi S: Selective stripping operation based on Doppler ultrasound findings, in: Sakaguchi S (ed): *Advances in Phlebology 86*. London, John Libbey & Co Ltd, 1987, pp 165–167.

4. Large J: Surgical treatment of saphenous varices, with preservation of the main great saphenous trunk. *J Vasc Surg* 1985; 2:886–891.
5. Ludbrook J: Primary great saphenous varicose veins revisited. *World J Surg* 1986; 10:954–958.
6. Moore DJ, Himmel PD, Sumner DS: Distribution of venous valvular incompetence in patients with the postphlebitic syndrome. *J Vasc Surg* 1986; 3:49–57.
7. Munn SR, Morton JB, Macbeth WAAG, et al: To strip or not to strip the long saphenous vein? A varicose vein trial. *Br J Surg* 1981; 68:426–428.

50   Acute Superficial Thrombophlebitis

A 48-year-old man is seen for a three-day history of increasing pain and redness of the medial knee region. He has had modest varicose veins in the leg for years, without symptoms. Examination reveals erythema and induration in the upper calf in the region of several varicosities, and a tender cord extending several centimeters above the knee in the presumed location of the saphenous vein.

Consultant: John D. Corson, M.B., Ch.B., F.R.C.S.(Eng.), F.A.C.S.

DISCUSSION

The case described is a classic example of acute superficial thrombophlebitis. This is a clinical entity that is much neglected, poorly understood and often mismanaged, despite the fact that superficial thrombophlebitis is a common complication of older patients with varicose veins. Other less common causes of thrombophlebitis in superficial veins include direct mechanical or chemical trauma, ionizing radiation, bacterial or fungal infections, blood dyscrasias, and immune reactions.

Treatment of this classic case is dependent on several factors which include the proximal extent of the thrombotic process, the state of the superficial and deep veins, the number of previous episodes of phlebitis, and the general health and ambulatory status of the individual.

VARICOSE VEINS AND SUPERFICIAL THROMBOPHLEBITIS

Varicose veins are a common affliction of our civilized society and are thought to affect at least one in five females and one in fifteen males over the age of 45 years. A frequent and bothersome complication of this condition is acute superficial thrombophlebitis which develops following minor trauma to a superficial varix. Although it appears inflammatory in nature, there is no infectious basis for its development. Following the initiating trauma to the vein, a thrombophlebitis develops. The thrombus formed at that site rapidly becomes adherent to the vein wall.

341

More proximally, a tail of thrombus may form that initially is not adherent to the vein wall for several days. This thrombus may extend five to ten centimeters proximal to the site of inflammation of the vein. Hence, there may be a clinically obvious area of acute superficial thrombophlebitis with a silent tail of phlebothrombosis extending more proximally. This tail of thrombus may propagate more proximally either extending into the deep venous system by overflowing at the juncture of the superficial vein within the deep system, or by propagation through perforating veins, or it may break loose and embolize to the lungs. Although rare, there are several documented cases of fatal pulmonary emboli associated with acute superficial thrombophlebitis without deep venous thrombosis. Hence, there remains a real need to emphasize that acute superficial thrombophlebitis of primary varicose veins may have all the dire sequelae of thrombosis in the deep venous system including the potential for pulmonary emboli. In addition, due to destruction of the valves of thrombosed perforating veins, there is a similar potential for postphlebitic ulcerative sequelae due to the superficial venous hypertension in the lower leg.

Occasionally, patients will develop an episode of superficial thrombophlebitis in collateral veins that have developed around an occlusion of a major vein. A good example of this is a patient whom we recently saw who had developed an axillary vein thrombosis following a Saturday night alcoholic binge and who had two subsequent episodes of superficial thrombophlebitis in the collateral veins on his anterior chest wall. It was learned that he traumatized these veins at work when he used an air hammer pressed against the involved shoulder.

Presentation and Diagnosis

Superficial thrombophlebitis is a frequent complication of varicose veins associated with pregnancy. Postpartum, there is usually spontaneous and prompt resolution of the problem. In a similar manner, much of the problem associated with acute superficial thrombophlebitis will depend on the severity of the underlying varicose vein process.

The long saphenous vein is more frequently involved with superficial thrombophlebitis than is the short saphenous vein. However, the veins below the knee are involved more frequently than those above the knee. Due to the superficial nature of the disease process, the entity is usually easy to diagnose. There is an erythematous, tender, easily palpable cord with associated swelling along the longitudinal axis of the involved vein segment. Proximal to that point, the vein appears normal by palpation. In the thigh area there may be quite marked swelling along the medial aspect overlying the long saphenous vein. In a lean thigh the diagnosis is not difficult since the tender cord is easily palpated. In obese limbs, however, the entity may be confused with an underlying cellulitis. Lymphadenitis and lymphadenopathy are not associated features of thrombophlebitis. A leukocytosis is rarely present with acute superficial thrombophlebitis and, if present, is frequently associated with a coincidental infectious process, such as a urinary tract infection. A mild febrile response, however, is common in acute superficial thrombophlebitis.

The presence of ankle edema should alert one to the possibility of deep venous thrombosis. The presence of erythema nodosum, nodular vasculitis, various manifestations of panniculitis, insect bites, and foreign body trauma all may serve to confuse the examining physician. When the diagnosis is in doubt, a biopsy of the lesion may provide invaluable information.

Although the diagnosis can usually be made clinically, I feel all patients with acute superficial thrombophlebitis should also be evaluated in the vascular laboratory by noninvasive venous tests. The purpose of these studies is to define the proximal extent of thrombus in the superficial system and to determine any involvement of the deep venous system from associated or propagated thrombus. B-mode imaging is valuable in determining the level of thrombus in the superficial veins (Figs 50–1A and 50–1B) and also in defining the status of the deep veins. We perform complementary venous Doppler studies in association with a standard venous duplex study. Patients with negative studies of the deep system who have documented superficial thrombophlebitis are restudied serially to determine any superficial propagation and confirm the absence of any significant deep venous thrombi. Only with very equivocal results from noninvasive studies is ascending venography required.

Treatment

Ambulatory Nonsurgical Treatment   Ambulatory patients without evidence of deep venous thrombosis and no clot extension to the midthigh can usually be treated nonoperatively. The inflamed area is treated symptomatically with local heat either from an electric pad or with warm wet towels. A firm compression bandage should be applied to the involved leg and the patient is encouraged to ambulate as much as possible. When recumbent, the leg should be elevated 20 cm to ensure optimal venous drainage. Although anti-inflammatory agents such as Phenylbutazone have been recommended for the management of this entity for many years, the data supporting their use appear lacking. Some authorities use aspirin for both its analgesic and its antiplatelet effect.

When first seen, the upper limits of the area of thrombophlebitis should be clearly marked on the leg and the patient instructed to return if proximal migration occurs. It is advisable to reexamine the patient after a couple of days to check for proximal extension. Proximal migration and the presence of clot above the midthigh level may necessitate an urgent surgical approach.

Routine anticoagulants have no place in the management of ambulatory patients with acute superficial thrombophlebitis. Hence these patients can easily be managed on an outpatient basis. However, patients with underlying deep venous thrombobosis should be treated as inpatients with conventional anticoagulation utilizing intravenous heparin initially followed by oral Coumadin therapy.

Ambulatory Surgical Outpatient Treatment   In Europe many of these problems are managed in the acute phase using local anesthesia and incising

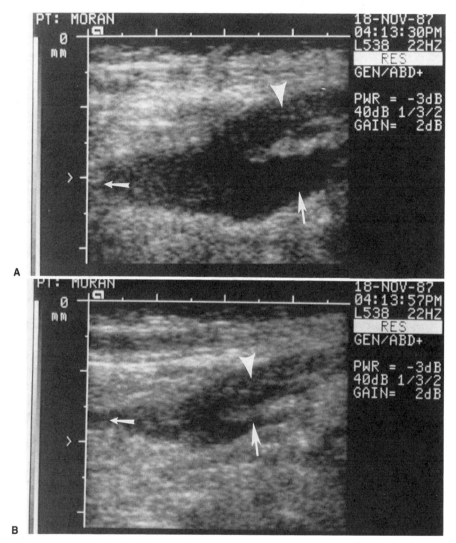

FIG 50–1.
This elderly white female with polycythemia presented with superficial thrombophlebitis of the lower leg. The patient's head is to the left. **A,** Duplex venous studies at the popliteal level demonstrate thrombus in the short saphenous vein (arrowhead). Thrombus extends into the popliteal vein. **B,** The large white arrow clearly shows normal compression of the distal popliteal vein, but no compression of the proximal popliteal vein or short saphenous vein.

with a No. 11 blade over the acutely phlebitic vein, expressing or extracting the clot manually. The leg is then wrapped with a compression bandage and the patient is managed on an outpatient basis. Underlying residual varicosities are treated electively at a later date. This approach has not been a common practice in the United States but would seem to have a place in those patients who have minimal varicosities for surgical management, and who present in the acute phase. Such incisional treatment would be similar to that of treating an acute thrombosed external hemorrhoid surgically.

Surgical Inpatient Treatment   A surgical approach is usually reserved for patients who demonstrate proximal propagation of clot into the deep venous system or who have evidence of clot migrating past the midthigh area. In the case of acute superficial thrombophlebitis of the long saphenous vein, the saphenofemoral junction is exposed in order to isolate the thrombosed segment. The saphenous vein is divided flush with the common femoral vein following removal of any thrombus extending into the deep system. This propagation may occur in up to one third of such operated cases. The deep vein may have, on occasion, to be controlled to ensure safe and complete extraction of any contained thrombus without embolization. Clot extending up the short saphenous vein toward the popliteal vein may require a similar aggressive surgical approach to prevent clot spilling over into the popliteal vein.

Selected patients who for other reasons cannot be heparinized, but who have associated clot in the deep system distally, may require superficial femoral vein ligation to protect against embolization. This would be an uncommon circumstance.

The best results following the surgical management of acute superficial thrombophlebitis are obtained by high saphenofemoral ligation and radical excision of the affected varicose veins. The involved phlebitic vein segment is excised or stripped along with any associated varices. The removal of the thrombosed vein segment shortens the convalescence and mitigates against later recurrence. Up to 14% of patients who undergo varicose vein surgery have some previous ongoing problem related to superficial thrombophlebitis which, frequently, has not resolved 30 days after its presentation.

Patients who have had previous episodes of superficial thrombophlebitis and who have underlying varicose veins should have surgical management of their varicose veins, with removal of the involved phlebitic segment. The incidence of recurrent superficial thrombophlebitis after this procedure is less than 4%.

There is some controversy in the literature regarding the prophylactic use of anticoagulants in patients undergoing varicose vein surgery who have had a previous venous thrombotic event process. Usually we would not give prophylactic anticoagulants to such patients, but would encourage rapid postoperative active ambulation and early discharge from the hospital. Others have suggested prophylactic anticoagulation for all patients undergoing varicose vein surgery who have had a previous venous thromboembolic event. We reserve anticoagulation only for that group who we find at operation to have an adherent clot in the deep veins.

ACUTE SUPERFICIAL THROMBOPHLEBITIS WITHOUT VARICOSE VEINS

Acute superficial thrombophlebitis in the absence of varicose veins has a more sinister connotation, as these episodes are more frequently associated with deep venous thrombosis in up to 25% of cases and also because they are associated with other significant lesions. In the paraneoplastic syndrome, which commonly presents in the older patient, the phlebitic event may antedate the more serious pathology by several years. In the classic example of thrombophlebitis migrans a short segment of superficial vein, often on the arm, becomes phlebitic and resolves and is frequently followed by a similar episode in a different area a month or two later. The malignancies associated with the paraneoplastic syndrome are usually mucin-secreting tumors and the majority involve the body and tail of the pancreas. Other malignancies have been reported with this entity including gastric, breast, lung, colon, ovary, prostate, and gallbladder cancer. In addition, it may be seen with myeloproliferative disorders and blood dyscrasias, as well as collagen vascular disease, sarcoid, secondary syphilis, typhoid and Ricketsiosis. Patients with severe dehydration from sepsis due to pneumonia, tonsillitis or severe viral episodes may also develop thrombophlebitis. Historically, gouty phlebitis was a condition of concern at the turn of the century. When varicose veins are not present, one should search carefully for some other pathology and look very carefully for thrombosis in the deep veins.

Behcet's Syndrome   Superficial thrombophlebitis is a common presentation of this syndrome which has other vascular manifestations including Budd-Chiari and arterial aneurysm formation. The phlebitic lesions appear as crops of hard indurated cordlike lesions on any site of the body. They may be linear or oval in shape. The syndrome, first reported in 1887, consists of recurrent orogenital ulcers associated with relapsing iritis. It is a chronic multisystem disease with a relapsing course. The etiology is unknown and the diagnosis is made on a clinical basis supported by the finding of HLA B5 antigen. Phenformin and ethylestronol may be useful in controlling the thrombophlebitis in this syndrome.

Buerger's Disease (Thromboangiitis Obliterans)   Stricter diagnostic criteria have limited the diagnosis of this entity in the United States over the past few decades; however, in Japan, it appears to be a more common vascular problem. It can be defined as a segmental obliterative disease of small- and medium-size arteries of the extremities, predominantly affecting young adults who smoke cigarettes. It involves an associated inflammation of the arteries and veins. Up to 10% of reported cases are not noted to be female. Jewish people seem to be affected more frequently. Approximately one third of cases present with recurring migratory superficial thrombophlebitis. The acute symptoms in the veins last seven to 18 days, and veins of the upper or lower extremities may be involved. Short segments of vein are frequently involved and often these are tributary veins of the dorsum of the hand, wrist, or foot.

wrist, or foot. Hence, focal and episodal bouts of thrombophlebitis in young people who smoke cigarettes should arouse suspicion of Buerger's disease and mandate the cessation of cigarettes smoking while the diagnosis is being clarified. Biopsy of the involved vein shows perivenous and venous inflammation as opposed to the bland thrombosis found in patients with the paraneoplastic syndrome.

Mondor's Disease   This clinical curiosity appears to be an acute superficial thrombophlebitis of the thoracoepigastric veins and their branches. It may be induced by trauma or possibly lymphatic infection. It more commonly affects females but is also found in males. Diagnosis is made by the finding of a palpable inflamed cord over the involved vein. No specific treatment is required and the entity is self-limiting. Its importance lies in the fact that it may simulate a significant underlying pleuro-pulmonary disease.

Hypercoagulable States   Thrombocythemic and polycythemic patients have a higher incidence of thrombotic events, as do patients with antithrombin III and protein C or S deficiency. The yield from screening patients is very low (1% to 2%) and is an expensive proposition. Certain groups should be evaluated more selectively, such as those patients with thromboembolic disease under 35 years of age, recurrent venous thrombosis developing on heparin therapy, deep venous thrombosis in early pregnancy, patients with a strong family history of leg thrombosis, pulmonary emboli or visceral vein thrombosis. A critical analysis of these problems is beyond the scope of this chapter but suffice it to say that the expertise of a skilled hematologist is required to titrate the individual antithrombotic therapy in each of these particular circumstances.

CONCLUSION

Acute superficial thrombophlebitis is a common entity. Usually it occurs secondary to underlying varicose veins. In the absence of varicose veins, there is a more sinister connotation as there is a higher incidence of associated deep venous thrombosis and other pathology. The treatment in the former situation is usually the treatment of the underlying varicose veins. In the latter situation, it is important to try to make a diagnosis and define any underlying pathology. In the patient presented, I would treat him with conservative ambulatory outpatient therapy if this was the first episode and there was no deep venous thrombosis.

BIBLIOGRAPHY

1. Cranley JK: Operation for acute superficial and deep femoral vein thrombosis, in: Ernst CB, Stanley JC (eds): *Current Therapy in Vascular Surgery*. Toronto, BC Decker Inc, 1987, pp 419–421.

2. Edwards EA: Migrating thrombophlebitis associated with carcinoma. *N Engl J Med* 1949; 240:1031–1035.
3. Edwards EA: Thrombophlebitis of varicose veins. *Surg Gynecol Obstet* 1983; 36:236–245.
4. Lofgren EP, Lofgren KA: The surgical treatment of superficial thrombophlebitis. *Surgery* 1981; 901:49–54.
5. O'Duffy JD, Lehner T, Barnes CG: Summary of the third international conference on Behcet's disease. *Brit Med J* 1979; 1:1766–1767.
6. Thaler E, Lechner K: Antithrombin III deficiency in thromboembolism. *Clin Haematol* 1981; 10:369–390.

51   Acute Deep Venous Thrombosis

A 54-year-old executive is seen with a one-day history of increasing swelling and pain in the left calf. Two days previously he had taken a six-hour flight from London after a business trip.

Consultant: Alfred V. Persson, M.D.

Patients with pain in the calf, with or without swelling, are seen in all branches of clinical medicine. Concerns are the presence of deep venous thrombosis and the threat of its complication—pulmonary embolus. Although deep venous thrombosis can occur in anyone, it is seen frequently in patients in a high-risk setting, when two or more of the following conditions are present: a postoperative period, especially after orthopedic and cancer surgery; dehydration; immobilization; advanced cancer; prior history of deep venous thrombosis; varicose veins; and obesity. Deep venous thrombosis is particularly associated with obesity, probably because of the sedentary manner of obese patients.

DIAGNOSIS

Physical examination is unreliable as a means of diagnosing deep venous thrombosis, being only 50% accurate under the best of conditions. Because of this inaccuracy, it is imperative to establish the diagnosis by using one of a number of objective tests available. Venography is definitive but expensive and not readily available (especially on nights and weekends). Furthermore, most physicians are reluctant to perform invasive tests when noninvasive tests are available.

Noninvasive Testing

Several reliable noninvasive tests are useful in the diagnosis of deep venous thrombosis. Impedance plethysmography and phleborheography have been used for more than 15 years. Both tests are reliable in patients without a prior history of deep venous thrombosis. Normal results with these noninvasive procedures indicate the absence of obstruction in the popliteal or more proximal veins, i.e., the patient does not have a clot of a size that would cause embolization and mortality. However, impedance plethysmography and phleborheography are not useful in diagnosing clots isolated in the tibial veins.

The hand-held Doppler is also an accurate noninvasive diagnostic instrument, but it requires skill to use. In our experience, if the Doppler examination and either the impedance plethysmography or phleborheography give positive results, a greater than 95% chance exists that the patient has deep venous thrombosis. When a noninvasive examination results in unequivocally positive findings, definitive therapy is given without obtaining confirmatory venography.

In recent years, the duplex ultrasonic scanner has been used to diagnose acute deep venous thrombosis. The duplex scanner is a B-mode scanner with a pulsed Doppler and permits visualization of the Doppler sampling site. It is of value if the clot involves the popliteal or superficial femoral veins. Semrow and associates have described use of the duplex scanner in defining thrombosis of the tibial veins, but this instrument is not commonly used for that purpose.

Recently, I have used angiodynography or the triplex scanner for the diagnosis of acute deep venous thrombosis. With the B-mode triplex scanner, gray-scale images are produced with Doppler information superimposed in color. Our experience to date with detection of popliteal and superficial femoral vein thrombosis has been good (Figs 51–1 and 51–2). The criteria used for a positive diagnosis by angiodynography are presence of a vein larger than normal (in most patients the vein and artery are approximately the same size); inability to demonstrate flow in the veins with the Doppler, i.e., the absence of a color image; no compression of the vein when the leg is compressed with the transducer; no flow demonstrated in the popliteal or superficial femoral veins after manual compression of the calf with the examiner's hand; and increased velocity noted in the saphenous vein (the major collateral pathway).

Severely ill or dehydrated patients are often difficult to examine. However, if these patients are rehydrated, which increases blood volume, and the test is repeated, the diagnosis of deep venous thrombosis can be made. This is true with all noninvasive tests. The diagnosis must be secure before embarking on the treatment of patients with acute deep venous thrombosis. All noninvasive tests have a small percentage of equivocal results. In such situations, venography is mandatory, especially if the patient is a high risk for anticoagulant therapy.

TREATMENT

Fibrinolytic Therapy

When fibrinolytic therapy is not contraindicated, as it would be in patients with gastrointestinal tract bleeding or who have recently had surgery, I believe that fi-

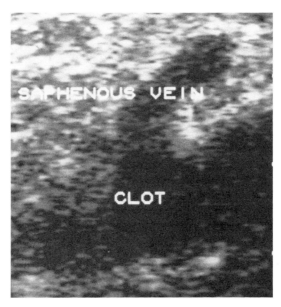

FIG 51–1.
Occluded common femoral and superficial femoral vein.

brinolytic agents (streptokinase or urokinase) are preferred in the treatment of patients with acute deep venous thrombosis. Fibrinolytic agents are administered through a peripheral vein, using what I have termed the "burst protocol"; this regimen consists of administration of 250,000 units of streptokinase during the first hour of therapy and then 100,000 units per hour for five hours. The infusion is then discontinued for 10 to 12 hours. After this time, 250,000 units mixed with 50 ml of normal saline solution is administered over a one-hour period, twice a day, usually at 9 AM and 6 PM. Urokinase is infused in a similar manner with the exact dose being determined by the patient's weight (see Bibliography No. 4 for details). Fibrinolytic therapy is monitored by partial thromboplastin time and serum fibrinogen studies three to four hours after the morning dose of the fibrinolytic agent. Blood studies are not used to regulate the exact dose; they are used to indicate the presence of a fibrinolytic state and to determine the patient's anticoagulation status.

In approximately 5% of our patients, a fibrinolytic state is not reached during fibrinolytic therapy. It is important to identify these patients because the existing clot will not lyse. These patients are also exposed to the possibility of extension of clot and pulmonary embolism. When a fibrinolytic state is not attained, even after adjustment of the dose of fibrinolytic agents, a program of intravenously administered heparin is instituted.

We have seen an objective improvement, defined as the return to normal of

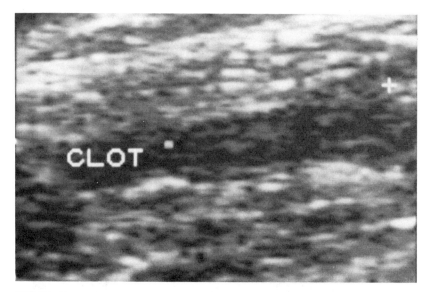

FIG 51–2.
Clot in distal popliteal vein.

the noninvasive examination within ten days, in approximately 70% of our patients treated for acute deep venous thrombosis with fibrinolytic therapy. When treating patients with heparin alone, only a few noninvasive examinations are normal at ten days. Most patients will have subjective clinical improvement regardless of the therapy used.

Heparin Therapy

Most patients with acute deep venous thrombosis are treated with continuous intravenously administered heparin. Conventional anticoagulation has long been regarded as standard treatment by most physicians. Even though I prefer fibrinolytic therapy, some patients have contraindications to fibrinolytic therapy, the most common contraindication being recent surgery. Our protocol for heparin therapy is administration of a loading bolus of 5,000 units followed by an initial infusion of 800 to 1,000 units per hour. The partial thromboplastin time is maintained at 1.5 to 2.0 times the normal control value.

Warfarin (Coumadin) Therapy

Within hours of ingestion, warfarin (Coumadin) blocks production of the protein-based coagulation factors in the liver. Several days are necessary for the prothrombin time to reach therapeutic range because of the half-life of the circulating clotting factors. For this reason, intravenous heparin must be continued during this interval. However, these clotting factors can be eliminated by a single bolus of a fibrinolytic agent. Therefore, the management of patients who undergo fibrinolytic therapy and are switched to warfarin therapy is slightly different from that of patients treated with heparin. Warfarin, 10 mg, is given the evening before the last day of fibrinolytic therapy; 12 hours later, the last bolus of fibrinolytic agent is given. The prothrombin time is usually in or near therapeutic range within 24 hours of the administration of warfarin.

For patients treated with intravenously administered heparin, warfarin is usually begun within 24 hours of the start of the heparin therapy. The average dose is 10 mg every day for three days, then 5 mg daily. It usually takes five to seven days to achieve a prothrombin time of 1.5 times the normal control value. When the prothrombin time is within therapeutic range, the heparin can be discontinued. Patients with acute deep venous thrombosis take warfarin for three to six months. Patients at high risk for recurrent deep venous thrombosis take the medication longer.

Treatment of Edema

Edema associated with acute deep venous thrombosis must also be controlled. Patients are placed at bedrest with elevation of the affected limb. Usually the legs are not wrapped with elastic bandages for 24 hours because an affected leg is often too tender to tolerate elastic wraps. The legs are then wrapped from the toes to below the knee and rewrapped every eight hours. When the edema has subsided (usually in five to six days), the patient is fitted for elastic stockings. Elastic stockings are worn for three months if the edema does not recur and permanently if the edema persists. Diuretics are not prescribed for patients with acute deep venous thrombosis because the problem is not excess fluid but rather the body's inability to remove fluid from the diseased leg.

Indications for Vena Caval Interruption

The most common indications for insertion of a vena caval filter are documented pulmonary embolus while the patient is taking therapy, pulmonary embolus in a patient who has contraindications to anticoagulation, or recurrent pulmonary embolus. The mortality and morbidity rates associated with the insertion of a Greenfield filter are low. A recent report by Greenfield and his colleagues indicates that the incidence of occlusion of the filter over time is also low.

The filter is inserted as an operative procedure with the patient under anesthesia. Fluoroscopy is used to guide placement of the filter opposite L3 and L4. Two paper clips are taped on the patient's back over L2 and L4. A plain film is obtained to verify the position of the paper clips. They are easily seen, and used to assist in the placement of the filter. In most patients, the filter can be placed through the right internal jugular vein. Occasionally, it must be placed from below through the right femoral vein and up the iliac vein.

Patients whose noninvasive examination or venography reveal positive findings, and in whom anticoagulation is contraindicated, pose a therapeutic dilemma. If a clot extends above the knee, placement of a vena caval filter is usually recommended. This procedure does not stop progression of the deep venous thrombosis but does prevent the patient from having a major pulmonary embolus. This treatment of acute deep venous thrombosis is less than optimal, and the patient must be informed of the increased incidence of chronic postphlebitic syndrome. These patients should be kept hydrated to maintain the blood volume and increase the blood flow in the veins. The affected leg should be elevated and intermittent compression devices applied to both legs. A concern is that the compression device will cause movement of a clot, but we have not had an instance of pulmonary embolism. The regimen of hydration, elevation, and intermittent compression, although inferior to the anticoagulation or fibrinolytic therapy, has been useful in this difficult situation.

PROGNOSIS

The prognosis for patients with acute deep venous thrombosis depends on several factors: prior history of deep venous thrombosis, extent of the clot, and general status of the patient. The greater saphenous vein is the major collateral vessel in patients with acute deep venous thrombosis of the superficial femoral and popliteal veins. With time, smaller branches of the deep femoral system also dilate. Unfortunately, as the branches dilate, the valves often become incompetent. This is the reason many patients with acute deep venous thrombosis do not have signs and symptoms of chronic deep venous insufficiency until several years after the acute event.

Deep venous thrombosis that extends beyond the point where the saphenous vein empties into the common femoral vein in the groin is associated with a high incidence of postphlebitic syndrome. Such patients have fewer unaffected veins to use as collateral vessels and more extensive valvular damage.

The postphlebitic syndrome also commonly develops in patients with recurrent acute deep venous thrombosis because the second clot occurs in one of the vessels used as a collateral. With regard to prognosis as well as treatment, it is important to establish that a new clot has developed in a patient with a history of deep venous thrombosis, along with new symptoms. Often some of these patients do not have new clots but have taken on a general increase in body fluids; this fluid is retained in the diseased leg due to impaired emptying of this extra fluid. The syndrome of pain and swelling in patients with recurrent deep venous thrombosis can be identical to that in patients with retained fluid but no new clots.

Because many patients with acute deep venous thrombosis in the superficial femoral vein often present later with new symptoms, they are studied in the non-invasive laboratory before discharge and again at six to eight weeks. The triplex scanner and hand-held Doppler are used to establish the extent of the clot and to determine which veins are being used as collateral vessels. Patients with acute deep venous thrombosis commonly have positive findings on impedance plethysmography or phleborheography whenever these studies are performed. These examinations are therefore more valuable in assessing patients who have deep venous thrombosis for the first time than they are in assessing patients suspected of having recurrent disease.

When the unaffected veins have been identified after a single episode of deep venous thrombosis, it is possible to assess whether the symptoms associated with the second episode are the result of a second thrombosis. The prognosis and treatment of patients with retention of fluid versus recurrent thrombosis are obviously different.

CONCLUSION

Acute deep venous thrombosis is commonly seen in medical practice. A definitive objective diagnosis must be established before embarking on therapy. Without contraindications, fibrinolytic therapy is instituted first, followed by three to six months of warfarin therapy. Control of edema and establishing the extent of thrombosis are important in the long-term management of these patients.

BIBLIOGRAPHY

1. Greenfield LJ, Peyton R, Crute S, et al: Greenfield vena caval filter experience: Late results in 156 patients. *Arch Surg* 1981; 116:1451–1456.
2. Kakkar VV, Corrigan TP: Detection of deep vein thrombosis: Survey and current status, in: Sasahara AA, Sonnenblick EH, Lesch M (eds): *Pulmonary emboli*. New York, Grune & Stratton, 1975, pp 45–55.
3. Messmer JM, Greenfield LJ: Greenfield caval filters: Long-term radiographic follow-up study. *Radiology* 1985; 156:613–618.
4. Persson AV, Persson CA: Thrombolytic therapy for deep vein thrombosis. *Am J Surg* 1985; 150:50–53.
5. Persson AV, Ekdahl KE: Treatment of acute deep venous thrombosis with fibrinolytic agents. *Med Clin North Am* 1986; 70:1325–1332.
6. Persson AV, Powis RL: Recent advances in imaging and evaluation of blood flow using ultrasound. *Med Clin North Am* 1986; 70:1241–1252.
7. Persson AV, Ekdahl K: Burst therapy: A method of administering fibrinolytic therapy. *Pract Cardiol* 1986; 12:162–172.
8. Semrow CM, Friedell M, Buchbinder D, et al: Characterization of lower extremity ve-

nous disease using real-time B-mode ultrasonic imaging. *J Vasc Tech* 1987; 11:187–191.

9. Sullivan ED, Peter DJ, Cranley JJ: Real-time B-mode venous ultrasound. *J Vasc Surg* 1984; 1:465–471.

10. Wheeler HB: Diagnosis of deep vein thrombosis. Review of clinical evaluation and impedance plethysmography. *Am J Surg* 1985; 150:7–13.

52 Pulmonary Embolism on Anticoagulant Treatment

A 68-year-old woman is found to have swelling on the right leg four days after a total hip replacement. Venography confirms a deep venous thrombosis, and she is begun on heparin therapy. The following morning she complains of some pleuritic chest pain.

Consultant: Lazar J. Greenfield, M.D.

The sequence of events reported in this case is not unusual given the propensity for elective orthopedic surgical patients to develop deep vein thrombosis (DVT) and its sequelae. Patients undergoing hip procedures or knee reconstruction are at greatest risk of developing DVT, at rates ranging from 45% to 70%. The incidence of subsequent pulmonary thromboembolism (PE) has been reported as high as 20% following hip surgery with a 1% to 3% incidence of fatal thromboembolism. Before approaching the management of the complication, we should consider the options available for prophylaxis. Considerable progress has been made in prophylactic regimens using either anticoagulants or mechanical techniques.

PROPHYLAXIS OF VENOUS THROMBOEMBOLISM

In 1986 a Consensus Development Conference on prevention of venous thrombosis and pulmonary embolism was held under the auspices of the National Heart, Lung and Blood Institute to review epidemiologic and statistical data in order to provide specific recommendations for prophylaxis. It should be recognized that the committee accepted the assumption that DVT is a reliable marker for PE which is generally supported by trials indicating a significant reduction in fatal PE when DVT is brought under control. However, unless sensitive screening tests are applied to detect early DVT, there may be no signs or symptoms of the disorder and fatal PE can occur because the DVT remains clinically silent. Therefore, the value of a reported prophylactic regimen for PE depends on the sensitivity and specificity of tests used to monitor the incidence of DVT in patients at high risk.

The most effective prophylactic regimen for thromboembolism as well documented in multiple trials, consists of low dose subcutaneous heparin administered two hours prior to surgery and every 12 hours postoperatively. Using this regimen, there is a net decrease in the incidence of detectable DVT from 25% to 10% of patients. Unfortunately, low dose heparin is less beneficial in orthopedic patients where only warfarin and dextran have been demonstrated to reduce the incidence of DVT by a factor of approximately two. These agents add their own risk of complications including hemorrhage and the risk of allergic reaction with dextran. The use of lower dose Coumadin will reduce the incidence of hemorrhagic complications and may be just as effective, although supporting data are limited. A more attractive approach to prophylaxis that is free of complication is external pneumatic compression which has been demonstrated to significantly reduce the incidence of DVT. Other mechanical approaches such as elevation of the foot of the bed or pressure gradient elastic stockings are probably of value, but cannot be relied on alone to provide adequate protection. The combination of heparin with dihydroergotamine adds the potential benefit of venoconstriction and may improve the results seen with subcutaneous heparin alone in orthopedic patients.

DIAGNOSTIC STUDIES

The patient described underwent a venogram to confirm the presence of deep vein thrombosis which is obviously the most accurate diagnostic approach. Standard venography, however, usually demonstrates only that the iliofemoral system is occluded without providing any information about the proximal extent or character of the thrombus. Our studies and the work of Jarrell, et al, indicate that the geometry of the proximal thrombus can provide useful information about the likelihood of embolism in the face of adequate anticoagulation. The presence of a free-floating proximal tail to the thrombus that is 5 cm in length or longer indicates that the patient has a mechanical predisposition to embolism that is ten times greater than the situation where the thrombus is circumferentially adherent to the vein wall. It may require retrograde venography to identify this feature of the proximal thrombus but in the future, a noninvasive approach, such as duplex scanning, should provide a less traumatic approach to characterizing the proximal thrombus. It is likely that duplex scanning will be utilized more at the bedside and will greatly reduce the need for contrast venograms. Both Doppler and impedance plethysmography now have sufficient accuracy exceeding 90% confidence to make the diagnosis of proximal DVT and justify a course of anticoagulation.

DIAGNOSIS OF PULMONARY EMBOLISM

The patient who develops chest pain or dyspnea while on anticoagulation for DVT should obviously be suspected of having sustained a PE, but the diagnosis requires accurate confirmation. The initial approach should include both electrocardiogram and chest X-ray to exclude myocardial infarction, pleural bleed, atelectasis or some other primary process in the lung. As long as the patient is hemodynamically stable, she would remain in the category of minor embolism (Class II) and be eligible for screening studies (Table 52–1). Under circumstances where the patient has been hypotensive, either transiently (Class III) or persistently with a requirement for vasopressors (Class IV), the approach should be more expeditious, proceeding directly to pulmonary arteriogram.

Since this patient falls into Class II and presumably has mild hypoxemia on arterial blood gas analysis, she is a good candidate for a screening ventilation perfusion lung scan. Although lung scans have a high rate of interobserver variability of interpretation, limiting them to about 65% accuracy, the finding of multiple large perfusion defects with normal ventilation would allow a diagnosis of pulmonary thromboembolism to be made with reasonable accuracy. Anything less than this, however, with either small defects or the presence of underlying pulmonary or cardiac disease, would render the scan unreliable and indicate the need for a pulmonary arteriogram. In fact, under most circumstances when a decision must be made about adding mechanical filter protection because of failure of anticoagulation, it is advisable to confirm the diagnosis by arteriography.

The other issue to be faced is whether the patient has had an adequate course of anticoagulation to justify adding mechanical protection. Although data are unavailable, it has been my experience that patients who sustain embolism initially on anticoagulation are likely to continue to embolize and increase the risk of fatal embolism as they progressively occlude their pulmonary vascular bed. The other consideration is the intrinsic risk of heparin itself, since it is the most common agent producing inhospital drug-related deaths. In the high-risk group of postmenopausal women, the risk of bleeding has been reported from 25% to 50%. Similar

TABLE 52-1.
Classification of Pulmonary Embolic Disease*

CLASS	SYMPTOMS	GASES	HEMODYNAMICS	PA OCCLUSION
I	None	Normal	Normal	<20%
II	Anxiety	PaO_2 <80 mm Hg	Tachycardia	20-30%
	Hyperventilation	$PaCO_2$ <35 mm Hg		
III	Dyspnea	PaO_2 <65 mm Hg	CVP ↑	30-50%
	Collapse	$PaCO_2$ <30 mm Hg	$\overline{PA}$ >20 mm Hg	
IV	Shock	PaO_2 <50 mm Hg	CVP ↑	>50%
	Dyspnea	$PaCO_2$ <30 mm Hg	$\overline{PA}$ >25 mm Hg	
			C.O. ↓	
V	Chronic Dyspnea	PaO_2 <50 mm Hg	$\overline{PA}$ 30-40 mm Hg	>50%
	Syncope	$PaCO_2$ 30-40 mm Hg		

*From Greenfield LJ: Intraluminal techniques for vena caval interruption and Pulmonary Embolectomy. *World J Surg* 1978; 2:46. Used by permission.

excess risk is associated with continued oral anticoagulation with Coumadin. Of course, the patient may not have been adequately anticoagulated to begin with, since often a house officer will assume that the same standard dose of 5,000 units of heparin used to anticoagulate a patient in the absence of thrombosis will suffice for the patient with DVT. This failure to appreciate the requirement for increased heparin to neutralize circulating thrombin leads to undertreatment and is readily apparent when the activated PTT fails to reach the therapeutic range of twice normal. This can be avoided by an initial dose of 100 to 150 units heparin per kilogram and careful monitoring of the APTT.

DECISION FOR MECHANICAL PROTECTION

Assuming that the patient has a documented embolic event while on adequate anticoagulation, she becomes a candidate for Greenfield filter insertion. Failure of anticoagulation to protect the patient from PE is the second most common indication for filter insertion, accounting for 28% of our experience. The most common indication is a contraindication to anticoagulation which accounts for 37% of our experience. The remaining indications include an anticoagulant complication forcing it to be discontinued; pure prophylaxis where the patient has not yet sustained PE but has a free floating thrombus, following open or catheter pulmonary embolectomy; and after failure of another device.

Since the procedure of filter insertion can be performed under local anesthesia with no significant risk to the patient, it is the appropriate option for the patient who requires mechanical protection. Long-term follow-up experience that now exceeds 14 years confirms a persistent patency rate of 95% and has allowed the filter to be inserted in any major vein where thrombus control is necessary. This includes the suprarenal vena cava when control of pelvic and gonadal vein sources is required or in the circumstance where the vena cava is thrombosed to the level of the renal veins. In very rare circumstances, the filter has also been inserted in the superior vena cava for control of innominate vein thrombi. Sepsis is not a contraindication to filter insertion since the filter is inert stainless steel and any infected thrombus within it can be sterilized with a two-week course of antibiotics.

TECHNICAL CONSIDERATIONS

The technique of filter insertion has been improved by routine use of a guidewire which can be manipulated past the troublesome areas of the eustachian valve in the right atrium and the orifice of the right renal vein. Use of the guidewire also minimizes the time that the carrier catheter must spend in the patient and facilitates axial orientation of the filter when it is discharged from the jugular approach. If the jugular vein is too small or if there is an open wound of the neck, the right femoral vein approach can be used and the guidewire should also be employed to facilitate exiting the pelvis into the inferior vena cava. The guidewire should be pulled back, however, before the filter is discharged from below, since pulling back against the filter in a direction opposite to the hooks could impart a tilt to the filter and reduce its effectiveness. The left axillary vein and the right atrium have also been used for access to insert the filter.

The insertion technique has been adapted to a percutaneous approach by some radiologists using dilators up to 24 French in order to accommodate the carrier. Although this can be performed safely in many circumstances, it can also lead to significant hemorrhage, hematoma formation, and venous thrombosis. Our current research is directed to the development of a titanium version of the filter which will allow it to be compressed into a size 12 French carrier which will obviously make percutaneous insertion both easier and safer. Another percutaneous device, the bird's nest filter which consists of a random jumble of wires, has been tested experimentally and clinically. Problems of caval thrombosis and fixation of the bird's nest device have been seen after thrombus capture with subsequent embolism of the device into the right ventricle and pulmonary artery in both the experimental comparison we reported and clinically. The Greenfield filter remains the only device available that has FDA approval, since the Mobin Uddin umbrella has been withdrawn. The use of vena caval plication or clipping has an unacceptable rate of caval occlusion, in addition to the fact that it requires a general anesthetic and laparotomy.

BIBLIOGRAPHY

1. Alexander JJ, Gewertz BL, Lu Ct, et al: New criteria for placement of a prophylactic vena caval filter. *Surg Gynecol Obstet* 1986; 163:405–409.
2. Burke PE, Michna BA, Harvey CF, et al: Experimental comparison of percutaneous vena caval devices: Titanium Greenfield filter vs. bird's nest filter. *J Vasc Surg* 1987; 6:66–70.
3. Denny DF, Cronan JJ, Dorfman GS, et al: Percutaneous Kimray-Greenfield filter placement by femoral vein puncture. *Am J Roent* 1985; 145:827–829.
4. Hoffman MJ, Greenfield LJ: Central venous septic thrombosis managed by superior vena cava Greenfield filter and venous thrombectomy: A case report. *J Vasc Surg* 1986; 4:606–611.
5. Jones TK, Barnes RW, Greenfield LJ: Greenfield vena caval filter rationale and current indications. *Ann Thoracic Surg* 1986; 42:S48–S55.
6. Norris CS, Greenfield LJ, Barnes RW: Free-floating iliofemoral thrombus: A risk of pulmonary embolism. *Arch Surg* 1985; 120:806–808.
7. Radowski JS, Jarrell BE, Carabasi RA, et al: Risk of pulmonary embolus with inferior vena cava thrombosis. *Am Surg* 1987; 53:97–101.

53 Chronic Venous Insufficiency

A 49-year-old construction worker is referred for chronic swelling of the left leg and recent development of ulceration around the left ankle. He denies a known history of prior venous thrombosis. Examination reveals a swollen left leg, with hyperpigmentation and brawny induration of the lower calf and ankle region. There is a 2 cm. dirty ulceration just above the medial malleolus.

Consultant: Thomas F. O'Donnell, Jr., M.D.

This patient is typical of patients who present with advanced chronic venous insufficiency (CVI). CVI affects 25% to 30% of the population in industrialized countries, but in contrast to arterial occlusive disease, CVI most commonly involves the younger working patient, as in the present case. An open leg ulcer may prevent an active construction worker from performing his job and place him on prolonged disability. The direct and indirect costs to society of advanced CVI are considerable. Although the approach to this man's leg ulcer has been largely nonsurgical in the past, consisting of compression and wound care, my preferred approach is based on defining the anatomic and functional venous abnormalities by an aggressive workup. Surgical reconstruction may then be carried out in selected patients.

CLASSIFICATION

Clinical

The clinical picture of chronic venous insufficiency ranges from mild ankle swelling, as in the early phases of this patient's disease process, to frank tissue breakdown with leg ulcer. Table 53–1 summarizes the classification of CVI into three clinical categories, based on history and physical examination. Mild CVI (Stage 1) is defined by symptoms of mild ankle swelling and limb heaviness and on clinical examination by dilated superficial veins. The skin and subcutaneous tissue are normal. With progression of the disease to Stage 2 the patient complains of a greater

TABLE 53–1.
Classification of Chronic Venous Insufficiency

GRADE	SYMPTOMS	PHYSICAL FINDINGS
I	Mild swelling Heaviness Vein dilation	Ankle edema <1 cm. Dilated superficial veins Normal skin and subcutaneous tissue
II	Moderate to severe swelling Heaviness Varicosities Skin changes	Edema >1 cm. Multiple dilated veins ICPV (mild) Pigmentation (mild) Liposclerosis (mild)
III	Severe swelling Calf pain +/− claudication	Edema >2 cm Multiple dilated veins ICPV (severe) Multiple vein varicosities Marked skin pigmentation Severe liposclerosis Ulcer

degree of swelling that is not as promptly relieved by limb elevation as with Stage 1. Varicosities are more pronounced and moderate skin changes develop. On physical examination the subcutaneous tissue is firm, and light brown skin pigmentary changes are noted in the submalleolar area. In Stage 3 disease the patient usually presents with an ulcer or has healed one in the past. The subcutaneous tissue is indurated and firm, while the skin, as in this case, is darkly pigmented and edematous. This patient is an example of progression of the disease from Stage 2 to Stage 3.

Anatomic and Functional Classification

The anatomic classification of chronic venous insufficiency is important, because it relates to the etiology and clinical management of CVI. CVI is generally divided anatomically by the systems involved: (1) superficial venous system (primary varicosities), (2) deep venous system, or (3) a combination of both. Incompetence of the perforating (communicating) veins is generally classified with the superficial venous system. The anatomic level affected is also important. For example, chronic deep venous insufficiency may involve the inferior vena cava, iliofemoral, popliteal, or tibial peroneal veins.

Functional classification of CVI by noninvasive hemodynamic studies is also of great value. Like the classification of arterial occlusive disease by Doppler pressure and pulse volume recording amplitude, noninvasive assessment of CVI allows objective determination of the severity of the disease. Our recent review of nearly 400 limbs with chronic venous insufficiency showed, by noninvasive assessment, that over 60% had deep system involvement, and this incidence increased with clinical severity. In a British study of nearly 500 consecutive patients examined with phlebography and noninvasive studies, Darke and Andress showed that only 25% of patients had complex disease (deep venous involvement). Obviously, the proportion of patients with CVI and deep system involvement is important, because this group represents those patients who may require more complex deep venous reconstruction.

PATHOPHYSIOLOGY

A detailed review of this aspect is beyond the scope of this discussion, but recent studies have deepened our understanding of the *cellular* changes associated with chronic venous insufficiency. The principal hemodynamic alterations in CVI occur during the systolic phase of the calf muscle pump cycle. Due to damage of the normally one-way flow valves within the perforating (communicating) veins, blood flows paradoxically from the deep to the superficial venous system. Thus, the high pressure developed within the deep venous system during the systolic phase of the calf muscle pump cycle is transmitted directly to the superficial venous system. Studies in our vascular laboratory have shown that superficial venous pressure can reach 150 to 160 mm Hg during calf muscle compression in limbs with Stage 3 chronic venous insufficiency. In contrast to the deep veins that are encased within tight muscle-fascial envelopes, the superficial veins are surrounded by loose areolar subcutaneous tissue. Dilation and lengthening of the superficial veins occur. Deep venous occlusion or valvular incompetence may further compound these adverse pressure changes. Occluded deep venous segments increase resistance to venous flow so that deep venous pressure may increase during exercise. By contrast, deep venous valvular incompetence permits an unchecked column of blood to exert its gravitational effects on the venous system in the upright position.

While these large vessel hemodynamic changes have long been recognized, the work of the St. Thomas' Surgical Unit has focused attention on alterations which occur at the cellular level. In a series of clinical and experimental studies, Burnand and Browse demonstrated a sequence of microscopic changes in the limb with CVI. On biopsies obtained from the pigmented and liposclerotic area, venous capillaries were noted to have undergone extensive proliferation which appeared related to the level of superficial ambulatory venous pressure. More extensive capillary proliferation occurred in limbs with elevated superficial ambulatory venous pressures. In addition, capillary permeability was altered due to widened interendothelial cell pores so that transcapillary leakage of osmotically-active particles occurred, in particular fibrinogen. While normal veins possess fibrinolytic properties that lyse fibrin and prevent pericapillary fibrin cuffing, in CVI the venous fibrinolytic capacity is altered. Thus, extravascular fibrin is not broken down so that fibrin coats the capillary, and prevents the normal exchange of oxygen and nutrients to the surrounding cells. Alterations in both subcutaneous tissue and skin occur.

DIAGNOSTIC WORKUP

Noninvasive Assessment

Patients with Stage 2 or Stage 3 CVI, like the patient under discussion, undergo a sequence of noninvasive screening studies. The purpose of these studies is twofold: (1) to assess the severity of the hemodynamic deficit, and (2) to define the anatomical components involved by the disease process. Such information has an important bearing on the type of therapy selected. As shown in Figure 53–1, our patients undergo initial evaluation with quantitative photophlethysmography by light reflection rheography (LRR), which assesses valvular competence in both the deep and superficial systems. LRR is a rapid and simple technique to perform and provides objective hard copy evidence of venous function. A probe is affixed to the lower medial calf area. Three diodes within the probe head emit light that reflects off the red blood cells contained within the subdermal venous plexus. The degree of light reflection is proportional to the red blood cell content of these vessels, so that light reflection will vary as red blood cell content changes during the phases of the calf muscle pump. Studies in our noninvasive laboratory with LRR have demonstrated an excellent correlation between both venous refill time and ambulatory venous pressure.

In patients such as the one under discussion with severe Stage 3 disease, venous refill time is usually less than ten seconds. Since the deep venous system is commonly involved with advanced Stage 3 CVI, the venous refill time is usually unimproved by tourniquet compression of the greater/lesser saphenous or perforating veins. Tourniquet compression permits a delineation of the systems involved: superficial alone, deep alone, or a combination of both venous systems (Table 53–2). If tourniquet compression shows improvement in the venous refill time, then surgical removal of the long saphenous and lesser saphenous veins by saphenectomy might improve venous function. In our series of patients with venous ulcer, superficial CVI occurred in approximately 12% of limbs. Certainly, lack of involvement of the deep venous system should be confirmed by ascending phlebography in such cases. Bidirectional Doppler examination is employed to assess valvular competence and patency of the superficial and deep venous systems, because the presence of valvular incompetence or obstruction and its anatomic level have important implications for therapy.

The presence of obstruction and/or valvular incompetence within the deep and superficial systems can be substantiated anatomically by the use of B-mode ultrasound. For example, an occluded venous segment is usually highly echoic and no blood flow is detected within it. Valvular function can be scrutinized directly in the superficial and deep veins by B-mode imaging. Hemodynamic function of the deep venous valves as assessed by Doppler spectral analysis with calf muscle compression may further verify valvular insufficiency by demonstrating valvular reflux.

For our patient, ascending phlebography is the next part of preoperative evaluation. The technique of ascending phlebography is different in the limb with CVI than that employed for detection of acute deep venous thrombosis. Multiple tour-

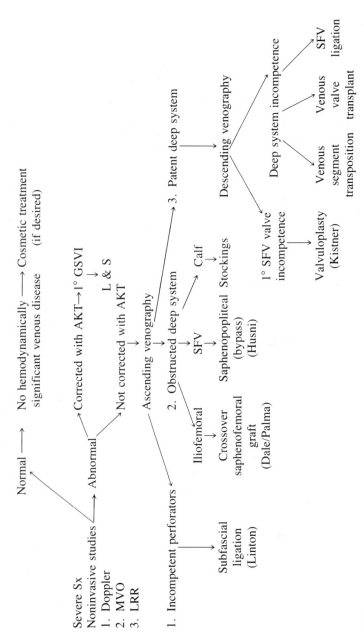

FIG 53–1.
Flow diagram for management of severe CVI. (From O'Donnell TF: Chronic Venous Insufficiency, in: Jarrett F, Hirsch S (eds): *Vascular Surgery of the Lower Extremity*. St Louis, CV Mosby, 1985.)

TABLE 53–2.
Comparison of Clinical, Hemodynamic and Anatomic Results of Venous Reconstruction

TYPE OF PROCEDURE	NUMBER OF LIMBS	HEALING OF ULCER (%) EARLY	LATE	HEMODYNAMICS IMPROVED (%)	ANATOMIC PATENCY (%)
Valvuloplasty	93	84	63	93	88
Venous Segment Transfer	26	65	--	71	80
Femoral Vein Transplant	67	82	66	67	95
Popliteal Vein Transplant	10	100	100	30	100

niquets are used to occlude the superficial venous system and prevent its filling. Visualization of dye within the superficial system indicates flow into it via incompetent perforating veins. In addition to detecting the presence and site of incompetent perforating veins, ascending phlebography is essential for defining anatomic signs of chronic deep venous disease such as recanalization, occlusion or avalvular segments. When no obstruction is observed in the deep system by ascending phlebography, the patient is next referred for descending phlebography. The purpose of this study is to demonstrate valvular function within the deep venous system. With the patient on the tilt table at 70 to 90 degrees a Valsalva maneuver is performed and the furthest level to which the contrast descends within the deep venous system is assessed. Surgery for valvular incompetence of the deep system is usually reserved for those limbs with reflux of dye to the below-knee popliteal or calf vein segments. This sequential method of evaluation allows the patient with CVI to be selected for the appropriate form of surgical treatment: (1) superficial venous surgery—ligation and stripping alone or with interruption of incompetent perforating veins, or (2) for deep venous reconstruction—bypass for venous obstruction, direct valvular reconstruction for valvular incompetence.

THERAPY

Therapy for the patient under discussion has two aims: (1) to cover or promote epithelialization of the venous ulcer, and (2) to correct the hemodynamic abnormality which led to the ulceration. Nonsurgical therapy may eventually accomplish one of these goals, coverage of the ulcer, but "conservative" treatment is unable to correct the underlying hemodynamic abnormalities. Certainly elastic compression of limbs with CVI reduces edema and appears to promote healing of venous ulcers. Elastic stockings have been the major method for treating CVI. In an effort to determine what effect custom fitted elastic stockings might have on venous hemodynamics, we measured venous pressure at rest and with exercise in limbs with the postthrombotic syndrome (Stage 3 disease). Venous pressure was measured with and without elastic stockings. Although the venous refill time and the ambulatory venous pressure (percent drop in venous pressure with exercise) were not improved by elastic stockings, the peak systolic pressure or that pressure achieved with activation of the calf muscle pump was reduced. Thus, the major hemodynamic effect of elastic compression is to reduce systolic hypertension that develops in the superficial veins during ambulation.

Skin Care

Depending on their severity, cutaneous infections are treated by oral or intravenous antibiotics. Scrapings of the skin are obtained if fungal infection is suspected, and oral agents are prescribed as indicated (Griseofulvin R). In patients with venous eczema, topical steroid creams are applied to the affected area, but direct application to the ulcer is avoided. If the ulcer bed is not clean and granulating, betadine wet-to-dry dressings are employed directly over the ulcer. Care must be taken to protect the surrounding nonulcerated skin from betadine, because it is quite drying. If no gross infection is present, saline wet-to-dry dressings are utilized and are changed three times daily.

SURGICAL THERAPY

Noninvasive and invasive assessment of the patients with CVI should delineate which systems are involved so that venous surgery can be carried out. A rational therapeutic approach to venous stasis is based on the tenet that as many systems as necessary must be corrected to restore the extremity to a compensated state of venous function. Superficial venous incompetence can be treated by greater and lesser saphenous vein ligation and stripping, while perforating vein incompetence requires subfascial ligation. We prefer the posterior stocking seam approach for the latter. Dependent on the type of pathology involving the deep system, bypass is carried out for obstruction as in the iliofemoral segment, or reconstruction is performed for valvular incompetence. If the noninvasive studies and phlebography demonstrate deep venous system involvement, usually by valvular incompetence, then surgery for superficial perforating vein incompetence alone does not appear rational.

In a previous study we examined ulcer recurrence in limbs which had undergone subfascial ligation for incompetent perforating veins. The limbs were divided into two groups based on the status of their deep system as defined by a preoperative ascending phlebogram. In those 18 limbs with a normal deep system only one ulcer occurred, but in the 23 limbs with an abnormal deep system as defined by phlebography, all had recurrent ulcer by five years postoperatively. In another study subsequent to this phlebographic study, ambulatory venous pressure was measured before and after surgery to the superficial system. While those limbs with saphe-nous vein incompetence had normalization of their venous pressure tracings, the limbs with deep venous insufficiency had insignificant improvement with subfascial ligation of incompetent perforating veins.

SPECIFIC SURGICAL PROCEDURES

A detailed description of the various surgical procedures for deep venous recon-structions is beyond the scope of this discussion. Figure 53–1 demonstrates how we select the appropriate procedure for our patients. We feel that candidates for deep venous reconstruction would have advanced CVI, usually with ulcer or venous claudication. In addition, the majority of these patients have failed attempts at the management of ulcer by conservative means. In our experience, the patient with venous obstruction, particularly of the iliofemoral segment will present more fre-quently with swelling and venous claudication than with venous ulcer. In the face of iliofemoral obstruction venous ulcer usually signifies concomitant valvular in-competence.

The patient under discussion is typical because he has no known previous his-tory of actue deep venous thrombosis. Approximately 40% to 60% of patients pre-senting with venous ulcer failed to have documented history of DVT. Detailed descending phlebograms have shown that 30% to 40% of patients with venous ulcer have primary valvular incompetence rather than loss of valvular function due to postthrombotic changes within the deep system. Defining valvular anatomy and the type of pathologic changes in the deep system is important, because primary val-vular insufficiency is amenable to valvuloplasty. In this procedure the floppy cau-liflower-like valves are "reefed up" so that venous valves that did not coapt prior to surgery become functional and coapt. By contrast, if typical postthrombotic changes are noted on ascending and descending phlebography, the patient would not be a candidate for valvuloplasty but rather for an alternative procedure. Of the options available, I prefer vein valve transplantation. Rather than transplanting to the superficial femoral vein, I utilize the popliteal vein segment as the recipient site of the valve transplant. The popliteal vein segment is used because the popliteal vein valve plays a critical role as a gate keeper mechanism above the calf muscle pump. In addition, I prefer the axillary vein as the donor segment because it has a better size match to the popliteal vein than a brachial vein. Venous transposition has sometimes led to late failure by dilation when the saphenous vein was used as the transposed segment. Kistner now prefers to use the profunda femoris vein as the transposed segment to avoid this problem. Our results with popliteal vein valve transplantation are summarized in Table 53–2 and show healing of venous ulcer in all limbs. Table 53–2 also summarizes the results from the surgical literature on other methods of direct venous reconstruction. We concur with Kistner's concept that treatment of deep venous valvular insufficiency alone without correction of perforating valve incompetence is destined for failure. Therefore, we ligate incompetent perforating veins which have been demonstrated on phlebography at the time of the deep venous reconstructive procedure.

BIBLIOGRAPHY

1. Burnand KG, O'Donnell TF, Thomas ML, et al: The relative importance of incompetent communicating veins in the production of varicose veins and venous ulcers. *Surgery* 1977; 82:9–14.
2. Burnand KG, Whimster IW, Clemenson G, et al: The relationship between the number of capillaries in the skin of the venous ulcer bearing area of the lower leg and the fall in foot vein pressure during exercise. *Br J Surg* 1981; 68:297–300.
3. Darke SG, Andress MR: The value of venography in the management of chronic venous disorders of the lower limb, in Greenhalgh RM (ed): *Diagnostic Techniques and Assessment Procedures in Vascular Surgery*. London, Grune & Stratton, 1985.
4. Johnson HD, Queral LA, Flinn WR, et al: Late objective assessment of venous valve surgery. *Arch Surg* 1981; 116:1461–1466.
5. Kistner R: Surgical repair of the incompetent femoral vein valve. *Arch Surg* 1975; 110:1336–1343.
6. Lea TM, McDonald LM: Complications of phlebography of the leg. *Br Med J* 1978; 2:307–315.
7. Moore DJ, Himmel PD, Sumner DS: Distribution of venous valvular incompetence in patients with postphlebitis syndrome. *J Vasc Surg* 1986; 3:49–57.
8. O'Donnell TF: The post-thrombotic syndrome: Classification, diagnosis, and treatment. *J Vasc Surg,* in press.
9. O'Donnell TF, Burnand KG, Browse NL: Is interruption of incompetent perforating veins really important to the management of chronic venous insufficiency: *Surgery* 1977; 82:9–14.
10. O'Donnell TF, Mackey WC, Shepard AD, et al: Clinical, hemodynamic, and anatomic follow-up of direct venous reconstruction. *Arch Surg* 1987; 122:474–482.
11. O'Donnell TF, Shepard AD: Chronic venous insufficiency, Jarett F, Hirsch J (eds): *Vascular Surgery of the Lower Extremity*. St Louis, CV Mosby Co, 1985.
12. Raju S, Fredericks R: Valve reconstruction procedures for nonobstructive venous insufficiency: Rationale, techniques, and results in 107 procedures with 2-8 year follow-up. *J Vasc Surg,* in press.
13. Schanzer H, Peirce EC: A rational approach to surgery of the chronic venous stasis syndrome. *Ann Surg* 1982; 195:25–29.
14. Taheri SA, Pendergast DR, Lazar E: Vein valve transplantation. *Am J Surg* 1985; 150:201–202.
15. Wesolowski SA, Greenfield H, Sawyer PN, et al: Diagnostic value of phlebography in venous disorders of the lower extremity. *J Cardiovasc Surg* 1965; 8 (suppl):133–151.

Miscellaneous

54 Spontaneous Atheroembolism

A 64-year-old male presents with a two-day history of a painful, blue toe. The patient is a heavy cigarette smoker, but denies any previous symptoms of extremity ischemia. Examination of the foot reveals a cyanotic, tender 4th toe on the right foot with several mottled areas on the sole and heel of the foot. Pedal pulses are easily palpable.

Consultant: Richard F. Kempczinski, M.D.

The above case is characteristic of patients with spontaneous atheroembolism. This condition is being seen with increasing frequency by vascular surgeons and represents one of the most challenging and frustrating problems in their clinical practice. Although the history is often quite typical, allowing a presumptive diagnosis to be made solely on the basis of the clinical features of the patient's presentation, precise localization of the lesion responsible for the embolus may be quite difficult. Furthermore, the patient, who is asymptomatic except for his painful digit, may have difficulty accepting the necessity for a major vascular reconstruction to treat his problem. Nevertheless, because of the tendency of atheroemboli to recur with progressively increasing vascular obliteration, an aggressive diagnostic and therapeutic approach is essential in their management.

CLINICAL FEATURES

The term "atheroemboli" is somewhat of a misnomer since similar emboli can originate as a result of traumatic arterial injuries or fibromuscular dysplasia. However, the term is so well entrenched in the medical literature that the more precise but cumbersome alternative, "arterio-arterial emboli," is unlikely to gain widespread acceptance.

Depending on the size of the embolus liberated and its precise point of impaction, atheroembolism can mimic a variety of systemic and extremity syndromes. *Macroscopic atheroemboli* consist largely of white thrombus which may, on occasion, even contain a portion of the atheromatous plaque from which it originated. Such emboli typically occlude major arterial branches. Patients suffering from such an event present with symptoms indistinguishable from emboli or cardiac origin. Only the absence of a legitimate cardiac source and a high index of suspicion will lead to recognition of the true nature of the problem.

Microscopic emboli consist of fibrinoplatelet aggregates or cholesterol crystals. Such emboli characteristically lodge in more peripheral vessels, ranging in size from 150 μ to 1,100 μ (average diameter, 460 μ). Since vessels of this size are typically muscular or dermal arterioles, peripheral pulses are usually intact, as they are in the case presented, and the patient complains of the sudden onset of painful cyanosis at the tip of one or more digits, a condition commonly referred to as the "blue toe syndrome."

The classic "blue toe" occurs in only a small percentage of patients suffering dermal atheroemboli. A typical lesion develops suddenly, is localized to the tip of a finger or toe, is tender, deeply cyanotic, and may be surrounded by erythema or mottling of the skin (Fig 54–1). Adjacent digits on the ipsilateral or contralateral extremity may exhibit similar lesions and there may be areas of tender lividity on the proximal forefoot. In patients with extensive lower extremity atheromatous embolization, the skin below their knees may manifest a condition known as "livedo reticularis" which appears as a fixed, reticulated cyanosis. Patients with such diffuse microembolization may also have low-grade fever, eosinophilia, myalgia, muscle tenderness and an elevated erythrocyte sedimentation rate. They are frequently misdiagnosed as having collagen vascular disease, polyarteritis nodosa, systemic bacterial endocarditis, vasculitis, or a wide variety of other systemic disor-

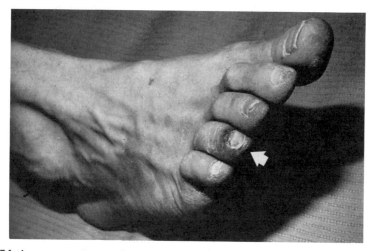

FIG 54–1.
Tender cyanosis at the tip of the right 4th toe (arrow) in a patient with easily palpable pedal pulses is typical of atheroembolism.

ders. Occasionally, skin nodules may also be present, thus further confusing the diagnosis with polyarteritis nodosa.

Although most cases of atheroembolism occur spontaneously, they can be precipitated by blunt trauma, aortic surgery, or intraarterial catheterization for angiography or cardiac catheterization.

DIAGNOSIS

In an elderly male smoker with palpable pedal pulses and the sudden onset of a painful, cyanotic digit, the diagnosis is fairly obvious. However, in many patients, it may be much less apparent and a high index of suspicion is essential if an accurate diagnosis is to be made and effective treatment initiated. This is especially true in instances of macroembolization where the signs and symptoms may be indistinguishable from emboli of cardiac origin. In a case such as the one under consideration where the diagnosis is fairly obvious, the surgeon may proceed directly to aortography. However, in other situations when the diagnosis is less clear, additional tests may prove helpful.

Noninvasive Vascular Testing

In patients with the "blue toe syndrome," noninvasive testing may be useful in identifying clinically occult, proximal stenosis and certainly will help in focusing subsequent angiography. In a recent report by Wingo and associates documenting the hemodynamic findings in 67 patients with the "blue toe syndrome," segmental limb pressures and ankle pressure indices were normal in 53% of the limbs examined. However, an abnormal toe/ankle pressure index was found in 43% of these. The noninvasive tests proved useful in sorting out the relative contribution of proximal versus distal arterial occlusive disease in these patients. When arteriography was subsequently performed, there was good correlation with the noninvasive testing, with an overall sensitivity of 84% and specificity of 100%. However, the negative predictive value of 68% emphasizes the importance of proceeding to angiography despite apparently normal noninvasive studies.

Pathologic Diagnosis

When the appearance of a cyanotic skin lesion is atypical and the diagnosis is unclear, biopsy of suspicious cutaneous lesions may be helpful in establishing the diagnosis. Similarly, random muscle biopsies from the lower extremities have been used to confirm the diagnosis of atheroembolism (Fig 54–2). These will usually be positive in patients who have suffered atheromatous embolization despite the absence of any focal muscle tenderness, thus emphasizing the diffuse nature of microscopic atheroemboli even when there are no obvious clinical symptoms. When digital amputation is required because of gangrene, pathologic examination of the

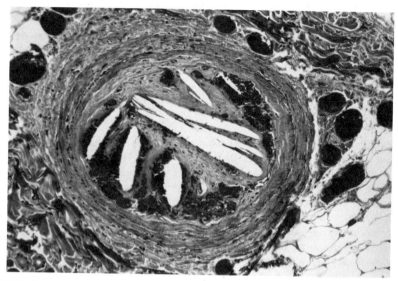

FIG 54–2.
Small, subdermal artery occluded by recent thrombus containing cholesterol crystals.
Such lesions are typically found in areas of cutaneous gangrene or livedo reticularis.

surgical specimen is rarely diagnostic, since the amputation is usually performed distal to the point at which the embolus impacts and the digital arteries are found only to contain propagated thrombus.

Arteriography

High quality, biplanar arteriography of the abdominal aorta and infrainguinal arterial tree is the cornerstone of diagnosis in spontaneous atheroembolism, and should be performed in all patients who would otherwise be reasonable operative candidates if an appropriate lesion were documented. The precise focus and extent of the angiograms will be determined by the location of the patient's symptoms and the results of the noninvasive vascular studies. In addition to the usual anterior-posterior and lateral views, oblique projections may occasionally be necessary to demonstrate small ulcerative lesions on the posterolateral wall of the aorta. In such cases, traditional views of the aorta may be surprisingly normal. Since aortic and peripheral aneurysms are a common source of atheroemboli, CT scans of suspicious sites within the arterial tree may occasionally be helpful, especially if angiograms of these vessels fail to confirm the diagnosis. However, this step would not usually be necessary. The location of previous embolic episodes may give additional clues as to the responsible source. For example, in patients who have suffered both upper and lower extremity emboli, the ascending aorta and transverse arch will have to be carefully inspected for an appropriate lesion. On the other hand, the most common source of bilateral lower extremity emboli is the infrarenal aorta. On those rare occasions when angiograms of this area are normal, it may be necessary to examine the thoracic aorta.

Patients with multiple atheroemboli from a diffusely diseased aorta are at significant risk of suffering iatrogenic emboli during arteriography unless great care is exercised and extensive manipulation with intraarterial catheters is avoided. In such cases, it may be appropriate to consider translumbar aortography, despite its limited versatility, rather than the more traditional Seldinger technique.

In general, in order to indict a proximal lesion as the source of distal emboli, a patent vascular channel must be demonstrable from the lesion to the point of impaction. Although microscopic cholesterol emboli can theoretically traverse the intervening collateral network around an arterial occlusion and impact in a distal arterial bed, this occurs only rarely.

PROGNOSIS

Despite the deceptively benign appearance of an isolated "blue toe" and the reassuring presence of palpable pedal pulses, atheroembolism is characterized by a tendency to recur with an increasing risk of tissue loss. In Wingo's series of such patients, only 44% of the affected extremities had an uncomplicated course without surgery. Thirty-eight percent of patients suffered tissue loss as a result of the initial embolic episode, and 14% had recurrent emboli. Twenty-two percent of the patients ultimately suffered amputation. During the seven years of follow-up in this study, the cumulative amputation rate was 32%, and the mortality rate was 52%.

TREATMENT

Medical

When macroembolization occurs, the patient should be systemically anticoagulated to prevent propagation of thrombus. The use of anticoagulation in patients with microembolization is less well established. Although anticoagulation during the acute major embolic event may be appropriate, the chronic use of anticoagulants in preventing recurrent embolization is generally unsuccessful. In fact, several reports have actually suggested that anticoagulation may favor repetitive embolization by preventing the formation of a protective thrombus over the eroded ulcerative plaque. Although platelet antiaggregating drugs, such as aspirin or dipyridamole have been useful in reducing the frequency of transient ischemic attacks in patients with carotid artery atherosclerosis, there is no data to support similar treatment in lower extremity atheroembolism.

Surgical

The most important challenge facing the surgeon treating a patient with spontaneous atheroembolism is to identify the source of the emboli. Once the responsible lesion is located, it can be removed directly by a local procedure or excluded from the circulation using bypass techniques. If the lesion is clearly focal and the adjacent artery is relatively normal, thromboendarterectomy, with or without patch angioplasty, may be perfectly adequate in preventing recurrent embolization. This type of treatment is generally used in the management of patients with localized disease at the aortic bifurcation.

When multiple, tandem lesions are present on the symptomatic side, precise localization may be impossible. Under such circumstances, we generally follow several principles in selecting the appropriate operation: (1) If stenotic lesions are of unequal severity, the most severe lesion should be treated first; (2) if they are of equal severity, then the more proximal lesion should be treated; (3) if an arterial aneurysm is identified, it should be replaced promptly because of its potential for rupture and/or thrombosis.

When emboli have arisen from an arterial aneurysm, that entire arterial segment must be replaced with an appropriate prosthetic graft. Bypass grafts, without exclusion of the native vessel, will not remove the embolic source and may permit further aneurysmal expansion and/or rupture.

The surgeon operating on patients for spontaneous atheroembolism must be particularly cautious during operative manipulation of the diseased arterial segment. Often such vessels are filled with loose, friable material that may be easily dislodged during dissection. In particularly worrisome cases, distal vascular clamps may be applied prior to dissection of the diseased segment to prevent showering the circulation with atheroma. Finally, once the arterial reconstruction is complete, but prior to release of the vascular clamps, the graft should be carefully flushed to prevent material proximal to the clamp from embolizing distally.

Atheromatous embolization during aortic or iliac reconstruction may result not only in distal extremity ischemia, but also has been reported to cause spinal cord ischemia, renal infarction, and buttock necrosis. Once such diffuse embolization has occurred, there is no effective form of medical or surgical treatment, and amputation and/or death may be inevitable. This fact reemphasizes the importance of careful intraoperative technique to *prevent* iatrogenic embolization. When embolization has resulted in chronic cutaneous ischemia that will not be immediately corrected by proximal bypass grafting, an adjunctive lumbar sympathectomy may be useful to increase skin blood flow and reduce tissue loss.

CONCLUSIONS

Spontaneous atheroembolism is a particularly challenging problem for the vascular surgeon. Because of its tendency to recur with increasing risk of tissue loss, precise diagnosis and appropriate treatment must be promptly instituted. A high index of suspicion is essential in this regard. Thorough biplanar arteriography remains the cornerstone of diagnosis and will usually localize the responsible lesion. Subsequent treatment can be planned based on the extent of disease and the quality of the surrounding vessels. For localized lesions, thromboendarterectomy and vein patch angioplasty may be perfectly suitable. However, for more diffuse disease or for emboli originating from arterial aneurysms, prosthetic graft replacement is essential. In such patients, the responsible arterial segment must be completely excluded from the circulation to prevent either further aneurysmal expansion or recurrent embolization. Once the responsible lesion is satisfactorily removed, the likelihood of recurrent embolization is small and a durable revascularization will usually result.

BIBLIOGRAPHY

1. Karmody AM, Powers SR, Monaco VJ, et al: "Blue toe" syndrome. An indication for limb salvage surgery. *Arch Surg* 1976; 111:1263–1268.
2. Kempczinski RF: Lower-extremity arterial emboli from ulcerating atherosclerotic plaques. *JAMA* 1979; 241:807–810.
3. Wagner RB, Martin AS: Peripheral atheroembolism: Confirmation of a clinical concept, with a case report and review of the literature. *Surgery* 1973; 73:353–359.
4. Wingo JP, Nix ML, Greenfield LJ, et al: The blue toe syndrome: Hemodynamics and therapeutic correlates of outcome. *J Vasc Surg* 1986; 3:475–480.

55 Upper Extremity Ischemia

A 51-year-old carpenter is seen for a painful index finger of the right hand. This began approximately one week ago, and now is too painful for him to work. He denies direct trauma to the finger. Examination reveals a tender, discolored fingertip with blistering and signs of early tissue necrosis.

Consultant: James S.T. Yao, M.D.

This case represents a form of occupational vascular injury. History taking must include whether the patient has used his hand to strike hard objects during his work. Repetitive use of the palm of the hand in activities which involve pushing, pounding, or twisting may cause injury to the ulnar artery. Inquiry also must include the frequency of use of the arm in an overhead position during work as a carpenter. The latter may stress the thoracic outlet and cause arterial damage. Physical examination should include palpation of the palm of the hand to look for a pulsatile mass indicating the presence of an aneurysm. An Allen test to determine patency of the palmar arch should be done in all patients with hand ischemia. Examination for thoracic outlet syndrome is mandatory in the evaluation of any patient suspected of having hand ischemia.

DIFFERENTIAL DIAGNOSIS

Unlike lower extremity ischemia, the potential etiological factors for hand ischemia are multiple. Diagnosis is aided by history taking and physical examination. History taking must include occupational, pharmacologic and medical aspects. Table 55–1 shows the various causes of hand ischemia. In general, a careful history will help guide diagnostic workup. In this case, the possibility of arterial injury is either due to repetitive trauma to the hand, causing the hypothenar hammer syndrome or thoracic outlet compression. A careful clinical examination including evaluation of the thoracic outlet, coupled with noninvasive tests and arteriography, will help establish the diagnosis.

TABLE 55-1.
Etiology of Upper Extremity and Digital Ischemia

I. Atherosclerosis
   A. Arteriosclerosis obliterans
   B. Embolization
      1. Cardiac
      2. Atheromatous emboli
      3. Arterial bypass graft
II. Arteritis
   A. Collagen disease
      1. Scleroderma
      2. Rheumatoid arteritis
      3. Systemic lupus erythematous
      4. Polyarteritis
   B. Allergic necrotizing arteritis
   C. Takayasu's disease (autoimmune disorder)
   D. Buerger's syndrome
   E. Giant cell arteritis
   F. Behcet's disease
III. Blood Dyscrasias
   A. Cold agglutins
   B. Cryoglobulins
   C. Polycythemia
IV. Drug Induced Ischemia
   A. Ergot poisoning
   B. Dopamine infusion
   C. Chemotherapeutic agents
   D. Beta-blockers
   E. Drug abuse
V. Occupational Trauma
   A. Vibratory white finger
   B. Hypothenar hammer syndrome
   C. Electrical burns
   D. Acro-osteolysis
VI. Thoracic Outlet Syndrome
VII. Congenital Arterial Wall Defects
VIII. Trauma
   A. Iatrogenic catheter injury
      1. Cardiac catheterization
      2. Arterial blood gas and pressure monitoring
      3. Arteriography
IX. Renal Transplantation and Related Problems
   A. Azotemic arteriopathy
   B. Hemodialysis shunts
X. Aneurysms of the Upper Extremity

OCCUPATIONAL VASCULAR INJURIES

Arterial injury of the hand in the form of occupational trauma includes vibration-induced white finger, hypothenar hammer syndrome, electrical burns, acroosteolysis, and athletic injuries. Diagnosis of vibration injury is simple if patients have been exposed to vibrating tools. Similarly, workers exposed to polyvinylchloride may present with digital artery occlusion and bone absorption collectively called "occupational acroosteolysis." Electrical burns causing arterial injury are uncommon and occur only in high voltage (>1000 V). Athletic injury is of interest. This may occur as a result of direct trauma to the hand (catchers, handball and frisbee players) or due to thoracic outlet compression such as seen in baseball pitchers.

A carpenter or electrician who uses his hand as a hammer may develop the so-called hypothenar hammer syndrome in which occlusion of the ulnar artery occurs as a result of repetitive trauma. Of the types of employment in 32 patients with hypothenar hammer syndrome reported by Pineda and colleagues, two were carpenters by profession (Table 55–2). Many of these workers used their hand as a hammer to strike hard objects.

The anatomical location of the ulnar artery in the area of the hypothenar eminence places it in a vulnerable position. The terminal branches of the ulnar artery (deep palmar branch and superficial arch) arise in a groove called Guyon's tunnel, bound medially by the pisiform and hook of the hamate and dorsally by the transverse carpal ligament. Over a distance of 2 cm, the ulnar artery lies quite superficially in the palm, being covered only by skin, subcutaneous tissue, and the palmaris brevis muscle (Fig 55–1). When this area is repeatedly traumatized, ulnar or digital arterial spasm, aneurysm formation, occlusion, or a combination of these lesions can result. Embolization from an aneurysm may cause multiple digital artery occlusions distally. The type of arterial abnormality observed will often depend on the nature of the damage to the vessel. Thus, intimal damage often results in thrombotic occlusion while injury to media causes palmar aneurysms (Fig 55–2).

TABLE 55–2.
Type of Employment in 32 patients with Hypothenar Hammer Syndrome (Modified from Pineda, et al)

Mechanic/Auto repair	15
Lathe operator	3
Fitter and turner	2
Tire braider	2
Carpenter	2
Engineer	2
Machinist	2
Painter	1
Butcher	1
Gardener	1
Tool and die worker	1
Bus conductor	1

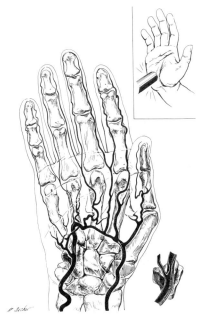

FIG 55–1.
Mechanism of injury to the ulnar artery in patients with hypothenar hammer syndrome. (From Yao JST: Occupational Vascular Problems, in: Rutherford R (ed): *Vascular Surgery*, ed 3. Philadelphia, WB Saunders, Co, in press. Used by permission.)

Clinically, the patient presents with symptoms of Raynaud's phenomenon, namely, numbness, paresthesias, stiffness, coldness, and blanching of one or more digits of the dominant hand. In the series of patients described by Conn, et al, the ring finger was the most commonly involved digit. The traditional triphasic color (white-blue-red) changes and thumb involvement are uncommon. Physical examination may disclose a prominent callus over the hypothenar eminence, coldness or mottling of the involved fingertip, along with atrophic ulceration. A positive Allen test, indicating ulnar artery occlusion, is a common finding. Occasionally, the presence of aneurysm can be detected as a pulsatile mass in the palm.

THORACIC OUTLET COMPRESSION

Carpenters' overhead hammering activities may subject the subclavian artery to compression, resulting in hand ischemia. Such a possibility is enhanced if bony abnormality such as cervical rib or abnormal first rib is present. In the absence of history of direct trauma to the hand, determining the cause of ischemia must include a careful examination of the thoracic outlet. The best positional test for evidence of thoracic outlet compression is adduction-external rotation. Obliteration of upper extremity pulses and the presence of a subclavian bruit in that position is diagnostic for compression to the subclavian artery. Compression of the subclavian artery by a cervical rib or abnormally large anterior scalene muscle may cause stenosis or aneurysm formation. The potential hazard of such aneurysmal degeneration is em-

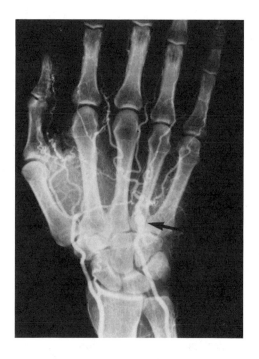

FIG 55–2.
Aneurysm of the terminal branch of the ulnar artery (arrow) due to hypothenar hammer syndrome. (From Flinn WR, et al: Aneurysms of secondary and tertiary branches of major arteries, in: Bergan JJ and Yao JST (eds): *Aneurysms: Diagnosis and Treatment.* New York, Grune & Stratton, Inc, 1982, p 452. Used by permission.)

bolization, leading to possibly severe arterial ischemia of the upper extremity, hand, or digit (Fig 55–3). Not infrequently, palpation of the supraclavicular space will reveal a cervical rib or a pulsatile mass. It is well known that a cervical rib may cause arterial damage, and this possible association should be suspected in young patients who present with unilateral hand ischemia symptoms. In occupational injuries, thoracic outlet compression is seen in athletes who engage in sporting activities requiring exaggerated shoulder activities. Injuries to the subclavian artery have been reported in baseball pitchers and oarsmen, among others.

DIAGNOSIS

Noninvasive Tests

Plethysmography or transcutaneous Doppler ultrasound flow detection are now available to establish the diagnosis of hand ischemia more accurately. Wave-form recording of symptomatic fingers by plethysmography helps to separate vasospastic

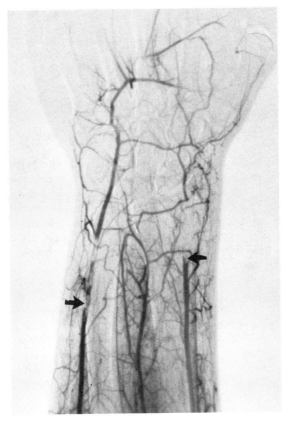

FIG 55–3.
Arteriogram of the hand in a carpenter with thoracic outlet compression. Filling defects (arrow) represent embolization from the damaged subclavian artery. (From Yao JST, Mc-Carthy WJ: Hand ischemia in young carpenter. *Contemp Surg* 1987; 30:83–87. Used by permission.)

from occlusive disease. The use of Doppler technique is simple, especially the recordings of systolic pressure. The Doppler finger systolic pressure is of particular value in detecting digital artery occlusions.

The Doppler technique is also useful to determine the patency of palmar arch more objectively, especially in uncooperative patients. Recently, the use of B-mode scan has helped detect a small aneurysm of the terminal branch of the ulnar artery in the palm. For thoracic outlet compression, the use of duplex scan and finger systolic pressure measurement provides a comprehensive examination of the thoracic outlet and the upper extremity.

For definitive diagnosis, arteriography is necessary, especially if surgical intervention is contemplated. Because thoracic outlet compression may be the cause of hand ischemia, arteriographic examination should include the subclavian artery. This would certainly be true of this patient, a carpenter. The preferred arteriographic approach is a retrograde catheter study with Seldinger's technique via the femoral artery. This approach allows a complete examination of the proximal artery as well as the arteries of all fingers. Positional or pharmacologic arteriography is often needed to complete the arteriographic examination.

TREATMENT

Surgical treatment is indicated if there is evidence of either thoracic outlet compression with damage to the artery or an aneurysm of the terminal branch of the ulnar artery. A patient with thrombus of the ulnar artery alone is seldom a candidate for surgery. In patients with digital artery occlusion without major arterial occlusion, a trial of calcium channel blocking may help to relieve Raynaud's symptoms. An ulnar aneurysm, if present, must be resected to eliminate the source of emboli. Restoration of arterial flow can be done by end-to-end anastomosis or by the use of an interposed vein graft.

For thoracic outlet compression, we prefer the combined supraclavicular and infraclavicular approach. The supraclavicular approach allows a detailed examination of the outlet. Also, the division of anterior scalene muscle facilitates exposure and also eliminates a possible cause of compression. A cervical rib, if present, must be removed. Arterial bypass is done to restore continuity if there is an aneurysm or occlusion of the artery. If a bypass graft is needed, we have found the additional infraclavicular incision helps to facilitate the performance of distal anastomosis. For graft material, we prefer saphenous vein harvested from the thigh.

Treatment of hypothenar hammer syndrome is largely conservative with the exception of aneurysm. Excellent long-term follow-up by this approach has recently been reported by Vayssairat and his colleagues. Because of the occupational hazards, avoidance of repetitive trauma or a change of profession may be necessary to prevent further injury.

BIBLIOGRAPHY

1. Conn J, Bergan JJ, Bell JL: Hypothenar hammer syndrome: Post-traumatic digital ischemia. *Surgery* 1970; 68:1122–1128.
2. Fields WS: Neurovascular syndromes of the neck and shoulders. *Seminars Neurol* 1981; 1:301–309.
3. Fields WS, Lemak NA, Ben-Menachem Y: Thoracic outlet syndrome: Review and reference to stroke in a major league pitcher. *AJNR* 1986; 7:73–78.
4. Kamienski RW, Barnes RW: Critique of the Allen test for continuity of the palmar arch assessed by Doppler ultrasound. *Surg Gynecol Obstet* 1976; 142:861–864.
5. Little JM, Ferguson DA: The incidence of the hypothenar hammer syndrome. *Arch Surg* 1972; 105:684–685.

6. Pineda CJ, Weisman MH, Bookstein JJ, et al: Hypothenar hammer syndrome: Form of reversible Raynaud's phenomenon. *Am J Med* 1985; 79:561–570.

7. Scher LA, Veith FJ, Haimovici H, et al: Staging of the arterial complications of cervical rib: Guidelines for surgical management. *Surgery* 1984; 95:644–649.

8. Sumner DS: Noninvasive assessment of upper extremity ischemia, in: Bergan JJ, Yao JST (eds): *Evaluation and Treatment of Upper and Lower Extremity Circulatory Disorders*. Orlando, Grune & Stratton, 1984, pp 75–95.

9. Vayssairat M, Debure C, Cormier J, et al: Hypothenar hammer syndrome: Seventeen cases with long-term follow-up. *J Vasc Surg* 1987; 5:838–843.

10. Yao JST: Preoperative assessment of upper extremity ischemia, in: Greenhalgh RM (ed): *Diagnostic Techniques and Assessment Procedures in Vascular Surgery*. London, Grune & Stratton, 1985, pp. 359–378.

11. Yao JST, McCarthy WJ: Hand ischemia in a young carpenter. *Contemp Surg* 1987; 30:83–87.

12. Yao JST: Occupational vascular problems, in Rutherford R (ed): *Vascular Surgery*, ed 3. Philadelphia, WB Saunders, Co, in press.

56 Vasospastic Disease

A 39-year-old waitress is seen for complaints of episodic cold numb fingers of both hands. Such symptoms have been present for several years, but are getting worse. When she handles cold glasses or plates, her hands and fingers become pale, numb, and sensitive. Rewarming may take up to one hour. She is having difficulty working. She gave up cigarette smoking six months ago, without much benefit.

Consultant: John M. Porter, M.D.

The history is typical for Raynaud's syndrome (RS). RS defines a clinical condition characterized by episodic digital vasospasm induced by cold exposure or emotional stimuli. The hands and fingers are most frequently affected, although the feet and toes may be involved in occasional patients. RS has classically been associated with a triple color digital response consisting of pallor, followed by cyanosis and rubor. During an attack, the hands feel cold and numb, and fine motor movements may be difficult to impossible. In my experience, most patients do not describe the classic triple color response, but develop only digital pallor or cyanosis during attacks. The attacks may subside spontaneously, or may persist until the patient enters a warm area or applies local heat to the part. Critical to the definition of RS is the observation that the affected part is normal between attacks. Persistent cyanosis of one hand or finger caused by acute or subacute arterial insufficiency should certainly not be termed RS.

A physician encountering a patient with RS has a need to establish the diagnosis; determine whether the patient has obstructive or spastic RS; conduct a search for associated diseases; and recommend treatment. A logical approach to the care of patients with RS requires an understanding of the pathophysiology of the condition.

PATHOPHYSIOLOGY OF RAYNAUD'S SYNDROME

Abundant evidence indicates that RS exists in two discrete forms, obstructive and spastic. Patients with obstructive Raynaud's have diffuse obstructive disease of the

388

palmar and digital arteries of diverse etiologies. In my experience, the most frequent are arteritis associated with autoimmune disease, hypersensitivity angiitis, atherosclerosis, and Buerger's disease. The presence of diffuse arterial obstruction results in diminished finger arterial pressure. In this setting, a normal digital artery vasoconstrictive response to cold is sufficient to overcome the diminished intraluminal distending pressure and cause arterial closure. Patients with spastic RS have unobstructed palmar and digital arteries and normal digital arterial pressure. In these patients the induction of a digital vasospastic attack requires an abnormally forceful cold-induced digital arterial constrictive response to overcome the normal arterial distending pressure and produce arterial closure. To date no consistent abnormalities in central nervous system function have been documented in patients with RS. The cause of the abnormally forceful digital arterial contraction in patients with spastic RS appears to reside in the arterial wall itself, a condition that has been termed ''local vascular fault.''

In the individual patient it is important to categorize the RS as obstructive or spastic, as this categorization has both prognostic and therapeutic implications. Patients with spastic RS have patent hand arteries and a low incidence of associated diseases. For most of these patients the RS represents merely a life-long incidental nuisance condition which does not proceed to finger gangrene. Additionally, spastic RS has a higher likelihood than obstructive RS of responding favorably to drug treatment. Patients with obstructive RS always have an associated disease that in certain patients is sufficiently serious as to shorten survival. With time, some of these patients will develop finger gangrene.

ESTABLISHING THE DIAGNOSIS

In most patients the diagnosis of RS is established by the patient's history of episodic digital ischemia manifested by numbness and pallor or cyanosis induced by cold exposure or emotional stimuli. Many patients, however, present an atypical history. For these patients, as well as additional patients with legal or compensation claims, a vascular lab diagnostic test to objectively document the presence of RS is clearly needed. Of the dozens of tests proposed, the only one sufficiently accurate to be clinically useful is the digital hypothermic perfusion test described by Nielsen and associates, and this is the one that I use routinely. While this test has an accuracy of over 90%, it is time consuming, requires relatively expensive equipment, and is quite technician dependent.

In addition to documenting the presence of RS, the vascular lab is essential in differentiating obstructive from spastic RS. Digital photophlethysmography is performed bilaterally on the index, long, and ring fingers, and digital pressures are obtained by the use of small proximal pneumatic cuffs in addition to PPG. Both the arterial waveforms and digital pressures are used to establish the presence or absence of arterial obstruction. A representative digital PPG tracing is shown in Figure 56–1. Digital BP more than 15 Torr below brachial or more than 15 Torr

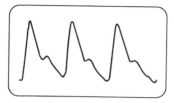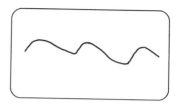

FIG 56–1.
The photoplethysmographic finger arterial waveform (digital PPG) has proved to be an extremely simple and important test in the evaluation of patients with RS. The left tracing is normal with rapid upstroke and descent, sharp peak, and clean dicrotic notch. The right tracing indicates severe stenosis or obstruction of both proper digital arteries and shows slow upstroke and descent, rounded peak, and absence of dicrotic notch.

below other fingers, or an absolute digital pressure less than 70 Torr is indicative of arterial obstruction.

As noted, one of the frequent causes of obstructive RS is generalized arteriosclerosis. The vascular lab may be helpful in this regard if peripheral arterial or cerebrovascular testing confirms widespread arterial disease in a patient suspected of having palmar and digital artery obstruction due to arteriosclerosis.

ASSOCIATED DISEASES

In the course of a detailed prospective evaluation of over 900 patients with RS we have found significant associated diseases in about 60%, with autoimmune disease present in about 40%. Only about 40% of patients had primary or vasospastic RS without an associated disease. This is summarized in Table 56–1. Thus, the investigation of any patient with RS must include a detailed evaluation for the presence of associated diseases, especially autoimmune diseases. The laboratory tests which we have found to be the most helpful are listed in Table 56–2. Scleroderma, the most frequent associated autoimmune disease, is usually associated with sclerodactyly, skin tightening, and calcinosis. A careful clinical exam for these features and hand x-ray for calcinosis are obtained routinely.

Based on the clinical exam, vascular lab digital plethysmography waveforms and pressures, and serologic lab screening tests, the presence and type of associated disease is clearly established. As noted, an associated disease is present in every patient with obstructive RS.

Arteriography has a limited role in the evaluation of patients with RS. It should be performed in patients suspected of having a proximal arterial lesion that may be amenable to surgical therapy. Patients most likely to have a proximal arterial lesion are those with diminished or absent elbow or wrist pulses, or patients with unilateral finger ischemia associated with palmar and digital artery obstruction in whom the arterial obstruction may be the result of embolization from a proximal arterial le-

TABLE 56–1.
Associated Disorders in 631 Patients' with Raynaud's Syndrome
1970-1987

Idiopathic (pure vasospasm with no associated disease)	236 (37.4%)
Connective Tissue Disease (CTD)	235 (37.2%)
Scleroderma, CREST	
Undifferentiated connective tissue disease	
Suspected CTD	
Mixed connective tissue disease	
Rheumatoid arthritis	
Systemic lupus erythematosus	
Hypersensitivy Angiitis (rapid onset vascular occlusion)	22 (3.5%)
Myeloproliferative Disorders	1 (0.2%)
Abnormal	13 (2%)
Atherosclerosis Obliterans	35 (5.5%)
Buerger's Disease	12 (1.9%)
Frostbite	25 (4%)
Trauma/Vibration Injury	10 (1.6%)
Medication Induced	10 (1.6%)
Embolization	5 (0.8%)
Other	9 (1.4%)
Miscellaneous	18 (2.9%)
Total Number of Patients	631 (100%)

TABLE 56–2.
Laboratory Evaluation of Raynaud's Syndrome

ROUTINE SCREENING TESTS	ADDITIONAL TESTS (SELECTED PATIENTS)
Complete blood count	Serum protein electrophoresis
Erythrocyte sedimentation rate	Extractable nuclear antibody
Chemistry profile	Antinative DNA antibody
Urinalysis	HEP-2 ANA
Rheumatoid factor	Cryoglobulins
Antinuclear antibody	Hepatitis B screen
	Anticentromere antibody

sion. On the other hand, patients with diffuse ischemia of all fingers, or at least multiple fingers on both hands, are unlikely to have bilateral simultaneously embolizing proximal arterial lesions, and in these patients arteriography does not appear indicated. In my experience patients with simultaneous bilateral finger ischemia invariably have diffuse intrinsic palmar and digital obstruction associated with a systemic disease process. Representative arteriograms of patients with spastic and obstructive RS are shown in Figures 56–2 and 56–3.

TREATMENT

Over 90% of patients with RS do well with simple cold and tobacco avoidance and careful attention to wearing warm clothing. Drug therapy is only occasionally effective. The most effective drugs in the management of the 10% of patients with RS not adequately improved by other measures are the calcium channel blockers, especially nifedipine, and occasionally diltiazem. The usual dose of nifedipine is 10 to 20 mg daily. Drug therapy has a higher likelihood of benefit in patients with spastic RS as opposed to obstructive RS. Unfortunately, up to 50% of patients with RS begun on nifedipine develop intolerable medication side effects including headache, lassitude, or ankle edema, leading to voluntary discontinuation of the drug.

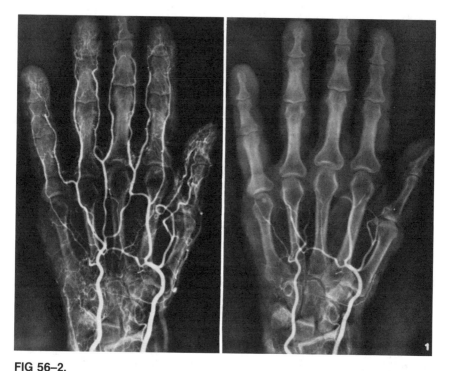

FIG 56–2.
Representative hand arteriogram of patient with vasospastic RS. The left film is at room temperature and the right film is following hand immersion in ice water. The marked vasospasm is obvious. The hand arterial anatomy is normal.

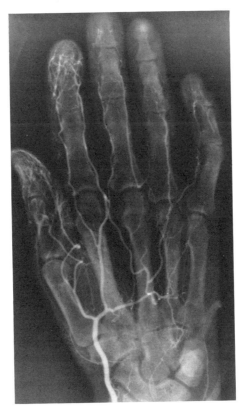

FIG 56–3.
Hand arteriogram of patient with obstructive RS. The ulnar artery and superficial palmar arch are occluded, as are a number of proper digital arteries.

Our overall experience is that only about 25% of patients started on drug therapy anecdotally derive significant benefit without severe side effects. Unfortunately, there is currently no vascular lab test which accurately detects drug benefit. This drug efficacy evaluation remains anecdotal, with all the drawbacks implicit in this method of drug assessment.

Historically, thoracic sympathectomy has been recommended frequently in the treatment of RS. My review of the published data includes several problems. In the first place the assessment of benefit is anecdotal since there is no objective test for this purpose. Additionally, the anecdotal assessment of benefit is invariably recorded by the operating surgeon, hardly a disinterested observer. Despite this built-in prejudice in favor of surgery, available data indicate inconsistent benefits, especially in patients with obstructive RS. I rarely recommend sympathectomy in the treatment of RS, and never in patients with obstructive RS. Our only recommendation for sympathectomy is in rare patients with severe spastic RS refractory to drug therapy who face loss of employment because of cold sensitivity. To date this group has included only individuals who must work outside, such as timber fallers and construction workers. The patient presented at the beginning of this section worked as a waitress. To date this has not been an occupation for which we have recommended sympathectomy.

CASE DISCUSSION

A detailed analysis of this case may now be considered, based on the preceding information. The symptomatic onset of RS in a 37-year-old smoking female is of interest. Most patients with RS are female but the onset in a large majority of these patients is in the second and third decade of life. The slightly older than usual onset and the history of smoking suggest the possibility of obstructive RS. I note the symptoms are symmetrical and bilateral and quite typical for RS. I recommend a vascular lab evaluation on this patient, including digital hypothermic perfusion test and digital blood pressure and plethysmography. This will undoubtedly confirm the presence of RS and will allow differentiation of spastic from obstructive RS. There is no indication of need for arteriography as the symptoms and findings are bilateral.

A hand x-ray is recommended for evidence of calcinosis suggesting scleroderma or CREST syndrome. Routine laboratory tests would include CBC and platelet count, antinuclear antibody, rheumatoid factor, erythrocyte sedimentation rate, chemistry profile, and urinalysis. Additional serologic testing may be requested depending on the results of the screening tests. Based on the results of these tests I will be able to diagnose most associated autoimmune disease processes. Certain combinations of findings may indicate the need for additional testing. For example, if the patient had diffusely obstructive palmar and digital circulation but no evidence of autoimmune disease, I would obtain a lower extremity vascular lab exam including toe plethysmography to determine if the patient had generalized arterial occlusions, which if present may suggest diffuse arteriosclerosis or Buerger's disease. At this point the evaluation should have confirmed that the patient has RS, indicating whether the RS was spastic or obstructive, and screened for the most frequently associated disease processes.

The next issue is treatment. Since the patient works indoors and has already stopped smoking, the usual recommendations of cold and tobacco avoidance are already being observed. Accordingly, I would recommend nifedipine 10 mg bid together with diltiazem 30 mg bid. As noted above, only about 25% of patients are significantly improved by drugs. Fully one half discontinue medication because of headache, lassitude, or ankle swelling. If the patient either cannot tolerate drugs or is unimproved, second line drugs including prazocin 1 mg bid, or guanethidine 10 mg qd, may be tried. If the patient continues unimproved by these drugs, additional drug therapy is unlikely to be of benefit.

Next we come to a series of ifs. If the patient has spastic RS with no associated diseases, if she continues sufficiently symptomatic as to threaten her employment, and if she is unimproved on drug therapy, then I might recommend thoracic sympathectomy. I would inform the patient there was about a 50% likelihood of long term improvement. It is important to note that the presence of either associated disease or obstructive RS rules out any consideration of sympathectomy. I perform upper extremity sympathectomy through the transaxillary route with resection of a short portion of third rib, and removal of the second through fourth sympathetic ganglia. I do not remove the inferior pole of the stellate ganglion as I find this does not materially improve the results of sympathectomy and significantly increases the likelihood of Horner's syndrome. The occurrence of this complication, especially the ptosis, can be a devastating cosmetic problem in a female. Despite these precautions, the patient is obviously always warned clearly preoperatively about the possibility of Horner's syndrome.

The long term prospects for this patient will depend entirely on the results of the evaluation. If she has spastic RS without associated disease she will have the RS only as an incidental nuisance condition. If she has an associated disease, the natural history of the associated condition will determine her future course. In any case, the likelihood of her subsequently developing severe finger ischemia with tissue loss is remote.

BIBLIOGRAPHY

1. Gates KH, Tyburczy JA, Zupan T, et al: The non-invasive quantification of digital vasospasm. *Bruit* 1984; 8:34–37.
2. Holmgren K, Baur GM, Porter JM: The role of digital photoplethysmography in the evaluation of Raynaud's syndrome. *Bruit* 1981; 5:19–24.
3. Nielsen SL, Lassen NA: Measurement of digital blood pressure after local cooling. *J Appl Physiol* 1977; 43:907–910.
4. Porter JM, Taylor LM, Jr: Limb ischemia caused by small artery disease. *World J Surg* 1983; 7:326–333.
5. Rivers SP, Porter JM: Clinical approach to Raynaud's syndrome. *Vasc Diag Ther* 1983; 4:15–24.
6. Rosch J, Porter JM, Gralino BJ: Cryodynamic hand angiography in the diagnosis and management of Raynaud's syndrome. *Circulation* 1977; 55:807–814.

57   Thoracic Outlet Syndrome

A 30-year-old professional tennis player is seen for swelling of the right arm the morning after a hard match. For the past year he has noticed periodic discomfort and tingling in the arm, particularly when serving, which he had ascribed to muscle fatigue.

Consultants: Brent Steffen, M.D.
and Donald Silver, M.D.

Mild to moderate muscular edema is not unexpected after strenuous activity. Most often the edema regresses quickly and there are no sequelae. If the edema persists for more than 24 hours, obstruction to venous outflow should be suspected. Venous compression by various structures at the thoracic outlet may be responsible, possibly leading to subclavian-axillary vein thrombosis. A combination of edema and neurological symptoms in the upper extremity should make one suspect that the patient, like the one described above, has a thoracic outlet syndrome.

The thoracic outlet syndrome is caused by compression of the neurovascular structures of the upper extremity. Most patients present with symptoms related to compression of the elements of the brachial plexus. However, symptoms from compression or thrombosis of the subclavian vein, as suggested by the sudden onset of unilateral upper extremity edema in this patient, occur in 1.5% of patients. Additionally, 3% to 4% of patients present with symptoms related to arterial compression. Although most patients complain of symptoms that are either neural or vascular, some patients may manifest a mixture of symptoms. This may account for the history of paresthesias in this tennis player, prior to the onset of arm swelling.

Upper extremity deep vein thrombosis is usually associated with congestive heart failure, axillary or intrathoracic tumors, indwelling subclavian venous catheters, or hypercoagulable states. It may, however, occur in a large group of otherwise healthy patients. In these patients, the thrombosis occurs spontaneously, following minor trauma, or following episodes of strenuous exertion. This type of thrombosis of the axillary and subclavian vein has been variously termed "primary thrombosis," "spontaneous thrombosis," and "effort thrombosis." An increased understanding of the pathophysiology of the thoracic outlet syndrome has led to the realization that many of these "primary" and "spontaneous" upper extremity thromboses are caused by venous compression in the thoracic outlet.

ANATOMY AND PATHOPHYSIOLOGY

The major arteries and components of the brachial plexus are subject to compression in several well-defined areas as they pass from the neck and thoracic outlet into the arm (Fig 57–1). The usual sites of compression include: (1) the interscalene triangle (artery and nerves); (2) the space between the scalenus anticus and the clavicle (vein); (3) between the first rib and clavicle (nerve, artery, and vein); and (4) the costocoracoid fascia (nerve, artery, and vein). Additionally, neurovascular compression by the pectoralis minor tendon may occur (nerve, artery, and vein) during times of hyperabduction of the arm.

ETIOLOGY

Symptoms may be caused by anything that distorts or narrows the spaces through which the neurovascular structures pass. The most common causes of the thoracic outlet syndrome are a deterioration of posture and/or an increase in weight. Ap-

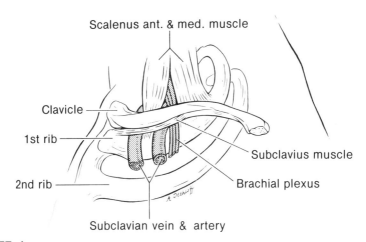

FIG 57–1.
The relationship of the scalenus anticus and medius muscles, the subclavius muscle, the clavicle and the first rib to the neurovascular structures are demonstrated.

proximately one third of the patients relate a history of trauma to the neck and shoulder regions prior to the development of symptoms. Trauma may produce muscular inflammation, edema, spasm, and fibrosis. The callous formation that occurs with healing of fractures may cause neurovascular compression. Neurovascular compression may also be caused by tumor encroachment on the various spaces. Occupations requiring heavy lifting or prolonged hyperabduction of the upper extremity (automobile mechanics, painters, and electricians) are associated with the thoracic outlet syndrome. In addition, strenuous exertion of the upper extremity that occurs in athletes such as tennis players and baseball pitchers leads to hypertrophy of the muscle mass and occasionally depression of the shoulder girdle, both predisposing to outlet compression.

Anatomic abnormalities within the thoracic outlet may cause neurovascular compression. Cervical ribs are present in approximately 1% of the population and produce symptoms of neurovascular compression in 10% of those individuals. The ribs may be unilateral or bilateral and frequently form an articulation with the first rib at the scalene tubercle. When a cervical rib is incomplete it frequently attaches to the first rib via a fibrous band. Long transverse processes of C7 may produce distortions similar to those produced by cervical ribs. These ribs and transverse processes elevate the vessels and inferior components of the brachial plexus.

Abnormalities of the scalene muscles may also produce compression. Such abnormalities include fibrous bands, incomplete muscular division, muscular fusion, fusion of muscle fibers to the perineurium of the brachial plexus, and the presence of a scalenus minimus. The contraction of these myofascial anomalies against the brachial plexus can cause a compression neuropathy.

DIAGNOSIS

General Considerations

The symptoms vary depending on whether nerves, arteries or veins are compressed. The symptoms are frequently multiple if more than one system is involved. All patients should be subjected to a thorough history and physical examination. The history should indicate the structures compressed, e.g., neural (paresthesias, weakness); arterial (coolness, pain, ulcers) and/or venous (edema, venous distention). The history should also detail changes in posture, weight, positions of sleep and positions required by occupation or physical activities. The physical examination should include a careful evaluation of the neurologic and vascular status of the upper extremities. Most often, the neurologic examination is normal even though the patient may complain of paresthesias and weakness. Occasionally a bruit will be heard in the supraclavicular space and, as in the patient described in this case, venous fullness and edema may be present. All patients should have a chest X-ray and cervical spine films to look for cervical ribs, foraminal narrowing, callous formation, and other structural abnormalities that may predispose to outlet compression.

Neural Compression

Compression of the brachial plexus is associated with pain, numbness, paresthesia, and weakness. Upper plexus involvement (C5, C6, and C7 nerve roots) results in pain, and/or paresthesias, in the side of the neck radiating to the ear, mandible, face, temple and occipital region. Hemicranial headaches may ensue. This pain also involves the rhomboid and pectoral regions and radiates down the outer aspect of the arm. The symptoms may mimic those of a C4 to C6 herniated disc; however, disc pain is usually constant, more severe, and radiates in a dermatomal distribution. Thoracic outlet symptoms usually are intermittent and aggravated by activity.

Lower plexus involvement (C8 and T1 nerve roots) tends to produce pain in the supraclavicular area, back of the neck, rhomboid and scapular regions and posterior axilla. This pain tends to radiate to the ulnar aspect of the arm and to the ring and small fingers. Again, hemicranial headaches and paresthesias may occur.

Pressure applied to the supraclavicular fossa may reproduce the symptoms. Tricep weakness may be present. Decreased grip, strength and interosseus weakness may also be present. Reflexes are normal. Lower plexus symptoms may mimic those produced by compression of the median nerve at the carpal tunnel and the ulnar nerve at the elbow. Electromyograms and nerve conduction studies are useful in identifying these peripheral compression syndromes, but are rarely specific for the thoracic outlet syndrome.

Physical maneuvers to diminish or obliterate radial pulses do not indicate brachial plexus compression as they are positive in 40% to 50% of the normal population. Similarly, arteriography and phlebography are not useful in patients with neural symptoms.

Venous Compression

Patients with venous compression or thrombosis are typically young, vigorous, healthy individuals who exhibit symptoms following periods of strenuous exertion or episodes of direct or indirect trauma. Venous compression was described in 1875 by Sir James Paget and subsequently in 1884 by von Schroetter, and for this reason this syndrome has been termed the Paget-Schroetter syndrome. Other names for this condition include ''spontaneous thrombosis,'' ''traumatic thrombosis,'' ''primary thrombosis'' and the ''effort syndrome.''

It is stated that microscopic intimal tears coupled with repetitive venous compression and stasis of flow predispose these patients to thrombosis. In the neck the subclavian vein is fixed by the internal and external jugular veins, while in the axilla the vein is anchored by the long thoracic, thoracodorsal, and subscapular veins. Thus, with motion of the arm and shoulder girdle, accommodation to movement of the vein occurs in the axillary-subclavian segment. This subjects the vein to stretching and shearing forces that may produce intimal injury.

Approximately two thirds of patients with venous compression symptoms present within 24 hours of the inciting event. These patients typically exhibit unilateral edema that increases from the shoulder to the finger tips. A feeling of tightness or an aching is usually present, and a prominent pattern of dilated superficial veins is seen on the hand, arm, neck, and anterior chest wall. Patients may exhibit cyanosis of the involved extremity. A few individuals may have a tender "cord" that is palpable in the axilla.

Phlebography is an important diagnostic modality in differentiating between thrombotic and nonthrombotic obstruction of the axillary-subclavian vein. If thrombotic obstruction is present the phlebogram will demonstrate prominent collateral veins, "first rib bypass collaterals," around the obstruction.

In most instances, these patients are managed with elevation of the extremity and anticoagulation with heparin for ten to 14 days followed by warfarin for three months. One is more likely to restore flow with lytic therapy, i.e., streptokinase, or urokinase, infused into a distal vein of the involved extremity in sufficient amounts until lysis has occurred. Lytic therapy should be followed by anticoagulant therapy. After the thrombus is lysed or recanalized, venous decompression will help prevent recurrence of the thrombosis. If lysis does not occur, bypass of the thrombosed segment with a saphenous vein graft may be necessary to provide adequate venous outflow from the involved upper extremity.

Arterial Compression

Compression of the second portion of the subclavian artery can cause turbulent flow and hemodynamic variations that may result in poststenotic dilatation and aneurysm formation. The arterial changes may contribute to distal embolization or even to thrombosis of the subclavian artery.

Signs and symptoms of arterial insufficiency include pain, weakness, and coolness of the involved extremity. In addition, the extremity may be easily fatigued and claudication may occur with use of the involved limb. Subungual splinter hemorrhages indicate peripheral embolization. Raynaud's phenomenon may also occur, with approximately one third of the patients with unilateral Raynaud's phenomenon having thoracic outlet compression. Advanced ischemia may lead to digital ulceration and gangrene.

Physical examination frequently reveals a supraclavicular bruit; a supraclavicular aneurysm may be palpable. The quality of the pulse from the subclavian artery to the radial artery should be evaluated and compared in the two arms, and the blood pressure of the two arms should also be compared. Maneuvers of arterial compression include the Adson maneuver in which the patient takes a deep breath, extends the neck, and turns the chin to the side being examined. A positive exam results in a reduction or disappearance of the radial pulse and a bruit may become audible in the supraclavicular fossa. The distal portion of the extremity may become cool and pale. The costoclavicular compression maneuver involves placing the patient in an exaggerated military brace position with the shoulders thrust downward and back. This may also reduce the radial pulse and produce a subclavian bruit.

With the hyperabduction maneuver, the radial pulse reduces or disappears as the arm is moved to a position of hyperabduction. During these maneuvers, brachial plexus compression, with resultant symptoms, may also occur. A large segment, 40% to 50%, of the normal population has findings of arterial compression during these maneuvers.

Arteriography is indicated in those patients with aneurysms, embolization, or arterial insufficiency. Arteriography is performed with the arm at the side and hyperabducted. Findings may include stenosis of the subclavian artery, at the first rib, with poststenotic dilatation or an aneurysm. Total occlusion of the subclavian artery and obstruction of the distal arteries by emboli may be demonstrated with arteriography.

MANAGEMENT

Management of the thoracic outlet syndrome requires reducing the compression of the neurovascular structures in the thoracic outlet and treating any complications of the compression, e.g., aneurysm, thrombosis, emboli, and the like. Many patients (50% to 60%) with neurologic symptoms will obtain relief of symptoms with a program designed to reduce the compression. The program usually consists of improving posture, weight reduction, avoiding positions of hyperabduction, sleeping supine without a pillow and with the arms by one's side, and physical therapy directed at shoulder girdle strengthening. Those patients who do not improve after four to six months of this program, especially those patients whose occupations require activities that preclude their compliance, e.g., painters, professional athletes, automobile mechanics and the like, are considered candidates for operative decompression of their thoracic outlet.

The several procedures for decompressing the thoracic outlet include some or all of the following: dividing or resecting a portion of the scalenus anticus and scalenus medius muscles; dividing and/or resecting any myofascial bands that cause neurovascular compression; resecting the cervical rib with its attachment to the first rib; resecting the first rib; and dividing the pectoralis minor tendon. Although we have previously utilized the transaxillary approach for decompression of the thoracic outlet, we now prefer the supraclavicular approach.

Operative Management

The patient is positioned with the neck extended and the head rotated to the opposite side. An incision 8 cm to 10 cm long is placed 2 cm above the clavicle in the supraclavicular space. The clavicular portion of the sternocleidomastoid muscle is divided, the scalene fat pad is mobilized (or resected) and the phrenic nerve identified as it crosses the scalenus anticus muscle and is protected. The scalenus anticus is freed from the subclavian vein anteriorly, and the subclavian artery and brachial trunks posteriorly, and a 1 cm to 3 cm segment of the muscle is resected. If a cervical rib is present, it and any fibrous bands that attach it to the first rib are resected sufficiently posteriorly to eliminate any possibility of distorting the neurovascular structures. The brachial trunks are gently mobilized and any myofascial bands that are found are divided or resected. The scalenus medius is identified posterior to the neurovascular structures and is carefully divided. If the first rib is felt to be contributing to the compression of the neurovascular structures, the anterior portion of the rib can be removed through this approach. The wound is irrigated to ensure that the pleura is intact. If the pleura is not intact, a small chest tube is inserted through the wound and removed later in the day. The wound is closed by approximating the platysma, subcutaneous tissues and skin. If upper extremity hyperabduction contributes to the patient's symptoms, another incision is placed inferior to the lateral half of the clavicle, and the pectoralis minor tendon is divided near its attachment onto the coracoid process.

We have compared our results with supraclavicular decompression of the thoracic outlet to those we had obtained with the transaxillary decompression. Both procedures offered good relief of symptoms with 93% and 81% of the patients having supraclavicular decompression and transaxillary decompression, respectively, experiencing significant improvement at two months, and 100% and over 90%, respectively, remaining improved at a mean follow-up of three years. However, there are fewer complications, decreased blood loss and shorter hospitalization in patients having supraclavicular decompression.

Although an adequate decompression will provide relief of symptoms in 85% to 95% of patients, it will not correct structural changes, e.g., aneurysm or ulceration of the subclavian artery, or relieve the obstruction of a subclavian vein thrombosis. Saphenous vein replacement or bypass of the subclavian artery will usually correct the arterial problem. When symptomatic venous thrombosis persists, saphenous vein bypass of the occluded segment usually provides relief of symptoms.

MANAGEMENT OF THIS PATIENT

In the patient described at the beginning of this report, a phlebogram would be most useful. If the axillary-subclavian vein is patent but compressed, decompression of the thoracic outlet is indicated because it is unlikely that the individual would change his profession. If the phlebogram demonstrated thrombosis of the axillary-subclavian veins, one could attempt a thrombectomy followed by decompression of the thoracic outlet or, more preferably, one could use anticoagulation (or lytic-anticoagulation) therapy for three to four months followed by decompression of the thoracic outlet. If the thrombosis did not resolve and symptoms of upper extremity venous hypertension persisted after the decompression of the thoracic outlet, bypass of the obstruction in the axillary-subclavian vein would be indicated.

SUMMARY

The thoracic outlet syndrome constitutes a complex of symptoms related to neurovascular compression at the thoracic outlet. In evaluating these patients one must ascertain whether symptoms are produced by neural compression, arterial compression, or venous compression. Brachial plexus involvement constitutes the most common type of thoracic outlet syndrome and is seen in approximately 95% of patients. Conservative management will be effective in 60% of these patients with the remainder requiring operative decompression of their thoracic outlet. Arteriography and phlebography are indicated only in those patients with specific signs and symptoms of vascular involvement. Operative management of patients with vascular involvement includes decompression of the thoracic outlet and associated vascular repair or bypass as necessary.

BIBLIOGRAPHY

1. Adams JT, DeWeese JA: "Effort" thrombosis of the axillary and subclavian veins. *J Trauma* 1971; 11:923–930.
2. Blank RH, Connar RG: Arterial complications associated with thoracic outlet compression syndrome. *Ann Thor Surg* 1974; 17:315–324.
3. Dale WA, Lewis MR: Management of thoracic outlet syndrome. *Ann Surg* 1975; 181:575–585.
4. Drapanas T, Curran WL: Thrombectomy in the treatment of "effort" thrombosis of the axillary and subclavian veins. *J Trauma* 1966; 6:107–119.
5. Glass BA: The relationship of axillary venous thrombosis to the thoracic outlet compression syndrome. *Ann Thorac Surg* 1975; 19:613–621.
6. Judy KL, Heymann RL: Vascular complications of the thoracic outlet syndrome. *Am J Surg* 1972; 123:521–531.
7. Priest JD, Nagel DA: Tennis shoulder. *Am J Sports Med* 1976; 4:28–42.
8. Roos DB: The place for scalenectomy and first-rib resection in thoracic outlet syndrome. *Surgery* 1982; 92:1077–1085.
9. Silver D: Thoracic outlet syndrome. *Hosp Physician,* Oct. 1983.

58   Role of Lumbar Sympathectomy

A 44-year-old man who is a heavy smoker is seen for a painful ulceration over the lateral aspect of the foot. Pedal pulses are absent, and arteriography shows patent femoral and popliteal arteries but extensive distal disease, with tapering and occlusion of all tibial branches above the ankle.

Consultant: Robert W. Barnes, M.D.

The case presentation suggests a patient with unreconstructible distal arterial occlusive disease and an ischemic ulcer on the foot. Such distal arterial disease may be the result of thromboangiitis obliterans (Buerger's disease), diabetes mellitus, thromboembolism, or collagen vascular disease. As the quality of angiography and the capabilities of vascular surgeons to extend grafts to the pedal arteries improve, fewer patients have "unreconstructible" peripheral arteries. If a preoperative arteriogram does not show excellent resolution of vessels in the lower leg and foot, including the plantar arch, operative arteriography should be performed to rule out reconstructibility. In this chapter I will assume that the aforementioned case is truly unreconstructible and therefore requires consideration of other means of surgical intervention to improve pedal blood flow to permit healing of the ischemic ulcer and limb salvage.

INDICATIONS FOR LUMBAR SYMPATHECTOMY

Table 58–1 depicts the current indications for lumbar sympathectomy. Prior to definitive arterial reconstructive surgery, lumbar sympathectomy was employed for a variety of vascular disorders of the lower extremity, with variable results. Currently, the two conditions that benefit the most from sympathectomy are hyperhidrosis and causalgia. Disabling hyperhidrosis usually involves the upper extremities. Causalgia, a chronic painful and disabling vasomotor reaction to mixed nerve

TABLE 58–1.
Indications for Lumbar Sympathectomy

A. Excess Sympathetic Tone
  1. Causalgia (major causalgia, reflex sympathetic dystrophy)
  2. Mimo-causalgia (minor causalgia)
  3. Hyperhidrosis
B. Vasospasm
  1. Raynaud's syndrome
  2. Livedo reticularis
  3. Pernio, chilblains
C. Arterial Occlusive Disease
  1. Unreconstructible pedal ischemia
    a. Ischemic rest pain
    b. "Blue toe syndrome" (digit microemboli)
    c. Ischemic ulceration (toes, forefoot)
    d. Minor gangrene (toes, forefoot)
  2. Frostbite (chronic, late symptoms)
  3. Thromboangiitis obliterans (Buerger's disease)
  4. Concomitant with aortoiliac reconstruction
    (multisegmental disease)

---

injury may be controlled with sympathetic nerve blocks or sympathectomy. Although Raynaud's disease may be improved with sympathectomy, such vasomotor disturbances of the feet are less common and less disabling than in the upper extremity.

Controversy continues to surround the role of lumbar sympathectomy for lower extremity peripheral arterial occlusive disease. The two conditions for which I most commonly perform a lumbar sympathectomy for vascular disease are microembolic "blue toe syndrome" and lumbar sympathectomy concomitant with aortoiliac reconstruction in patients with more distal (femoropopliteal or tibial) arterial occlusive disease. Patients with thromboangiitis obliterans will often have disease progression as long as they continue smoking, and sympathectomy is uncommonly of benefit. This is perhaps an important consideration in the patient described. Patients with advanced distal arterial occlusive disease associated with diabetes mellitus similarly are seldom improved by lumbar sympathectomy, particularly when autonomic neuropathy often accompanies this disease. Finally, patients with advanced unreconstructible arterial occlusive disease with signs of early rest pain, ischemic ulceration, or localized gangrene of the toes or distal forefoot may occasionally benefit from lumbar sympathectomy. This clinical situation seems most pertinent to our patient. However, the clinician should make every effort to rule out reconstructible arterial occlusive disease, even to vessels of the foot. Patients with advanced ischemia and ulceration or gangrene involving the mid- or hindfoot will not benefit from lumbar sympathectomy. Similarly, patients with claudication will not improve following lumbar sympathectomy.

ANATOMY AND PHYSIOLOGY

The sympathetic nervous system consists of afferent and efferent fibers that form a reflex arc. Afferent fibers originate in blood vessels and other structures in the skin, muscles and viscera and travel with the somatic nerves to cell bodies in the dorsal root ganglia of the spinal nerves. The central axons of these nerves synapse with the cell bodies of the efferent fibers that are located in the anteromediolateral columns of the spinal cord. These efferent fibers are myelinated and travel in the white rami communicantes as preganglionic fibers to ganglia in the sympathetic chain, to ganglia in the preaortic (celiac, renal, superior and inferior mesenteric ganglia), or to terminal ganglia near the urinary bladder and rectum. After synapsing in these ganglia, the postganglionic fibers that are unmyelinated, travel in grey rami communicantes to join the somatic nerves and innervate blood vessels (vasomotor), sweat glands (sudomotor) and erector pili muscles (pilomotor) of the skin, blood vessels of the skeletal muscles, and blood vessels and smooth muscles of the visceral organs.

The dominant effect of sympathetic innervation is vasoconstriction, particularly of the skin. Lumbar sympathetic block or sympathectomy will result in vasodilation with increase in cutaneous blood flow of the foot. Cutaneous circulation, however, gradually returns toward normal in three to six weeks, although never returning to baseline values.

Much of the increased blood flow in the feet passes through arteriovenous shunts. Although some investigators question whether any increase in nutritional blood flow to the skin actually occurs, the healing of ischemic ulcers, the growth of toenails, and the increase in blood flow by xenon washout studies all suggest that some improvement in nutrient circulation occurs. The return of cutaneous blood flow toward normal is probably the result of reestablishment of intrinsic cutaneous vasomotor tone, or the increased sensitivity of blood vessels to circulating catecholamines.

In addition, lumbar sympathectomy results in ablation of sweat gland function that is usually permanent. The loss of sweating results in the dry skin which is typical following lumbar sympathectomy.

DIAGNOSTIC EVALUATION

The decision to perform lumbar sympathectomy initially rests on the history and physical examination. Patients with isolated claudication are not candidates for sympathectomy. Patients with advanced ischemia including ulceration or gangrene of the mid- or hindfoot likewise will not benefit from sympathectomy. The ideal candidate has early ischemic rest pain of the toes or forefoot, with or without focal ulceration or gangrene of those areas. Patients with diabetes mellitus, particularly those with advanced neuropathy, are unlikely to benefit from lumbar sympathectomy.

Noninvasive diagnostic techniques can complement the clinical evaluation in assessing patients for lumbar sympathectomy. Doppler arterial waveforms of the pedal arteries, although abnormal, should be present if the patient is to improve after sympathectomy. Patients with unobtainable Doppler arterial velocity signals have too advanced ischemia to benefit from sympathectomy. The ankle/brachial systolic pressure index determined by ultrasound is usually less than 0.5 in patients with early rest pain. However, if the ankle pressure index is less than 0.30, the patient is unlikely to improve following sympathectomy, according to data of Yao and Bergan.

We have found digit plethysmography to be the most helpful predictor of response to lumbar sympathectomy (Fig 58–1). The normal digit pulse wave form mimics an arterial pressure pulse, with a rapid upstroke, a relatively sharp peak, and a dicrotic wave on the downslope. In the presence of arterial occlusive disease, the waveform is attenuated with a more gradual upslope, a rounded peak, and loss of the dicrotic wave. In advanced ischemia there may be no detectable waveform in the digit. The presence of sympathetic vasomotor tone may be assessed by noting the response of the digit pulse amplitude to a deep breath. Normally, the pulse amplitude is attenuated with such a maneuver, whereas patients with autosympathectomy (diabetes mellitus), surgical sympathectomy, or advanced ischemia may lose such a vasoconstrictive reflex. Finally, the ability of the digit circulation to increase in response to ischemia (reactive hyperemia) may be assessed by noting the pulse waveform response to temporary arterial occlusion induced by a pneumatic cuff on the proximal digit. Normally, the digit pulse amplitude should at least double in response to temporary (three-minute) digit ischemia. Patients with ad-

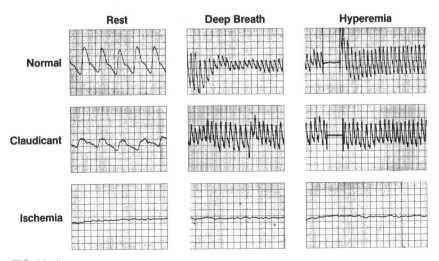

FIG 58–1.
Digit photoplethysmographic (PPG) tracings illustrating normal and abnormal pulse waveforms, sympathetic-mediated vasoconstrictive reflex and reactive hyperemia.

vanced occlusive disease may not have the capacity to further vasodilate. Such patients are unlikely to benefit from lumbar sympathectomy.

All patients being considered for lumbar sympathectomy should have had preoperative arteriography to rule out the possibility of arterial reconstruction. If the circulation is not visualized in the distal leg and foot, distal arteriography should be performed to document that the patient will not benefit from arterial reconstruction.

OPERATIVE TECHNIQUE

Unilateral or bilateral lumbar sympathectomy is performed with the patient in the supine position. No roll or lift under the flanks is necessary. The abdomen and sides are draped down to the table. A transverse lateral abdominal incision is made from the lateral border of the rectus, approximately four finger-breadths lateral to the umbilicus, to a point just anterior to the tip of the eleventh rib. The external oblique aponeurosis is incised in the direction of its fibers. The internal oblique and transversus abdominis muscles are incised in the direction of the skin incision. Care must be taken not to enter the peritoneum at the anterior extent of the incision, near the lateral border of the rectus sheath. The transversalis fascia is searched for and carefully incised deep to the transversus abdominis muscle, near the lateral extent of the incision. Just deep to this fascia, preperitoneal fat will be noted at the lateral abdominal wall. Blunt finger dissection should be initiated between the preperitoneal fat and the peritoneum at the lateral end of the incision. By gentle blunt dissection the peritoneum is stripped from the preperitoneal fat and transversalis fascia, and progressively mobilized toward the midline. The surgeon must be careful not to carry the plane of blunt dissection behind the quadratus lumborum or the psoas muscles. Once the blunt dissection is carried anterior to the psoas muscle, the surgeon should feel the vertebral bodies, with the pulsatile aorta on the left or the inferior vena cava on the right. The ureter and lower pole of the kidney should be retracted anterior with the intraperitoneal structures. Be sure to identify and leave the genitofemoral nerve as it obliquely crosses the psoas muscle. The surgeon should then carefully position two large Deaver or Harrington retractors at the medial end of the wound, angling both cephalad and caudad to maintain medial retraction of the peritoneum and its contents.

The next step is to palpate for the lumbar sympathetic chain that is usually located just anterior to the anterior border of the psoas muscle, closely adherent to the vertebral bodies. The sympathetic chain has a firm cordlike quality with nodular expansions of the sympathetic ganglia. A standard lumbar sympathectomy usually involves removal of one to three ganglia, usually L2 to L4. The second lumbar sympathetic ganglion can usually be found near the caudal end of the crus of the diaphragm. A Smithwick dissector is used to free the sympathetic chain from adjacent tissue. Care should be taken to identify lumbar arteries or veins, which should be individually ligated with metal hemoclips. Once a segment of the sympathetic chain has been dissected free, the nerve hook end of the Smithwick dissector is used to elevate the chain from adjacent tissue. This maneuver is important to differentiate the sympathetic chain from other structures such as the genitofemoral nerve, ureter, or lymph node chain. The sympathetic chain is the only structure that remains tethered to the vertebral bodies by the rami communicantes. The rami are transected with scissors. A metal hemoclip is placed across the sympathetic chain at the cephalad end of the dissection. The chain is grasped with a long tonsil clamp and the chain is transected by retracting on the tonsil clamp and dissecting along the sympathetic chain with a Smithwick dissector. The chain is mobilized in a caudad direction. The dissection is carried down to a point just cephalad to the common iliac arteries, where the caudal end of the chain is controlled with a hemoclip and transected. The sympathectomy usually encompasses two or three sympathetic ganglia. The excised specimen is sent for pathologic confirmation.

Concomitant lumbar sympathectomy at the time of aortoiliac reconstruction is best carried out after mobilization of the abdominal aorta and prior to systemic anticoagulation. The left sympathetic chain is approached lateral to the aorta and anterior to the psoas muscle, with care taken to avoid injury to the inferior mesenteric vessels. Likewise care should be taken to avoid undue retraction of the aorta that may lead to distal microemboli. The sympathetic chain is palpated against the vertebral bodies. Once identified, the sympathectomy is carried out in a fashion similar to that described above. The right sympathetic chain is approached by sharp and blunt dissection anterior to the inferior vena cava and posterior to the root of the small bowel mesentery, just caudad to the third portion of the duodenum. Once an areolar plane has been entered, the right lateral border of the inferior vena cava can be identified and retracted anteriorly. It is important to avoid injury to lumbar veins that should be individually ligated and divided. By maintaining anterior retraction of the inferior vena cava with a peanut sponge, the finger of the operating surgeon should be used to identify the sympathetic chain anterior to the right psoas muscle, against the vertebral bodies. Once identified, the sympathectomy can be carried out in a fashion similar to that described above.

With increasing use of retroperitoneal approaches for aortoiliac reconstruction, concomitant left lumbar sympathectomy is readily performed by this approach. Unfortunately, the technique limits access to the right sympathetic chain.

COMPLICATIONS

The most common minor sequela of lumbar sympathectomy is postsympathectomy neuralgia, which usually develops within one or two weeks following the procedure. A deep ache or boring pain on the anteromedial aspect of the thigh usually lasts for a few weeks or at the most three months. Its cause is unknown. Symptomatic treatment usually suffices, although severe cases may require diphenylhydantoin or carbamazepine. An expected side effect of lumbar sympathectomy is dryness and cracking of the skin of the feet, which may be treated with oils or lotions.

Postoperative ileus is managed with nasogastric suction. Impotence rarely, if ever, occurs unless bilateral resection of the first lumbar ganglia is carried out. Injury to the genitofemoral nerve, ureter, or retroperitoneal hematoma should be avoided by careful operative technique. Paradoxical gangrene has been described following sympathectomy but is unlikely to be a direct result of the procedure. The author feels that such cases most likely represent progression of arterial disease or emboli from a diseased abdominal aorta.

RESULTS

Lumbar sympathectomy may be curative of causalgia and hyperhidrosis. However, the response to sympathectomy in patients with advanced peripheral arterial occlusive disease is less gratifying. The literature suggests that approximately 50% of patients will obtain a salutary effect of sympathectomy for advanced limb ischemia. As previously stated, patients with claudication alone will not benefit from sympathectomy. In the author's experience, approximately 75% of carefully selected patients with advanced unreconstructible arterial disease will show at least a temporary benefit of lumbar sympathectomy, with relief of rest pain and healing of minor lesions. The author and his colleagues carried out the first published randomized trial of concomitant lumbar sympathectomy with aortoiliac reconstruction. The results of that study suggested that lumbar sympathectomy did not improve early or late graft patency but did significantly improve the circulation to the foot in the early postoperative period. It is for this reason that the author recommends concomitant lumbar sympathectomy in patients undergoing aortoiliac reconstruction for multisegmental arterial occlusive disease or with a past history of microembolic "blue toe syndrome." Fortunately, with recent advances in extended bypass vein grafts to the level of the pedal arteries, lumbar sympathectomy as a sole procedure for patients with "inoperable" arterial occlusive disease is becoming more uncommon.

SUMMARY

Lumbar sympathectomy continues to be a controversial but probably efficacious procedure for select patients with advanced peripheral arterial occlusive disease. While the procedure is most appropriate for patients with causalgia or hyperhidrosis, some patients may benefit from lumbar sympathectomy as a sole procedure, or in conjunction with aortoiliac reconstruction. The author prefers this procedure for patients with multisegmental arterial occlusive disease undergoing aortoiliac reconstruction or patients with a history of microembolic "blue toe syndrome." Although much of the increased blood flow associated with this procedure may pass through arteriovenous shunts, some nutrient blood flow may occur. Both clinical judgment and noninvasive diagnostic techniques, particularly digit photoplethysmography, are important for selecting patients who may benefit from lumbar sympathectomy. Patients with early foot rest pain and ischemic ulcers or gangrene, limited to the toes or distal forefoot, are candidates for the procedure. However, the procedure may be unnecessary if a more complete distal revascularization is possible. Between 50% and 75% of selected patients may notice subjective and objective improvement after operation. The procedure is becoming more infrequent as surgeons extend successful bypass vein grafts to the distal leg and foot.

BIBLIOGRAPHY

1. Barnes RW, Baker WH, Shanik G, et al: Value of concomitant sympathectomy in aorto-iliac reconstruction: Results of a prospective, randomized study. *Arch Surg* 1977; 112:1325–1330.
2. Ewing M: The history of lumbar sympathectomy. *Surgery* 1971; 70:790–796.
3. Imparato AM: Lumbar sympathectomy: Role in the treatment of occlusive arterial disease in the lower extremities. *Surg Clin N Am* 1979; 59:719–735.
4. Simeone FA: Intravascular pressure, vascular tone, and sympathectomy. *Surgery* 1963; 53:1–18.
5. Smithwick RH: Lumbar sympathectomy in treatment of obliterative vascular disease of lower extremities. *Surgery* 1957; 42:567–568.
6. van der Stricht J: Effect of lumbar sympathectomy on the lower extremity. *J Cardiovasc Surg* 1979; 20:279–306.
7. Yao JST, Bergan JJ: Predictability of vascular reactivity relative to sympathetic ablation. *Arch Surg* 1973; 107:676–680.

59   Diabetic Foot Sepsis

A 50-year-old diabetic woman is seen for a foot infection. Examination reveals a swollen foot, with pus draining from an ulceration on the plantar surface of the foot in the region of the third metatarsal head. Temperature is 102° and blood sugar 400 mg%.

Consultant: Gary W. Gibbons, M.D.

For the diabetic, foot infection continues to be the leading cause for hospitalization with astonishing emotional and financial cost to the patient and society. Amputation is the diabetic's greatest fear yet two thirds of the major amputations in the United States are performed on diabetics. Unfortunately, many of these could have been avoided by better patient and physician education and understanding, and by eliminating the misconceptions relating to treatment of foot infections.

THE PROBLEM

Unfortunately, this case typifies the diabetic with an infected foot: the patient is not seen until a potentially limb-threatening problem already exists. The etiology relates to three primary pathological situations that either singularly, or in combination, are responsible for the development of all diabetic foot problems. These are: neuropathy, vascular insufficiency, and infection. Patient and physician appreciation of these three entities correlate directly with both prevention of such lesions as well as successful treatment of established foot infections.

Neuropathy includes loss of the perception of touch, pressure and most importantly, pain. Loss of proprioception results in an altered position sense of the foot. There is denervation of the intrinsic and skeletal muscles of the foot and leg, resulting in atrophy and deformity. Autosympathectomy is not uncommon and results in a falsely warm foot, the skin of which is dry and very susceptible to cracks and fissures.

Peripheral vascular disease is 20 times more common in the diabetic population. Unique to the diabetic is a predilection for occlusive disease to involve the more distal vessels of the lower extremity and limited ability to develop collateral

412

circulation around blockages. A compromised local circulation delays the proper host response to infection, the delivery of antimicrobial agents to the infected area, and proper wound healing. In addition, the atherosclerotic plaque and media of diabetic arteries often contain extensive calcium, resulting in rigidity and noncompressibility. Handling these arteries requires expertise and experience and is not recommended for the occasional vascular surgeon.

Infection is poorly tolerated by diabetics, probably secondary to defects in the host defense mechanism. This may predispose them to some infections and certainly may alter their response to an infectious process. The primary defect is a variety of neutrophil dysfunctions including chemotaxis, phagocytosis, and bactericidal function. Certainly, uncontrolled diabetes affects infection and infection affects diabetic control. Most importantly, systemic signs and symptoms of a septic process often occur late, making unexplained and uncontrolled hyperglycemia the only reliable sign of a potentially serious limb threatening infection. It is not infrequent therefore, that hyperglycemia, odor, or circulatory collapse bring the patient to the hospital with a limb-threatening foot infection.

BASIC MANAGEMENT PRINCIPLES

While certain basic management principles are applicable to all diabetic foot infections, the severity of the infected ulcer will determine whether treatment requires immediate admission to the hospital or whether it can be initiated on an outpatient basis. It is a misconception to base treatment by the outside appearance of the ulcer. The severity of tissue destruction and sepsis may not be totally apparent from just looking at the ulcer or infected callus, especially in patients who have continued to bear weight on a painless area or who do not have the visual acuity to recognize a problem. A sterile probe, scissors, and forceps are essential equipment for the physician who evaluates and treats diabetic foot ulcers. Deep calluses must be debrided and all encrusted areas unroofed and inspected to determine the extent of deep tissue destruction and possible bone or joint involvement.

The decision for admission is easy in this case since there is a swollen foot with pus coming from a probable deep ulceration on the plantar surface of the foot in the region of the third metatarsal head. This patient also demonstrated systemic toxicity with a temperature of 102° and a blood sugar that is abnormally elevated. If the probe hits bone, then clinical osteomyelitis is present even if the X-ray is negative. Clear drainage coming from a wound that probes to or near a joint indicates probable joint involvement. Plain X-rays with or without magnification views are obtained, but are not pathognomonic for osteomyelitis. These films also help identify subcutaneous gas indicating anaerobic infection. Bone scans and gallium scans are contraindicated in our experience since they are costly and add no further information than that provided by clinical judgment and a plain X-ray. They may also delay needed operative intervention.

The wound is cultured aerobically and anaerobically with the initial debridement obtaining deep swabs and/or actual tissue whenever possible. Criteria for admission or initial treatment at home are outlined in Table 59–1. Early superficial ulcerations with minimal cellulitis may be treated at home, providing there is no evidence of any systemic toxicity, and that the patient is compliant, reliable, and has a vigilant support system. Limb threatening infections require immediate admission to the hospital and include those ulcers with more extensive cellulitis and necrosis, but not necessarily bone or joint involvement. It must be remembered that the absence of signs and symptoms of systemic toxicity do not exclude a limb threatening infection. Their presence, especially elevation of temperature, white blood count or pulse rate requires immediate admission. Immediate admission is also recommended for patients who cannot be compliant or who have no support system at home. Any patient with gangrene (a term we never use in front of the patient), diminished circulation, renal failure, or who is on immunosuppressive therapy following transplantation requires immediate admission. Despite increasing hospital cost constraints and DRGs, if there is any question as to the severity of the

TABLE 59–1.

Diabetic Foot Ulcer

MILD	LIMB THREATENING
Superficial	Deep ulcer
Minimal or no cellulitis	±Bone or joint
No bone involvement	>2 cm cellulitis
No systemic toxicity	±Systemic toxicity
Reliable and compliant patient	Noncompliance
Good support system	? Support system
	Gangrene or ischemia
	Immunosuppression
↓	↓
RX	RX
Rest of injured part	Immediate admission
Plain X-ray	Control blood sugar
Culture and sensitivities	Total rest injured area
Initial broad-spectrum antibiotic	Culture and sensitivities
Δbased on sensitivities and	Plain X-ray
response	Initial broad-spectrum intravenous antibiotics
Careful debridement	Specific antibiotic based on sensitivities and
Local dressings	response
Podiatric appliances and special shoes	Early surgical debridement, dependent
Careful follow-up	drainage and open amputation
	Local dressings
	Later selected revascularization and
	conservative amputations or revisions
	Podiatric appliances and special shoes
	Careful follow-up

infection, admit the patient to the hospital. Admission and treatment is still more effective and less expensive in the long run, especially if a major amputation is avoided.

No matter what the severity of the initial infection is, the injured area must be put to complete and total rest. Because of neuropathy, it is impossible for a diabetic to partially bear weight, despite belief by the patient that he is conforming to treatment. In my experience, continued trauma including any type of weight bearing prevents or prolongs healing 100% of the time. While total contact casting has become popular since it allows weight bearing, it is contraindicated except under the most unusual circumstances. In my experience, the complications of total contact casting far outweigh its usefulness.

While the exact role aerobic and anaerobic bacteria play in the deterioration of seemingly uncomplicated diabetic foot ulcers is unclear, bacterial invasion is certainly paramount to the septic complications that result. In our experience, polymicrobial infections (average 3.2 isolated per ulcer) are the rule. Certain bacteria may be more frequent in deeply ulcerated tissue and anaerobes are present in about two thirds of the patients with deep limb threatening infections. Any wound that has a foul fetid odor, crepitance on palpation, or gas by X-ray harbors anaerobes and requires urgent attention. Gas is not synonymous with clostridia and guillotine amputation. Peptostreptococcus, bacteriodes species and oblilate anaerobes are the most frequently cultured. Aerobic gram positive cocci (most commonly Staphylococcus and Streptococcus species) are encountered in over 90% of cases, while aerobic gram negative rods are found in over 50% of cases.

Broad-spectrum antibiotics are certainly justified and administered intravenously to assure adequate serum levels. The choice of an initial antibiotic regimen is influenced by several variables as outlined in Table 59–2. Careful monitoring of drug levels and toxicity is essential, particularly in the diabetic with impaired renal function. Antibiotic therapy is changed pending sensitivity reports and the response of the wound to therapy. Intravenous antibiotics are continued until the open wound is healing well and is clearly free from deep infection. While newer antibiotics are rapidly appearing, their use in serious infections must be questioned when com-

TABLE 59–2.
Initial Antibiotic Regimen

Likely Pathogens
Knowledge → 90% gram (+) cocci
→ 50% gram (−) enteric
→ 66% anaerobes
Gram staining
Odor, crepitance, gas, pus
Severity of infection
Local bacterial resistance patterns
Prior antibiotic therapy
Preexisting renal or hepatic dysfunction

---

pared to those antibiotics with established track records. Certainly, more experienced consultation should be sought when a wound is not responding or when questions arise as to proper antibiotic therapy.

There is no greater misconception relating to treatment of potentially serious foot ulcers than that related to surgical management. It is a fallacy to think that one can rely on intravenous antibiotics to solve the problem of a deep necrotic infection. It is still believed by many that diabetics can't heal big incisions, so that incisions are often kept small with inappropriate reliance on drains and soaks. Nothing could be further from the truth. Simply stated, diabetics do not tolerate undrained infection. This begins with the initial inspection and debridement to determine the severity of the infection. All calluses and encrusted areas must be debrided and carefully inspected for deeper necrotic destruction and bone joint or tendon sheath involvement. While medical stabilization is important, it should not be done at the expense of delaying needed and urgent surgical therapy. The blood sugar must be brought under immediate control, which most often requires the use of insulin and not oral agents. Proper broad-spectrum intravenous antibiotic therapy is initiated, as already mentioned, but systemic toxicity or shock will not be reversed until the septic process is arrested. This requires immediate surgical debridement of all necrotic tissue and dependent drainage of all areas involving pus. Small stab wounds and the use of drains and irrigations uniformly provides inadequate debridement and results in further progression of the infection.

This debridement must be done no matter what the circulatory status is, and the experienced vascular surgeon would never entertain the thought of performing a vascular reconstruction in a patient with an ongoing limb threatening infection. Because of neuropathy many of these procedures, especially the initial examination and debridement, can be done with little or no anesthesia, often times at the bedside.

While the initial surgical treatment must be radical enough to assure adequate debridement and drainage, it must be done with an expertise that will ensure later reconstruction or revision with the overall goal of limb salvage. This requires a knowledge and expertise of knowing where to place the incision yet conserving as much healthy tissue, such as small skin flaps, that may later be useful in reconstructing the foot. For infections involving the tendon sheaths, these areas need to be opened along the course of the tendon sheath and continued until there is no question as to viable and noninfected tissue. In general, any viable area should be left and protected since it may be vital in later reconstruction or revision. For the ischemic foot, rarely does the initial surgical debridement and drainage provide the definitive result.

Dressings begin with the initial surgical procedure. Again, there are great misconceptions and folklore. The important message is never to soak the diabetic foot. In my experience, heat in any form, soaks, or whirlpools have led to more complications than any other form of treatment. This also applies to the use of astringents, full strength solutions, and other harsh medications such as enzymatic debriding agents, since the majority of diabetics do not tolerate them. We prefer to keep dressings simple, using diluted, isotonic antiseptic solutions applied to plain gauze and packed into the wound one to three times per day. These can easily be done by the nursing staff, by the patient or his family, or by allied health professionals, depending on individual patient needs. We have tried all of the latest dressings and wound preparations and continue to revert to our old standard dressings that have given us the best results over the years. One should never rely on the dressings to debride a necrotic wound for the reasons mentioned earlier.

Dry, cracked areas or fissures can be effectively treated with Bacitracin ointment and covered by a small dry dressing. Dry skin and calluses can certainly be softened with Lanolin or Eucerin Cream, avoiding lotions and solution medications that contain alcohol and that actually dry the area more. It is also essential to pad the heel and cushion it against trauma while patients are lying in bed. A soft foam rubber pillow with the heels extended over it is invaluable to prevent pressure sore from developing on insensitive heels. A metal cradle over the end of the bed keeps sheets and blankets off the toes.

Once the infection is controlled vascular evaluation is essential. In my experience, clinical judgment continues to be most important in determining the severity of vascular insufficiency in the diabetic lower extremity. Because of the peculiarities of diabetic peripheral vascular disease previously described, noninvasive vascular laboratory results are only complementary to clinical judgment. New techniques such as transcutaneous measurement of tissue oxygenation hold promise for the future, but as yet there are no large series evaluating diabetic patients. No diabetic patient should be denied a more conservative distal amputation solely on the basis of unfavorable results of noninvasive testing.

Arteriography and appropriate vascular reconstructions are carried out once infection is controlled. Diabetics tolerate vascular reconstruction quite well, and results support an aggressive revascularization approach for the diabetic. Subsequent revision of an original surgical wound or a more conservative distal amputation can then be performed resulting in healing and limb salvage.

MANAGEMENT OF THIS CASE

For the diabetic, the location of the ulcer, the extent of the infection and its control, and the adequacy of the circulation will determine whether limb salvage will be successful. In general, it is advisable to try to save as much of the weight bearing surface as possible. However, the more ischemic the area is, the more important it is to close the amputated area primarily. The case presented serves as an excellent example. Admission is obvious since she has a limb threatening infection and systemic toxicity. Her blood sugar must be brought under immediate control and because she is septic, blood cultures are indicated. The plain X-ray must be carefully evaluated, looking for subcutaneous gas, osteomyelitis, and the etiology of the swelling. Most critical, however, is the immediate bedside exploration and probing of the third metatarsal ulcerated area to determine the extent of the infection.

If the ulcer is superficial or only moderately deep, and one can assure oneself that the pus is coming from the localized area with the swelling secondary to cellulitis, and not a deeper collection and if the X-ray is negative, then one could start dressings and broad-spectrum intravenous antibiotics following the guidelines previously mentioned. Because of the swelling, pus, and systemic toxicity, this area must be watched closely for a deep penetrating infection. If the blood sugar returns to normal, the wound responds, and the patient gets better, then conservative treatment may be all that is needed. If this is a first time ulcer with no previous callus or scar formation in the ulcer area, modification of the patient's footwear may be all that is needed to keep this area healed and pressure free. If this area has been a site of chronic callus formation or previous ulceration, and if there is a very prominent metatarsal head that is responsible for the problem, then an osteotomy carried out through a dorsal incision may release the metatarsal head and relieve the pressure in that area. This again is in the case of a neuropathic foot with good circulation.

If the ulcer is deep, extending to the metatarsal head or joint, and pus is coming from deep within the wound or from the tendon sheath, initial surgical drainage may allow some time to further stabilize the patient. Deep cultures should be taken from this area and again broad-spectrum intravenous antibiotics administered. The patient should then be taken to the operating room. In the neuropathic patient with good circulation, one may be able to control the sepsis and provide healing with an open amputation of the third toe plus metatarsal head and appropriate drainage and debridement. Again, the incision should be such that there is no necrotic tissue or undermining left. The skin should be opened further than the subcutaneous tissue, which is opened further than the deepest part of the wound. This incision can be carried down following the tendon sheath until one is assured of controlling the sepsis and debriding all necrotic tissue. The same infection in an ischemic foot may be best treated with the initial procedure as above, followed by selective revascularization. Depending on how improved the distal circulation is, this area may be revised or a closed transmetatarsal amputation may be indicated. Primary closure of a toe or a transmetatarsal amputation can usually be assured if all active infection has been controlled, the venous filling time is less than 25 seconds, there is little or no dependent rubor, and if there is no persistent rest pain in areas proximal to the amputation site. Needless to say, the preparation, technique and precision used in performing the amputation are equally important in achieving a successful outcome.

No matter what course of action is taken on the ulcer, absolute nonweight bearing is essential until healing is certain. It is tragic to see a marvelous initial surgical result lost because of too early weight bearing. Weight bearing is progressed slowly and under careful surveillance using podiatric appliances and modifications of footwear to protect sensitive high-risk areas. Progressing weight bearing too quickly may be responsible for recurrent breakdown or the development of an acute Charcot foot. Careful follow-up and continued education is essential.

Prevention is still the key to successful management of diabetic foot related problems. As with this patient, it is essential that any traumatic lesion or ulcer on the diabetic lower extremity be evaluated and attended to immediately. Even with the best treatment a limb threatening foot infection in our hospital carries a 25% risk of a major (below-knee or above-knee) amputation. Treating limb threatening infections is not for the uninterested physician or for the physician who sees only an occasional diabetic foot infection. Certainly one should never be afraid to seek more experienced consultation, especially if it means saving the diabetic's lower extremity.

BIBLIOGRAPHY

1. Bartlett FF, Gibbons GW, Wheelock FC Jr: Aortic reconstruction for occlusive disease: Comparable results in diabetics. *Arch Surg* 1986; 121:1150–1153.
2. Frykberg RG, Kozak GP: Neuropathic arthropathy in the diabetic foot. *Am Fam Physician* 1978; 17:105–113.
3. Gibbons GW, Wheelock FC Jr, Siembieda C, et al: Noninvasive prediction of amputation level in diabetic patients. *Arch Surg* 1979; 113:1253–1257.
4. Gibbons GW: Diabetic foot infections. *Diabetes Educ* 1982; 8:16–19.
5. Gibbons GW: Management of pre- and postoperative infection in the diabetic patient. *Host/Pathogen News* 1983.
6. Gibbons GW, Eliopoulos GM: Infection of the diabetic foot, in Kozak GP, et al (eds): *Management of Diabetic Foot Problems*. Philadelphia, WB Saunders, 1984, pp 97–103.
7. Wheelock FC Jr, Gibbons GW, Marble A: Surgery in diabetics, in Marble A, et al (eds): *Joslin's Diabetes Mellitus*. Philadelphia, Lea and Febiger, 1984, pp 712–732.
8. Wheelock FC Jr, Gibbons GW: Arterial reconstruction: Femoral-popliteal-tibial, in: Kozak GP, et al (eds): *Management of Diabetic Foot Problems*. Philadelphia, WB Saunders, 1984, pp 173–187.

60 Amputation Level Selection

A patient is admitted with painful gangrene of the entire first and second toes of the right foot. Two previous femoro-distal bypass grafts have failed. Repeat angiography shows a nonreconstructible-situation and amputation appears inevitable.

Consultant: Glenn M. LaMuraglia, M.D.

This case, involving gangrene of the forefoot, represents a typical example of an inevitable amputation. Appropriate amputation is the definitive therapeutic option in patients with significant tissue loss for the relief of pain and the restoration to a functional state. This scenario, however, poses a dilemma to the surgeon since the level chosen for amputation can have significant implications for the patient's longevity and lifestyle.

With continual improvement of health care, and the increasing number of the aged, problems associated with vascular disease such as gangrene are becoming more prevalent. The large experience developed in the treatment of these patients, along with careful selection and properly performed amputations have brought about substantially improved results. It is appropriate to regard amputation as a method of surgical reconstruction and rehabilitation rather than just as a means of resecting nonviable tissue.

Indications for amputation result primarily from complications associated with diabetes mellitus, ischemic vascular disease, and infection such as osteomyelitis and septic arthritis. The most prevalent group of patients are diabetics, because of their accelerated atherosclerosis, widespread distribution of small vessel disease, poor resistance to infection, and neuropathy. Since gangrene and ischemic ulceration in the lower extremity reflects systemic disease, it is not surprising that the prognosis of this patient population is poor. The need for contralateral amputation is about 50% within two years, and the mortality rate is about 50% at three years. Also, because these patients undergoing amputation usually have multiple medical problems and are not a resilient group, it is important to carefully plan their operation within the urgency of the clinical situation.

AMPUTATION PRINCIPLES

The aim of amputations is to resect the necrotic or nonhealing tissue, preserving as much function as possible, and provide a stable, healed extremity. Therefore, it is performed at the most distal level that is likely to heal. When feasible, the preservation of the ankle and the knee joint is important, primarily for postoperative rehabilitation of the patient. For example, the use of an above-the-knee prosthesis requires over 50% more energy than a below-the-knee prosthesis because of the loss of mobility and proprioception and the strain on the remaining musculature. Many elderly or debilitated patients may therefore not have the stamina to use a prosthesis, which may result in confinement to a bed or a wheelchair. Confinement carries a high mortality from pneumonia, debilitation and further ulceration. Even though a patient would clearly not be a candidate for rehabilitation and ambulation, the presence of a knee joint may be very useful for transferring to a chair, sitting upright and moving in bed. To make the proper decision in the individual patient, several factors need to be addressed.

Generally, there are accepted clinical criteria for enabling amputations to heal. Any infective process needs to be well controlled. Good collateral circulation for healing needs to be developed, as noted by a venous filling time of 20 to 25 seconds or less, no dependent rubor, and no temperature level through the area of the proposed amputation. The importance of attention to technical detail cannot be overemphasized when discussing amputations. Ischemic tissue that is compromised, often in malnourished patients, will not heal if not treated with the utmost care.

PREOPERATIVE ASSESSMENT

Like all vascular patients, proper assessment of the patient requiring an amputation requires both a careful systemic and local evaluation. Together, these will delineate the urgency of the problem at hand and therefore outline the optimal pathway for obtaining the best result for the patient.

Patient Evaluation

It is important to evaluate the patient's general medical health, with special attention to diabetes mellitus, tobacco smoking, hypertension, cardiac history, and chronic obstructive pulmonary disease. The history should also include the location and severity of pain, previous vascular procedures and their indications, medications that could be affecting circulation or healing, and the nutritional state and ability of the patient to heal.

Examination of the patient should pay particular attention to the distribution and quality of the pulses, level of palpable temperature demarcation, presence and extent of dependent rubor or infection, tenderness and quality of local tissues, especially the skin, and motor and sensory function. These criteria may quickly give the examiner a good idea of the required level of amputation since an amputation below the demarcation of rubor of palpable temperature change is often doomed to failure. Tenderness and the quality of the local tissue are more subjective; however, they may reflect the circulation to that level and the ability of the patient to heal.

The importance of this initial evaluation is to enable the clinician to determine the medical risk and anticipated survival of the patient, his rehabilitation potential, the presence of toxicity from necrotic tissue or an underlying infection, and the amenability of the patient to undergo an amputation.

Laboratory Evaluation

Besides clinical evaluation of the patient, several laboratory tests have been developed to help assess the likelihood of healing at a particular amputation level. When performing an amputation, there are several factors that determine a successful operative result. Probably the most important patient criteria is the adequacy of skin circulation to promote healing.

The most prevalent vascular laboratory tests remain Doppler segmental blood pressures and segmental pulse volume recordings. There is evidence to suggest that there is a minimal ankle pressure of 50 mm Hg (90 mm Hg in the diabetic), or an ankle/brachial pressure index of > 0.35 (> 0.45 for the diabetic), for adequate healing of amputations of the foot. Using corresponding criteria at higher levels of the leg, similar conclusions have been drawn regarding the success of amputation. However, I feel these criteria, especially in diabetics who may have medial calcinosis, have been the least helpful in determining the outcome of the amputation. Plethysmography or pulse volume recording has been more helpful, since if there is not at least a 5 mm pulsatile displacement at the level of planned amputation, it is unlikely to heal.

Transcutaneous; pO_2 measurements ($TcpO_2$) taken at various amputation levels of the leg with an oxygen electrode at 45° C can give useful data to determine healing. Good results at a proposed level can be predicted with $TcpO_2$ measurements that exceeded 40 mm Hg, with failure predicted with $TcpO_2$ measurements less than 20 mm Hg. Somewhat time consuming and cumbersome to perform, this test requires constant ambient temperature, normal skin at the site measured, and is not reliable in the presence of local infection or inflammation. The standard baseline chest $TcpO_2$ measurement is also a good indicator of the validity of the test, since if the value is low, the results of the extremity measurements may not reflect the true skin perfusion at that level. The author finds the test more useful as a positive indicator for success than a predictor for failure of an amputation.

Another method of determining skin blood flow is the use of ^{133}Xe clearance. After simultaneous intradermal injections of ^{133}Xe at various amputation levels, the various rates of radioactive decay are used to calculate the corresponding dermal blood flow. Successful healing with this technique has been predicted with blood flows > 2.6 ml per min per 100 gm tissue, with poor results < 2.0 ml per min per

100 gm tissue. The shortcomings of this invasive technique are similar to those of the $TcpO_2$, with the added necessity of nuclear medicine and computing capability.

Other modalities have been developed to help determine the selection of the level of amputation. These include digital or transmetatarsal photoplethysmography, radio-labelled skin blood pressure measurements, and skin fluorescence after intravenous fluorescein dye administration. Despite their various proponents, they are not generally available and all have their inherent complexity of use and fallibility without adding a significant amount of information to those discussed above.

Arteriographic Evaluation

Although this patient's angiogram has been described as nonreconstructible, it is imperative to review certain key points. Even though there may be no alternative to amputation to treat the local problem irrespective of vascular reconstructability, it is important to recognize that the level of amputation can be changed with a vascular procedure. Is there an inflow problem or a profunda femoris artery reconstruction that could be undertaken even though two outflow procedures have been previously undertaken in our patient and have failed? This could improve the circulation sufficiently to move the amputation level more distally. However, it is important to keep in mind that when these remote reconstruction procedures are undertaken, a sufficient amount of time is needed to permit the full collateral flow to develop before undertaking reevaluation and a more distal amputation.

ACUTE VS CHRONIC ISCHEMIA

An amputation for acute ischemia lends itself to more complicated issues and carries with it a higher morbidity and mortality. In the acute setting, loss of sensory-motor function, sepsis, systemic toxicity from the necrotic tissue, or overwhelming pain can mandate immediate amputation which may be life saving. However, if the presentation is delayed and no systemic compromise is evident, it is advantageous to permit collaterals to develop for clear demarcation of the gangrene. During the interim, the vascular situation can be improved with heparinization, local foot care, optimizing the fluid balance, reverse Trendelenberg, and when appropriate, revascularization or fasciotomy.

Observation of such a patient requires careful serial examination of the focal ischemic tissue and systemic systems. Special care should be used to monitor the cardiopulmonary system for evidence of congestive heart failure or angina from stress, and renal function for compromise from the liberation of myoglobin and other toxins.

With time, demarcation of the ischemic/necrotic tissue, and the recruitment of collateral circulation, it then becomes possible to make a better decision as to the proper level of amputation of the patient.

INFECTION AND AMPUTATION

In this patient, with gangrene involving his right first two toes, it is important to differentiate dry from wet gangrene. Dry gangrene denotes mummified tissue that is usually not infected and can be approached conservatively with careful observation. However, when there is involvement of a bone or joint, it eventually becomes necessary to proceed with amputation because of recurrent infections.

Wet or infected gangrene can be a life threatening problem, especially in the diabetic patient. It is important to proceed with blood cultures and, when available, to culture and gram stain the local wound exudate. An aggressive intravenous antibiotic regimen should be started that includes coverage of Staphlococcus, Streptococcus, gram negative organisms, and occasionally anaerobic bacteria. The choice of drugs should be predicated in part by the severity of the local wound involvement, the local flora of the area, and the hepatorenal function of the patient. Diabetics are particularly prone to anaerobic organisms, but they can be also readily cultured from older, debilitated patients. In all cases, careful, close observation is necessary to monitor the response to the antibiotics or progression of the sepsis. It is important to emphasize that although the antibiotics are started, it may also be essential, especially in diabetic patients, to perform local or radical debridement or drainage.

Open or guillotine amputations may be necessary to salvage the limb. These should be performed in a manner that provides adequate drainage and removes all necrotic tissue, but not necessarily all infected tissue. It is important to keep in mind the eventual, planned, definitive amputation so that those tissues can be preserved when possible. The soft tissue infection then needs to be fully controlled before a definitive, more proximal amputation can be performed. As a precaution, all amputations should be performed with antibiotic coverage, the drugs used and the duration of administration is predicated by the severity of the clinical problem.

SPECIFIC SITES OF AMPUTATION

Digital Amputation

Digital or button toe amputations involve intraphalangeal resection with lateral flap coverage. Indications include gangrene or soft tissue/bone involvement of the toe distal to the metatarsal phalangeal joint. Adequate skin at the base of the toe is imperative for the successful coverage of the toe. Involvement of the skin in the web space, forefoot sepsis, septic arthritis of the metatarsal phalangeal joint are specific contraindications for this procedure. The patient described in this case, having involvement of the entire first two toes of the right foot, would probably not fulfill this criteria and therefore digital amputation probably cannot be considered.

Postoperative management requires bed rest for at least the first week, and if healing is satisfactory, wheelchair privileges are granted and physical therapy strengthening exercises are instituted. Coumadin is usually started for deep venous thrombosis prophylaxis on the second postoperative day and chest physical therapy is continued throughout to avoid atelectasis and pneumonia. As with all amputations, the wound needs to be carefully observed for infection or nonhealing as it should, throughout its course. Ambulation progressing to full weight bearing is usually not started before two to three weeks, with careful attention to swelling that can precipitate wound breakdown. Sutures are usually removed no earlier than four weeks.

Transmetatarsal Amputation

Transmetatarsal amputations can be divided into single digit ray amputations or complete forefoot amputation. These involve resecting one or all toes, including the corresponding metatarsal phalangeal joint. The indications for this procedure are similar to that of digital amputation, except that there is involvement of the proximal phalanx, the digital web space, the metatarsal head, or other areas of the forefoot. Another factor, besides the technical feasibility and healing of the operation, is creating a stable foot that will not break down further with trauma. Patients, especially diabetics, with neuropathy and contracture of the extensor tendons, or with two involved metatarsal heads should undergo a complete transmetatarsal amputation.

In this patient, with two gangrenous toes, a complete transmetatarsal amputation would be the most appropriate. Clinical criteria that would indicate feasibility of this level of amputation include: control of active infection, good local skin and tissue, no dependent rubor, temperature level or pain proximal to this level, and a venous filling time of less than 20 to 25 seconds. Laboratory criteria predicting the success of this amputation include: a pulsatile pulse volume recording of the forefoot, an ankle/brachial pressure index of > 0.35 (> 0.45 for the diabetic), a transcutaneous pO_2 measurement of the forefoot exceeding 40 mm Hg, and a ^{133}Xe clearance of > 2.6 ml per min per 100 gm tissue.

Ankle Amputation

An ankle or Syme amputation has not developed popularity among surgeons treating patients with vascular disease. Its only inherent benefit is that it enables patients to ambulate for short periods of time without a prosthesis, i.e., not putting on a prosthesis when getting out of bed. The disadvantages include that the leg is several inches shorter than the other, and that it places all the pressure on the heel bed which can break down in the marginally vascularized patient. With the excellent quality of below the knee prostheses, I feel there is rarely an indication to proceed with this amputation.

Below-Knee Amputation

Because of the importance of the knee in the rehabilitation of the patient, every effort should be made to preserve it. Situations that preclude below-the-knee amputations include inadequate surrounding tissues, presence of joint contractures of the hip or knee, severe arthritis of the knee or leg rigidity. Neuropathy at this level is of concern but not a contraindication for this procedure.

Prevention of perioperative knee flexion contracture is important. A posterior knee brace and physical therapy exercise commencing around one week postoperatively are helpful to prevent this serious complication.

Above-Knee Amputation

Above-the-knee amputation is provided for patients who are prohibitive risks for surgery with questionable viability of tissue below the knee, or patients with an extensive amount of tissue loss or ulcers/gangrene that precludes below-the-knee amputation. The author will always attempt, if feasible, a below-the-knee amputation by intraoperatively examining the tissues and the amount of skin bleeding before proceeding with a definitive above the knee amputation.

Postoperative hip flexion contracture can complicate this procedure, but that can be avoided by early, careful physical therapy. If this amputation fails, a higher level can usually be performed. A hip disarticulation is the highest level of amputation possible, but is almost never necessary unless there is uncontrolled sepsis.

CONCLUSION

Determining the proper level of lower extremity amputation is an intricate balance between clinical judgment and laboratory testing. The urgency and associated treatments need to be incorporated with the most distal level of amputation that will remove the necrotic, infected and painful tissue, leaving the patient with the best functional result possible.

BIBLIOGRAPHY

1. Bodily KC, Burgess EM: Contralateral limb and patient survival after leg amputation. *Am J Surg* 1983; 146:280–282.
2. Gibbons GW, Wheelock FC Jr, Siembieda C, et al: Noninvasive prediction of amputation level in diabetic patients. *Arch Surg* 1979; 113:1253–1257.
3. Johansen K, Burgess EM, Zorn R, et al: Improvement of amputation level by lower extremity revascularization. *Surg Gynecol Obstet* 1981; 153:707–709.
4. Katsamouris A, Brewster DC, Megerman J, et al: Transcutaneous oxygen tension in selection of amputation level. *Am J Surg* 1984; 147:510–515.

5. Malone JM, Goldstone J: Lower extremity amputation, in: Moore WS (ed): *Vascular Surgery: A Comprehensive Review,* ed 2. Orlando, Grune & Stratton, 1986, pp 1139–1209.

6. Moore WS, Henry RE, Malone JM, et al: Prospective use of [133]Xenon clearance for amputation level selection. *Arch Surg* 1981; 116:86–88.

61　Popliteal Entrapment Syndrome

A 27-year-old healthy male is seen for symptoms of cramping in the left calf with exercise. He has had to give up jogging, but he also experiences problems when playing tennis or even walking briskly. He has no pain at rest. Examination of the extremity is unremarkable, with intact pedal pulses.

Consultant: Eugene F. Bernstein, M.D., Ph.D.

Young healthy males who present with calf claudication, or other evidence of lower extremity ischemia, must be suspected of having one of the lesions known to cause peripheral arterial disease in that population of patients. These conditions include cystic adventitial disease of the popliteal artery, cardiac embolism, trauma or bony abnormality, Buerger's disease, fibromuscular dysplasia, pseudoclaudication on a neurogenic basis, and the popliteal artery entrapment syndrome. None of these conditions is common in males under the age of 40, but the entrapment syndrome is the most common of the group. It is still considered relatively rare, with only a few hundred cases in the entire world's literature. Ninety percent of the patients are young, physically active, male patients. The condition usually presents with claudication, frequently in the foot as well as the calf. Occasionally, a patient will present with acute ischemia as a result of sudden occlusion of the popliteal artery. Pulse deficits, which are not present in the case presented, are variable with both time and the position of the extremity. The lesions are equally divided between right and left lower extremities and one third of the patients have bilateral lesions.

Additional clinical findings in these patients include the observations that claudication frequently begins after walking only a few steps and that foot paresthesias are common when the patient is sitting with the knee flexed. Symptoms are generally unilateral in young patients with no signs of premature generalized atherosclerosis. The condition may be associated with other congenital abnormalities.

Obstruction of the popliteal artery because of compression from a contracting muscle or tendon was first described in 1879 by T.P. Anderson Stuart, a medical student in Edinburgh who dissected the amputated leg of a 64-year-old man and described the anomaly of an abnormal popliteal artery deviating medially around the medial head of the gastrocnemius muscle. The vein, nerve, and muscle were all normal. The first clinical case was not reported until 1959 by Hamming, who described a 12-year-old boy in whom treatment was successfully accomplished by division of the muscle tendon. Love and Whelan coined the term ''popliteal artery entrapment syndrome'' in 1965.

In general, the entrapped popliteal artery courses abnormally around the medial head of the gastrocnemius muscle, has normal flow when the muscle is relaxed and in most positions of the leg. The artery is compressed when the muscle contracts, as with running, and in hyperextension of the knee joint. Focal trauma to the vessel from the compressing tendon will sometimes lead to intimal hyperplasia with smooth muscle proliferation. In addition, occasionally the condition may progress to sudden thrombosis or distal embolism (Fig 61–1).

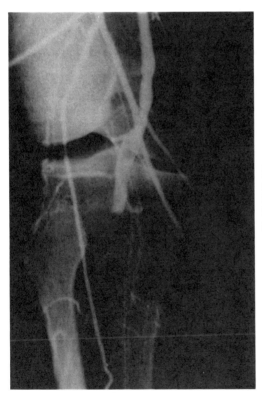

FIG 61–1.
Acute thrombosis of popliteal artery due to popliteal entrapment. Fresh thrombus is evident just proximal to the abrupt occlusion.

DIAGNOSIS

When a patient in the appropriate age group presents with symptoms suggesting popliteal entrapment, the first step is to perform a physical examination with the extremity in the normal supine resting position. If all pulses are present, it is then appropriate to reexamine the patient with the knee in hyperextension and with maximal passive dorsal flexion of the foot. These tests should demonstrate the obstructing mechanism. The patient should then be studied in each of these positions in the noninvasive vascular laboratory using segmental pressures and Doppler velocity information to document the obstruction with changing positions and to search for bilateral lesions. Commonly, these patients have arm/leg segmental pressure ratios which are 0.8 or less at the level of the ankle and which decrease to 0.5 or less with exercise. In addition, the initial examination should rule out neurogenic causes, primary muscle disorders, and psychoneurosis. A CT examination may define the anomaly.

Based on the physical examination and noninvasive vascular laboratory measurements, a decision should be made to proceed to angiography. Biplane films should be obtained with passive dorsal flexion and hyperextension of both lower extremities (Fig 61–2). While medial deviation of the popliteal artery is the first variant to be searched for, other forms of popliteal artery stenosis or obstruction may also be detected. These include entrapment by muscle slips or fibrous bands, venous entrapment (alone or with arterial entrapment), or an artery in the normal position with aberrant muscle or fibrous strips causing the stenosis.

Initially, the syndrome was classified with two major anatomic variations: Type I—the popliteal artery passing medial to the medial head of the gastrocnemius muscle, and Type II—the artery in its normal course compressed by an abnormal origin of the gastrocnemius muscle. However, in 1979, Rich added those anomalies in which an accessory slip of the gastrocnemius muscle compresses the artery, a fibrous band of the popliteus muscle causes medial deviation of the artery, and one in which both the artery and the vein are deviated around the medial head of the gastrocnemius muscle (Table 61–1). In addition to these lesions, a form of acquired popliteal artery entrapment syndrome has been described by Baker and Stoney following a femoropopliteal bypass in which the graft was placed medial to the medial head of the gastrocnemius muscle and acutely angulated when passing deep into the popliteal space.

TREATMENT

Based on the arteriographic demonstration of abnormalities that should delineate this condition from the other items mentioned in the differential diagnosis, operative therapy is generally considered to be appropriate. Both medial leg and posterior popliteal space incisions have been advocated, but my personal preference is for a posterior S-shaped incision that permits dissection of the abnormality and selective

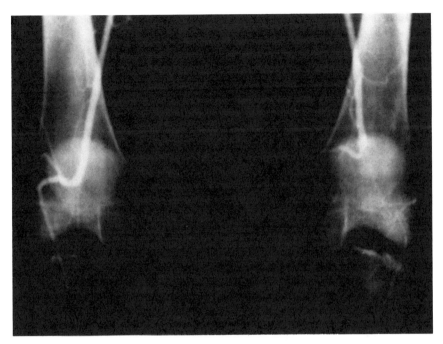

FIG 61–2.
Arteriogram of bilateral popliteal artery occlusion due to entrapment syndrome.

operative intervention, depending on the specific pathology encountered. Thus, when the artery is apparently normal on angiography and at operative inspection, an obstructing fibrous band or the medial head of the gastrocnemius muscle may be divided, permitting further evaluation and a decision for direct arterial surgery. If either external inspection or the angiogram (or both) indicate a significant arterial lesion, then resection of the artery with vein replacement is most appropriate. I have generally used proximal saphenous vein for end-to-end replacement of the excised segment. The use of autogenous tissue is particularly important in this young patient group. In addition, during the course of the procedure, a Fogarty catheter should be passed distally into the main branches of the popliteal artery to search for emboli, and the distal artery should be carefully inspected for evidence of a distal popliteal aneurysm (reported in four of 59 cases). Completion operative angiography is appropriate to assure the technical adequacy of the procedure.

The alternative surgical procedure is to perform a saphenous vein bypass of the popliteal artery utilizing a medial approach. If this is done, and it is appropriate in cases with popliteal thrombosis, I believe it is particularly important to divide the artery proximal to the site of the distal anastomosis to prevent emboli or thrombus from propagating down from the stenosing lesion.

TABLE 61–1.
Classification of Popliteal Entrapment*

TYPE 1	Popliteal artery deviated medially around the medial head of the gastrocnemius muscle. Vein and nerve in normal anatomic position.
TYPE 2	Popliteal artery compressed by abnormal attachments of the medial head of the gastrocnemius muscle to the posterior surface of the femur.
TYPE 3	Popliteal artery compressed by accessory slip of gastrocnemius muscle.
TYPE 4	Popliteal artery compressed by fibrous band or the popliteus muscle or the tibial nerve.
TYPE 5	Popliteal artery and vein both deviated around the medial head of the gastrocnemius muscle. The vein also may be entrapped in any of the types listed above.

*From Rich NM, Collins GJ, McDonald PT, et al: Popliteal vascular entrapment: Its increasing interest. *Arch Surg* 1979; 114:1377–1384. Used by permission.

CYSTIC ADVENTITIAL DISEASE

Patients with cystic adventitial disease of the popliteal artery are also primarily males (ratio of 5:1) but tend to be older (average age 42 with a range of 11 to 70 in the review by Flanigan, et al). They usually present with a more abrupt onset of calf claudication, and distal pulses typically disappear with knee flexion. Angiography in this condition demonstrates a midline scimitarlike stenosis, which is generally above the knee joint in patients essentially free of arteriosclerosis. Most of the described cases have been reported from Europe, although there have been a few from Australia and North America. These patients, with an embryonic cystic structure perhaps related to a ganglion or a popliteal bursa extension, can sometimes be treated by aspiration or evacuation of the cyst. Percutaneous aspiration with ultrasound or CT guidance has been reported. The alternative and more common approach is arterial resection, similar to the treatment for popliteal entrapment.

SUMMARY

Since these conditions generally occur in young, otherwise healthy patients with a normal arterial tree, the outlook following their appropriate identification and repair is excellent, providing the patient has been diagnosed and treated prior to distal destruction of the arterial tree by thrombosis or embolism.

BIBLIOGRAPHY

1. Baker WH, Stoney RJ: Acquired popliteal entrapment syndrome. *Arch Surg* 1972; 105:780–781.

2. Darling RC, Buckley CJ, Abbott WM, et al: Intermittent claudication in young athletes: Popliteal artery entrapment syndrome. *J Trauma* 1974; 14:543–552.
3. Flanigan DP, Burnham JJ, Goodrear JJ, et al: Summary of cases of adventitial cystic disease of the popliteal artery. *Ann Surg* 1979; 189:165–175.
4. Gibson MHL, Mills JG, Johnson GE, et al: Popliteal entrapment syndrome. *Ann Surg* 1977; 185:341–348.
5. Love JW, Whelan TJ: Popliteal artery entrapment syndrome. *Am J Surg* 1965; 109:620–624.
6. McDonald PT, Easterbrook JA, Rich NM, et al: Popliteal artery entrapment syndrome: Clinical, noninvasive and angiographic diagnosis. *Am J Surg* 1980; 139:318–325.
7. Muller N, Morris DC, Nichols DM: Popliteal artery entrapment demonstrated by CT. *Radiol* 1984; 151:157–158.
8. Podore PC: Popliteal entrapment syndrome: A report of tibial nerve entrapment. *J Vasc Surg* 1985; 2:335–336.
9. Rich NM, Collins GJ, McDonald PT, et al: Popliteal vascular entrapment: Its increasing interest. *Arch Surg* 1979; 114:1377–1384.

62　Vasculogenic Impotence

A 59-year-old man is referred by his internist for evaluation and possible treatment of impotence. He is a nondiabetic who, two years ago underwent successful femoropopliteal bypass for calf claudication. The patient had been a past cigarette smoker and stopped smoking for six months after operation. He has resumed cigarette smoking and now smokes a pack a day. He has noted increasing inability to achieve and sustain satisfactory erections. His internist feels this may be secondary to vascular disease and perhaps amenable to treatment.

Consultant: Ralph G. DePalma, M.D.

This presentation is typical of a patient with vasculogenic impotence, probably of arterial origin. Most of these men present in their mid or late 50s. The combination of claudication and impotence as chief complaints suggests an arterial inflow problem. Since this patient is nondiabetic, it is probable that impotence is not due to neuropathy or a refractory state of the corpora cavernosa on a metabolic basis.

In the recent decade there has been increasing interest in the diagnosis and treatment of men with this complaint. This case, as presented, is unusual in that this patient has undergone a femoropopliteal bypass for claudication. The presumption is that this is a highly motivated patient who required relief of work-limiting claudication. Similarly, motivation is an important factor in the steps required for proper diagnosis and ultimately effective treatment of vasculogenic impotence.

DIAGNOSTIC EVALUATION

The causes of impotence are psychogenic, hormonal, neurogenic, or vascular. Our experience with screening large numbers of men suggests that this patient has arteriogenic impotence. Historically, this is based on his increasing inability to achieve and sustain satisfactory erections. This dysfunction appeared in the absence of particular psychic trauma and persists in spite of a willing partner. Appropriate evaluations must be performed in an orderly fashion.

Physical examination with special attention to palpation of pulses and neurosensory evaluation is required. At this time, to be sure that the patient has not developed diabetes, fasting and two-hour blood glucose determinations are indicated. Serum testosterone levels and prolactin levels are obtained. These rule out the presence of abnormalities in testicular secretion or in the pituitary gland. It is quite rare, however, to detect endocrine abnormalities in patients who present like this. The most commonly detected occult metabolic abnormality is diabetes. In this case, it is verified that the patient is not diabetic.

Occult neural abnormalities may also be associated with impotence. Testing routinely done by our group consists of measurement of the bulbocavernosus reflex time. In normal men mean bulbocavernosus reflex time is 30.6 ± SD 1.9 milliseconds. Pudendal evoked potentials and posterior tibial nerve cortical evoked potentials are also measured. Both of these tests may generally be obtained in the hospital's clinical neurophysiology laboratory or through neurology consultation. In this case, in the absence of diabetes or complicating neurogenic factors such as disc disease or prior back injury, these values are returned as normal.

The causes of vasculogenic impotence are outlined in Table 62–1. As can be seen, these are many and complex and sometimes coexist. For example, cavernosal leak syndrome due to venous insufficiency can coexist with diffuse arterial disease in some instances. Investigations would be then directed to delineating a possible cause of vasculogenic impotence in this patient. Clinically, arterial insufficiency would be considered most likely.

In our noninvasive vascular laboratory measurements of the pulse volume recording and penile-brachial indices, as well as screening of the arteries of the lower extremities are done in all cases. We have found that abnormalities of penile perfusion correlate most strongly with the presence of large vessel disease and continued cigarette smoking. In cavernosal leak syndrome without complicating arterial inflow disease, pulse volume recordings and pressures are often normal. After noninvasive flow studies are done, the history of erectile dysfunction is reviewed in further detail with the patient and, if possible, the spouse. Four major historical points to be obtained are as follows:

TABLE 62–1.
Vasculogenic Impotence Provisional Classification

ARTERIAL
Large vessels: aorta and branches to division of internal iliac
Small vessels: proper pudendal and branches
Combined: embolization from aneurysm, ulcerated plaque or postoperative
CAVERNOSAL
Fibrosis: idiopathic or postpriapic
Peyronie's disease: deformity and/or venous leakage
Refractory states: diabetes, antihypertensive therapy, hormonal
VENOUS
Congenital: cavernous-spongious leak
Acquired: cavernosal leak syndrome (venous insufficiency)

1. Physiologic impairment: inability to obtain or maintain erection or some combination of these.
2. How firm does the penis become?
3. Is the impairment constant or episodic?
4. What life events were occurring when the dysfunction appeared?

We found it convenient to review noninvasive laboratory testing results and history and physical examination simultaneously so that the next step in the workup, artificial erection, can proceed at the first or second office visit.

If the pulse volume recording reveals, as it most likely would in this patient, decreased wave forms with prolonged upward stroke and penile-brachial pressure ratios of about 0.6, the next step would be artificial erection using intracorporal injection of papaverine. This injection is performed under close clinical observation to observe the response. In this man, with a history of failing erectile function and arterial insufficiency, an initial intracavernosal dose of 30 mg of papaverine would be chosen. The patient is observed in the clinic for one to two hours and then would be instructed to call back to describe the response after three to four hours. Failure of response to intracavernosal papaverine injection serves to select patients for highly selective pudendal arteriography or dynamic cavernosography. The algorithm used to select patients for arteriography is shown in Figure 62–1. In this instance intracavernosal papaverine injection resulted in a moderate erection which was self supporting and capable for use in intercourse. After this type of response about 20% of men will improve.

Should prolonged erection occur, it is necessary for the patient to return to the clinic to aspirate blood from the corpus cavernosum using a No. 18 needle. When flaccidity is obtained 0.1 mg to 0.2 mg of metaraminol in 10 ml saline is injected. In this case, the erection lasted two and a half hours and was adequate for intercourse with his wife who was available for this occasion. The patient subsequently reports improved function. This patient is then a candidate for continued medical treatment that would include the use of ixosuprine 10 mg QID and injections of a similar dose of papaverine at intervals of two to three months or as needed. Repeated intracorporal self injection of papaverine is not recommended by this author. Repeated injections may cause fibrosis of the corpora cavernosa or complications such as priapism or skin slough due to its misapplication. At the same time, this patient is advised to stop smoking cigarettes. Often the combination of several injections of papaverine, the use of ixosuprine, and complete cessation of cigarette smoking will alleviate impotence.

This patient does have atherosclerosis and may have other large vessel involvement. Particular attention should be given to aortic palpation and examination of the abdominal aorta by ultrasound examination even if an aneurysm is not palpable. Impotence can be a presenting complaint in occult aneurysms. In addition, local conditions such as Peyronie's disease may be disclosed during the use of artificial erection.

ALGORITHM

ARTERIAL IMPOTENCE

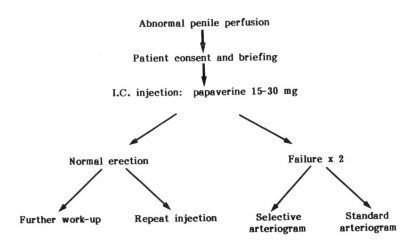

Abnormal penile perfusion

Patient consent and briefing

I.C. injection: papaverine 15-30 mg

Normal erection   Failure x 2

Further work-up   Repeat injection   Selective   Standard
                                            arteriogram   arteriogram

FIG 62–1.
Algorithm used to select patients with impotence for arteriography.

INVASIVE DIAGNOSTIC PROCEDURES

If papaverine injections of up to 60 mg fail to produce erection, either arterial or venous insufficiency is suggested. Flattened pulse waves and decreased arterial pressures suggest arterial insufficiency. Pure venous insufficiency or cavernosal leak syndrome will be accompanied by bounding arterial pulse waves. The use of nocturnal penile tumescence monitoring in the setting of a sleep laboratory can also be helpful. With arterial insufficiency, the patient becomes a candidate for highly selective pudendal arteriography. The only exception would be a diabetic patient, as such patients are generally poor candidates for small vessel revascularization procedures. This is currently done by our group using nonionic contrast media in a sedated patient. Sometimes the arteriogram is supplemented with a small intracavernosal injection of papaverine to better display reactivity of the penile vessels. Dynamic cavernosography to detect venous insufficiency is performed by measurement of corporal pressure and infusion of calibrated amounts of warmed heparinized saline while corpus cavernosum pressure is monitored. This procedure is carried out in the radiographic suite. A roller pump is calibrated to deliver increments of warmed heparinized saline. An abnormal dynamic cavernosography is noted when the infusion rate of 120 ml per min is exceeded without producing an erection. During the injection phase dilute renografin or nonionic contrast media is used to visualize cavernosal leaks. These leaks in the absence of arterial insufficiency are amenable to interruption of venous outflow.

OPERATIVE MANAGEMENT

Depending on the site of arterial obstruction, large vessel, small vessel, or combined, a variety of surgical options are available. With common iliac arterial occlusive disease, transluminal angioplasty can be safe and effective. In addition, angioplasty of stenotic external iliac arteries can alleviate pelvic steal.

The finding of high-grade stenosis or occlusive disease of the mainstem of one or the other of the internal iliac arteries is a situation amenable to extraperitoneal approach and direct endarterectomy. The approach to arterial lesions depends on optimal visualization of involved vessels. When aortic aneurysms or tortuous or ulcerated and severely atherosclerotic large vessels are found, the experienced angiographer will abandon selective catheterization of the internal iliac artery and its distal branches in order to avoid embolization. In such cases, it is likely that embolization to the pudendal vessels may have already occurred.

Before the patient is offered options of small vessel reconstruction, i.e., microvascular revascularization of the penile arteries or creation of arteriovenous fistula in the dorsal vein, it is important to recognize the limitations of these operations. These offer about a 65% to 70% success rate in the best of circumstances and may be age dependent as well. In addition, I would not personally recommend microvascular surgical procedures to a patient with diabetes.

The convenience of modern penile prostheses and the many prosthetic options that exist make initial insertion of penile prosthesis a valuable shortcut in some cases. The patient should be offered this option before small vessel reconstruction is planned. He should also understand that if small vessel reconstruction fails the next step will be insertion of an intracavernosal prosthetic device. The disadvantage of intracavernosal devices is that once one is inserted, vascular reconstruction is no longer possible. Prosthetic devices damage erectile tissues within the corpus cavernosum. Therefore, once a prosthesis is inserted one will always be needed.

All these men require careful consideration of various options to produce optimal results. Cessation of risk factors that promote vascular disease are most important in controlling not only the impotence but prolonging the patency of vascular grafts. This is perhaps one of the most important health steps that they can take. Normal sexual function provides a strong motivating factor contributing to dietary control and cessation of cigarette smoking. It must also be understood that sexual dysfunctions are treated in the setting of an interpersonal relationship. Before operative treatment is undertaken, it is important to understand the nature of that interpersonal relationship. If the patient cooperates, several interviews should be conducted with the couple as well. The wife should be made to understand that the erectile problem is physical. Cooperation between the couple and the treating physician or surgeon is essential if optimal results are to be achieved.

BIBLIOGRAPHY

1. DePalma RG, Emsellem HA, Edwards CM, et al: A screening sequence for vasculogenic impotence. *J Vasc Surg* 1987; 5:228–236.
2. Haldeman S, Bradley WE, Bhatia NN, et al: Pudendal evoked responses. *Arch Neurol* 1982; 39:280–283.
3. Levine SB: Marital sexual dysfunction: Erectile dysfunction. *Ann Int Med* 1976; 85:342–350.
4. Stauffer D, DePalma RG: A comparison of penile-brachial index (PBI) and penile pulse volume recordings (PVR) for diagnosis of vasculogenic impotence. *Bruit* 1983; 7:29–32.

63 Bleeding Esophageal Varices

A 48-year-old man is admitted for recurrent hematemesis. Two months earlier he had been treated successfully for a similar episode. Bleeding that time stopped spontaneously after transfusion of two units of blood. Endoscopy and upper gastrointestinal contrast studies demonstrated esophageal varices. Although he is a heavy drinker, his liver function studies are normal. Active upper gastrointestinal bleeding continues.

Consultant: Ronald A. Malt, M.D.

Two thirds of patients with bleeding varices stop spontaneously. The patients who require active therapy are a biased subset of those who have large varices, which are more likely to bleed irrespective of the portal pressure, and of those who have such poor liver function that they cannot clot or enlist the other mechanisms necessary for homeostasis. The chief determinant of the fate of this subset is the outcome of the episode of bleeding, because the death rate at that time is 50%, a statistic of magnitude never remotely approached by any other intercurrent catastrophe.

EMERGENCY TREATMENT

If the patient can tolerate it without orthostatic hypotension, the first form of treatment is to sit him upright. Variceal pressure will probably be less, and the likelihood of aspiration of blood into the bronchial tree certainly will be. But, obviously, the ability of the patient to tolerate this position is a selective element as well.

Persistent bleeding at a moderate rate, probably from rupture of intraepithelial venous channels, can usually be slowed with intravenous vasopressin at a rate of 0.4 IU per minute (made up as 10 ampules of 20 IU vasopressin per 500 ml of 5% dextrose solution). Torrential bleeding, from rupture of a major, deep venous trunk, demands placement of a Sengstaken-Blakemore tube (Minnesota modification, with a separate lumen for aspirating the secretions that pool above the esophageal balloon). It is no job for an amateur.

SENGSTAKEN-BLAKEMORE TUBE

In ideal circumstances the patient should be intubated with an endotracheal tube. The cuff should be inflated to effect a good seal before the balloon-tube is passed into either the nose or the pharynx. Although oral placement is easier, it is less comfortable and prevents proper securing of the external length of the tube. Like the Dutch boy's finger in the dike, the Sengstaken tube works by obturating the rent in a column of esophageal varices and to a lesser extent by compression of gastric varices. Traction is not required. In fact, it is contraindicated because traction of a pound or two can cause necrosis of the esophagogastric junction within a few hours. The tube is simply fixed to the nose with the piece of plastic foam supplied with it. More elaborately, it is attached to a plastic guard tied around the cheeks or is fitted to a football helmet. To the contrary, the Linton and Nachlas tubes must have traction applied to them, inasmuch as they have only a single, large balloon in the stomach and are meant to slow blood flow from the gastric-coronary circuit into esophageal varices only until a definitive procedure for arrest of bleeding can be done within 24 hours. Furthermore, continuous pressure on the esophagus and trachea between an inflated endotracheal tube cuff and a large-bore intraesophageal tube can cause a tracheo-esophageal fistula.

In passing the Sengstaken tube no local anesthesia is required; it never has time to work and it paralyzes pharyngeal reflexes. The balloons are collapsed and spiralled around the tube like the shrouds and canopy of a child's parachute rocket. The whole unit is then covered with surgical lubricant. It is passed through the nasopharynx, into the esophagus, and then down the stomach.

The pretested gastric balloon is inflated with about 450 ml of air and is pulled against the esophagogastric junction to be sure it is properly seated. The esophageal balloon port is connected in parallel to a manometer and a 50-ml irrigating syringe filled with air. Although the pretested balloon is inflated to 30 mm Hg initially, if that pressure does not arrest the bleeding, 40 mm Hg is used. The esophageal balloon is deflated for five minutes every six hours. Throughout the course of the tamponade treatment, the pressure must be regulated and aspiration prevented; hence, an attendant must be with the patient at all times.

The final precaution is to obtain a chest roentgenogram that includes the upper abdomen in its field to be sure that the gastric balloon lies beneath the diaphragm and that the position of the esophageal balloon is not compromised by the presence of a hiatal hernia. In an unintubated patient either of these situations can cause the tube to override the pharynx, causing asphyxiation. Instructions to the attendant include the order to cut the tube if there is any sign of respiratory distress. The esophageal balloon is thus deflated. When they are removed, tubes must be cut so they cannot be reused.

After tamponade and vasopressin, singly or in combination, have controlled the bleeding, as they almost always do, upper gastrointestinal endoscopy is in order to determine whether varices truly are the cause of bleeding. If they are, treatment should begin with sclerotherapy.

ENDOSCOPY

A patient like this one, with "fairly normal" hepatic function, is virtually certain to have his bleeding controlled by sclerosis for some period, usually for at least three days, when sclerosis can be repeated. Progressive obliteration of the varices with successive treatments argues for continued sclerotherapy. Nonetheless, despite the hope that most patients would respond satisfactorily and that sclerotherapy would decrease the need for surgery and the cost of care, these goals have not been realized. The longer the period of follow-up, the fewer the patients who are totally controlled by sclerotherapy, and the less the difference between the costs of portasystemic shunting and those of sclerotherapy. Sclerotherapy can never control gastric varices, of course, and disappointing results are more likely the worse for the hepatic function.

PORTASYSTEMIC SHUNTS

Failure of tamponade, vasopressin, and sclerotherapy to deal with the bleeding demands an emergency portasystemic shunt. Despite the attractiveness of esophageal devascularization and esophageal transection with reanastomosis as a means of getting to the problem directly and of avoiding portasystemic encephalopathy, these operations for patients with alcoholic cirrhosis have not met with the same success in the Western world as they have in Japan. Transesophageal ligation of varices alone is an obsolete procedure because the complication rate is high, and the results are good only in good-risk patients.

The portasystemic shunt most nearly certain to work is the end-to-side portacaval shunt. It is also the easiest. Except in hypercoagulable states or in cases of gross technical error, such as sewing the front and back walls of the shunt together, failure is all but unknown. There is no advantage in the more difficult side-to-side shunt—in fact, some potential harm, inasmuch as intrahepatic decompression can permit retrograde flow of portal venous or hepatic arterial blood from the liver through the cephalad limb of the shunt to the vena cava. I do not use a mesocaval shunt unless the portal vein is thrombosed. It has a clotting rate worldwide of 30% and offers no incontestable advantages.

Peripheral shunts such as the proximal splenorenal shunt (with splenectomy) and the distal splenorenal shunt (Warren) may also work well and have the advantage that they may be associated with a lower incidence of severe portasystemic encephalopathy. The trouble is that they are harder to perform and do not uniformly relieve the portal hypertension fast enough.

TABLE 63–1.
Scale for Predicting Operative Mortality

	POINTS ASSIGNED		
PREDICTOR	0	1	2
Bilirubin (mg/dl)	≤0.99	1.00–1.99	≥2.0
Ascites	None	Controlled (stable)	Uncontrollable
Operative urgency	Elective	Emergency	—

Score is the sum of points assigned for each predictor: 0 = minimum; 5 = maximum.

EMERGENCY SHUNTS

But is it fair to impose an emergency portacaval shunt on all patients with uncontrollable variceal bleeding? A valid and accurate assessment of the risk is possible. For two cohorts of patients over two chronologic intervals, only three variables had to be determined to predict the outcome (Table 63–1): the last serum bilirubin level before the shunt, the degree to which ascites could be controlled, and the urgency of the operation. These predictors (Fig 63–1) are more parsimonious than those involved in the Child's scale or its modifications because the bilirubin level reflects

OPERATIVE MORTALITY RATE

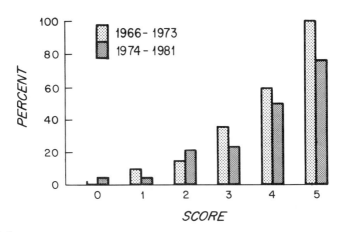

FIG 63–1.
Mortality rates by score (Table 63–1): comparison of two chronologic intervals. (From Lacaine F, LaMuraglia GM, Malt RA: Prognostic factors in survival after portasystemic shunts: Multivariate analysis. *Ann Surg* 1985; 202:729–734. Used with permission.) Annals of Surgery, ref. 5.

both the degree of hepatic dysfunction and the number of transfusions necessary; the difficulty of controlling the ascites reflects both the portal pressure and the serum oncotic pressure; and the urgency of the shunt adds an element of unique risk. Using the score from this scale, the surgeon may decide for himself where the acceptable cutpoint lies for him and his patient. Refusing to shunt certain poor-risk patients because of their near certainty of death is acceptable. On the other hand, when sclerotherapy quells acute bleeding and control persists, continued sclerotherapy is a reasonable option for some patients unless large gastric varices are present, since these cannot be controlled by sclerotherapy.

ELECTIVE SHUNTS

Instead, the range of shunting and nonshunting operations for elective control of portal hypertension is appropriate. I choose a shunting procedure preferentially. For the patient at the best risk, with flow of portal blood to the liver and appropriate anatomy (reasonable size, patent splenic and renal veins disclosed on the venous phase of a splanchnic arteriogram), a selective distal splenorenal shunt may be the best option. I temper the decision, however, by the facts that the reliability of assessing portal flow and volume by angiography is inexact and that in our small series of patients randomized between a proximal and distal splenorenal shunt (Malt and Ottinger, unpublished), the patient with the worst encephalopathy had a distal splenorenal shunt. Furthermore, any operation that takes more than average skill for satisfactory results to be achieved routinely and that requires devascularization of the pancreas at a remote time to maintain its effectiveness should not be a routine procedure except for those who are studying the operation physiologically and habitually. Renal venography is not an essential discriminant in the choice of either a proximal or a distal shunt because the number of anastomoses to the renal vein unable to be done because of aberrant anatomy is small. Neither is hypersplenism an indication for splenectomy. Any patient with an initial platelet count over 40,000 per mm will have a relative thrombocytosis after any kind of portal decompression.

CHOICE OF SHUNTS

In choosing between a portacaval and proximal splenorenal shunt, the bias of a referring internist helps. If he is certain that a splenorenal shunt is best for his patient, there is no reason not to do it, provided that the venous anatomy is suitable. When both are feasible, the abdominal approach is better than thoracoabdominal exposure, because it avoids the morbidity of splitting the costal margin and the diaphragm, and it protects against a transdiaphragmatic leak of ascites in the postoperative period. No one examining the results scientifically doubts that the results of splenorenal and portacaval shunting are the same in populations, although they may differ in any one individual. Because the proximal splenorenal shunt is an operation long done and done well here, it is appropriate for us to perpetuate its use and study the results. Otherwise, I am content with the end-to-side portacaval shunt. When the day comes that we understand which splanchnic compartments are drained by which portasystemic shunts, the selection will be more rational.

DEVASCULARIZATION

An operation of the Sugiura genre is reserved for bleeding in patients who have no veins usable for direct decompression. I prefer a one-stage thoracoabdominal approach involving devascularization of the esophagus and stomach, plus parietal-cell vagotomy and transection and reanastomosis of the esophagus with a circular stapler. Although a few long-term cures have been obtained in children and adolescents with extrahepatic portal hypertension, most offer protection for no more than two years in adults—and some for no longer than a few months.

BIBLIOGRAPHY

1. Cello JP, Grendell JH, Crass RA, et al: Endoscopic sclerotherapy versus portacaval shunt in patients with severe cirrhosis and acute variceal hemorrhage: Long-term follow-up. *N Engl J Med* 1987; 316:11–15.
2. Donovan AJ: Surgical treatment of portal hypertension: A historical perspective. *World J Surg* 1984; 8:626–645.
3. Henderson JM: Variceal bleeding: Which shunt? *Gastroenterology* 1986; 91:1021–1023.
4. Hosking SW, Johnson AG: What happens to esophageal varices after transection and devascularization? *Surgery* 1987; 101:531–534.
5. Lacaine F, LaMuraglia GM, Malt RA: Prognostic factors in survival after portasystemic shunts: Multivariate analysis. *Ann Surg* 1985; 202:729–734.
6. Ottinger LW, Moncure AC: Transthoracic ligation of bleeding esophageal varices in patients with intrahepatic portal obstruction. *Ann Surg* 1974; 179:35–38.
7. Smith JL, Graham DY: Variceal hemorrhage: A critical evaluation of survival analysis. Gastroenterology 1982; 82:968–973.
8. Spence RAJ, Terblanche J: Venous anatomy of the lower esophagus: A new perspective. *Br J Surg* 1986; 73:659–660.
9. Sugiura M, Futagawa S: Esophageal transection with paraesophagogastric devascularization (the Sugiura procedure) in the treatment of esophageal varices. *World J Surg* 1984; 8:673–682.
10. Villeneuve JP, Pomier-Layrargues G, Dugay L, et al: Emergency portacaval shunt for variceal hemorrhage: A prospective study. *Ann Surg* 1987; 296:48–52.
11. Warren WD, Millikan WJ Jr, Henderson JM, et al: Splenopancreatic disconnection: Improved selectivity of the distal splenorenal shunt. *Ann Surg* 1987; 204:346–355.

64   Lymphedema

A 25-year-old woman is seen in your office for a six-month history of a swollen right foot. She denies prior trauma. The painless swelling began insidiously and has increased. She now has difficulty putting on a shoe. Examination reveals non-pitting edema of the foot and ankle. There are no obvious venous abnormalities.

Consultant: Harry L. Bush, Jr., M.D.

This young woman presents with a classical clinical picture of primary lymphedema. While her management is straightforward, it is worthwhile to discuss the full spectrum of lymphedema so we can better understand her evaluation, treatment, and prognosis.

DIAGNOSIS AND STAGING OF DISEASE

The selection of therapy and the expectations of the patient depend on understanding the different manifestations of lymphedema. Lymphedema can be due to congenital abnormalities of the lymphatic system (primary lymphedema), or can be secondary to another process (acquired lymphedema).

Primary Lymphedema

Primary lymphedema is classified by the anatomical pattern visualized on lymphangiogram (Table 64–1). The patterns of lymphatic pathology include: (1) distal obliteration (hypoplasia, aplasia) of the lymphatic channels of the foot and lower leg; (2) proximal obstruction of the lymphatic channels and nodes of the inguinal and pelvic regions; (3) obstruction or aplasia of the thoracic duct; and (4) diffuse obliteration of the lymphatic structures.

(1) Distal obliteration. This is the most common and mildest form of the disease affecting 70% of the patients. The swelling of the lower extremity develops insidiously over several months, starting at the forefoot and ankle and progressing proximally. Only 2% of these patients progress to edema of the whole leg. A sim-

TABLE 64–1.
Anatomical Classification of Lymphedema

STAGE	INGUINAL NODES	THIGH LYMPHATICS	CALF LYMPHATICS
Primary			
Distal obliteration	normal	normal	abnormal
Iliofemoral obstruction	abnormal	normal	normal
Thoracic duct obstruction	normal	normal	normal
Combined Obliteration	abnormal	abnormal	abnormal
Acquired			
Early proximal obstruction	abnormal	normal	normal
Combined obliteration	abnormal	abnormal	abnormal

ilar but less severe process appears in the contralateral leg in about 70% of these patients. The patient is usually female (90%) and most commonly develops the edema during her teens at time of menarche, or in her twenties frequently with pregnancy.

(2) Proximal obstruction: The iliofemoral lymphatic structures draining a single leg are blocked and inguinal lymph nodes are usually palpable at time of presentation. The distal lymphatics are patent but are dilated (frequently termed hyperplasia) and dermal backflow is seen on lymphangiogram. There is no sex preference and the majority of these patients (82%) will progress to whole leg edema, although it usually remains unilateral.

(3) Thoracic duct obstruction. The absence or obstruction of the thoracic duct results in bilateral lymphedema. The lymphatic channels are normal except for dilatation and slow flow. This form of lymphedema is rare (7%) but can result in morbid, whole leg edema in 25% of the patients.

(4) Combined proximal and distal obliteration. Diffuse blockage of lymphatic structures of the leg and pelvis may occur as one extreme form of lymphedema. More commonly, it is thought to represent the late, untreated result of recurrent infections and perilymphatic fibrosis occurring in patients with acquired lymphedema or with the iliofemoral obstructive or thoracic duct obstructive forms of primary lymphedema. This form usually results in severe, whole leg edema that is difficult to control medically.

Acquired Lymphedema

Any condition that injures or distorts the normal structure and function of the lymphatics of the lower extremity can produce lymphedema. The degree and severity will vary with the extent of disruption of the normal lymphatics. Common examples of such conditions include pelvic or inguinal lymph node dissections, trauma, radiotherapy, neoplastic infiltration of the lymph nodes, and recurrent lymphangitis.

Although rare in this country, the most common cause worldwide is infestation with the parasite *Filaria bancrofti*.

Acquired forms of lymphedema are characterized initially by discrete obstruction of the lymphatic flow due to the underlying process. The distal lymphatic channels are initially distended with dermal backflow, but are otherwise normal. However, in time, fibrosis of the subcutaneous tissue results from the inflammation caused by the increased protein content of the interstitial fluid and by recurrent lymphangitis. The fibrotic process obstructs the otherwise normal lymphatic channels, resulting in further anatomical and functional abnormalities.

CLINICAL ASSESSMENT

A careful history and physical examination should provide the diagnosis of lymphedema in the majority of patients. The age and sex of the patient, the insidious onset and distribution of the edema, characteristics of the skin, and the presence of other medical conditions frequently provide the necessary information to diagnose and stage lymphedema. A careful history might elicit potential etiologies responsible for an acquired form of lymphedema. One of the most common problems in assessing early forms of primary lymphedema is the potential confusion with edema due to venous insufficiency or obstruction. In lymphedema, the edema is difficult to control and several days of elevation may be needed to reduce it. In contrast, the edema of venous insufficiency clears overnight. The soft, pitting, bilateral edema of congestive heart failure, renal insufficiency, hypothyroidism, or aldosteronism is rarely a diagnostic problem. The appearance of the skin is different in early lymphedema. Skin ulceration is rare in lymphedema since dermal capillary perfusion is normal, plus the brown pigmentation of venous hypertension is absent. Nevertheless, one may need to rule out venous insufficiency as the primary cause of the peripheral edema or as a concomitant process in patients who have a history of phlebitis or varicosities.

LABORATORY ASSESSMENT

A lymphangiogram is not routinely needed for diagnosis and therapy. The majority of patients have primary lymphedema of the distal obliterative type associated with a mild peripheral edema. Clinical evaluation is sufficient to plan therapy. In patients where venous obstruction or insufficiency is suspected, noninvasive vascular laboratory studies and occasionally ascending and descending venography may be indicated. However, in patients with acquired lymphedema and in the 30% of patients with primary lymphedema who have edema of the entire leg, lymphangiograms may be valuable in planning therapy. These patients frequently have more functional disability and are plagued by recurrent infections. Definition of a discrete level of obstruction may allow surgical intervention before the progressive obliteration of the distal lymphatic channels. While technically easier, radionuclide lymphangiography using a variety of radiocolloid agents has not proven clinically useful in staging. These techniques may play some role in the future in assessing the functional status of the lymphatic system initially and in following surgical intervention. Imaging techniques of the pelvis and inguinal region using computed axial tomography or magnetic resonance imaging are sensitive and specific techniques for defining the status of the retroperitoneum.

THERAPEUTIC APPROACH

Medical Management

The conservative nonoperative approach is always indicated when initially approaching the patient with lymphedema. Although the underlying pathology cannot be reversed, rigorous control of the subcutaneous edema and of recurrent infections will inhibit or delay the progression of further fibrotic obstructive injury to the lymphatic system. If these secondary forms of progressive injury can be avoided, the lymphedema will progress slowly during the first year of observation, and then stabilize. Control of edema, interstitial protein, and secondary infections are the important features. Elevation of the leg is necessary periodically during the day and at night. The interstitial fluid of lymphedema clears slowly, and additional assistance may be required using manual or mechanical massage techniques. Expensive but efficient devices for sequential pneumatic compression are currently available for refractory cases of lymphedema. Diuretic therapy is rarely of benefit and may be detrimental if used too vigorously. Once the extremity is relatively free of edema, tight, elastic stockings must be worn during the day to continue the compression therapy. In general, I prescribe knee-length elastic stockings, as edema is usually limited to or most troublesome in the distal calf, ankle, and foot regions. In addition, patient compliance is often poor in wearing thigh length stockings. Thigh length stockings or those with a leotard design may be necessary in the few patients with significant lymphedema of the entire extremity. If swelling is not too severe, a pressure gradient of 30 to 40 mm Hg or 40 to 50 mm Hg is prescribed. If severe edema is present that responds poorly to lighter weight stockings, a truly heavy weight support with 50 to 60 mm Hg compression at the ankle may be required.

    Hygiene of the skin and nails of the foot and toes must be maintained. Although skin perfusion is normal, any portal of entry for infection, such as skin cracks in hyperkeratotic areas or around nail beds, must be prevented. Prophylactic antibiotics are rarely indicated. However, at the first indication of acute lymphangitis or cellulitis, hospitalization with bedrest, continuous elevation, and systemic antibiotics should minimize further injury to the subcutaneous tissue. Understanding and compliance by the patient are essential. These principles must be adhered to for life, even in patients who require surgery. The therapeutic goals are to maintain healthy skin and to delay progression of disease by minimizing edema and recurrent infections.

Surgical Management

Surgery is required infrequently and is only palliative in nature. Indications for surgical intervention include severe functional impairment and recurrent lymphangitis. Since the surgical procedures currently available cannot restore the limb to a normal appearance, cosmetic indications are rarely valid even when there are psychological difficulties. Surgery should never be considered unless the patient has complied with a maximal regimen of medical management. Two basic approaches are offered, depending on the philosophy of the surgeon and the stage of the disease. The first approach consists of excision of the diseased subcutaneous tissue and deep muscle fascia. The skin and subdermal lymphatics (which are normal) are preserved intact as flaps, or are excised and replaced as an autogenous full-thickness skin graft.

The second approach is to provide alternative lymphatic channels to bypass the obstructed portion of the lymphatic system. Three such surgical approaches that have some support include: (1) an attempt to create new subcutaneous lymphatic channels along a network of monofilament sutures, (2) creation of microlymphatic-venous anastomoses using either dilated lymphatic channels or lymph nodes anastomosed to adjacent superficial veins, or (3) use of a pedicle of omentum or ileal mesentery to form a bridge of intact lymphatic channels across the obstruction. While these procedures are more physiological in concept, they are still experimental and have not proven to provide consistent clinical benefit. The ileal mesentery bridging operation appears to have the greatest potential for a discrete group of patients with pelvic or iliofemoral nodal obstruction in both primary and acquired lymphedema. It has no role in patients with progressive obliteration of the distal lymphatics, nor in patients with thoracic duct obstruction (i.e., proximal to the mesenteric lymphatic drainage).

In my opinion, excisional techniques modified from the original Charles operation effectively remove the diseased tissue, reduce the size and weight of the leg, and restore reasonable function, and decrease the incidence of cellulitis and lymphangitis that normally accelerate the progression of the lymphedema. I feel that subcutaneous excision with autogenous, full-thickness skin grafts placed directly on the muscle provides the most reliable procedure with the best functional benefit for severe end-stage lymphedema. The more physiological operation using a lymphatic bridge of ileal mesentery may be considered for patients with primary or acquired obstruction in the pelvic or inguinal regions.

EXPECTATIONS

Lymphedema is a physical sign indicating a chronic derangement in the lymphatic circulation. Successful nonoperative therapy will palliate this disease by avoiding secondary lymphatic injury and therefore progression of the underlying disease. In spite of effective medical therapy, patients with lymphatic abnormalities proximal to the extremity may have progressive edema resulting in functional disability or repeated infection. These patients frequently require surgical intervention to achieve palliation of the disease.

SUMMARY COMMENT ON THE SPECIFIC CASE

This 25-year-old woman who presents to us with early lymphedema should have a favorable prognosis. In the absence of an underlying disease of the right pelvic or inguinal region causing an acquired form of lymphedema, she probably has primary lymphedema of the distal obliterative type. Her edema therefore should remain relatively mild and should be easily controlled with nonoperative therapy. She has a very small risk of the disease progressing to whole leg edema or to the contralateral leg. While the disease will not reverse itself, she has an excellent chance to avoid functional disability and recurrent infection if she complies with a sound medical regimen. Surgical intervention would be potentially necessary only if she is in the 2% of patients who are noncompliant or have disease progression. Since current surgical techniques cannot restore her leg to its normal appearance, cosmetic indications for surgery should not be considered.

BIBLIOGRAPHY

1. Chilvers AS, Kinmonth JB: Operations for lymphedema of the lower limbs. *J Cardiovasc Surg* 1975; 16:115–119.
2. Degni M: Surgical management of selected patients with lymphedema of the extremities. *J Cardiovasc Surg* 1984; 25:481–488.
3. Kinmonth JB, Hurst PAE, Edwards JM, et al: Relief of lymph obstruction by the use of a bridge of mesentery and ileum. *Br J Surg* 1979; 65:829–833.
4. Richmand DM, O'Donnell TF, Zelikovski A: Sequential pneumatic compression for lymphedema. *Arch Surg* 1985; 120:1116–1119.
5. Wolfe JHN, Kinmonth JB: The prognosis of primary lymphedema of the lower limbs. *Arch Surg* 1981; 116:1157–1160.
6. Wolfe JHN: The prognosis and possible cause of severe primary lymphedema. *Ann Roy Coll Surg* 1984; 66:251–257.

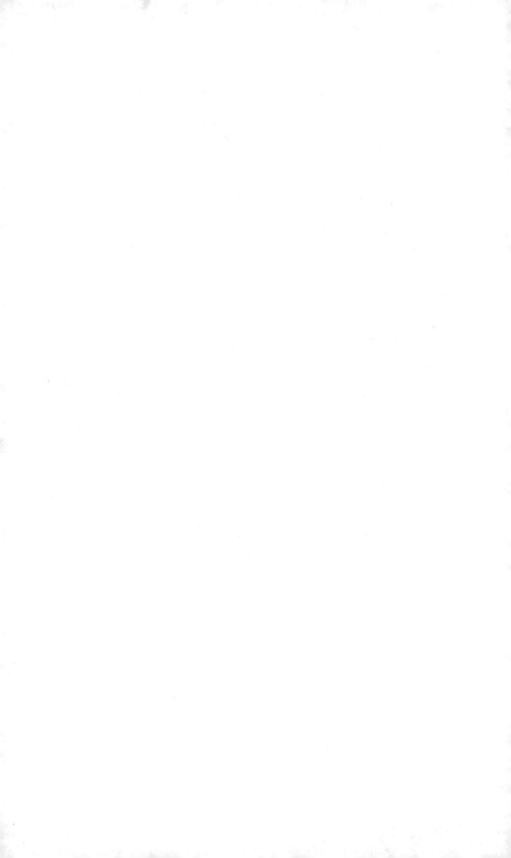

Index

453